Environmental Influences on Dietary Intake of Children and Adolescents

Environmental Influences on Dietary Intake of Children and Adolescents

Special Issue Editor
Jessica Sophia Gubbels

MDPI • Basel • Beijing • Wuhan • Barcelona • Belgrade • Manchester • Tokyo • Cluj • Tianjin

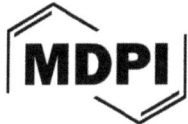

Special Issue Editor
Jessica Sophia Gubbels
Maastricht University
The Netherlands

Editorial Office
MDPI
St. Alban-Anlage 66
4052 Basel, Switzerland

This is a reprint of articles from the Special Issue published online in the open access journal *Nutrients* (ISSN 2072-6643) (available at: https://www.mdpi.com/journal/nutrients/special_issues/Environmental_Influences_Dietary_Intake?authAll=true).

For citation purposes, cite each article independently as indicated on the article page online and as indicated below:

LastName, A.A.; LastName, B.B.; LastName, C.C. Article Title. *Journal Name* **Year**, *Article Number*, Page Range.

ISBN 978-3-03936-533-3 (Hbk)
ISBN 978-3-03936-534-0 (PDF)

© 2020 by the authors. Articles in this book are Open Access and distributed under the Creative Commons Attribution (CC BY) license, which allows users to download, copy and build upon published articles, as long as the author and publisher are properly credited, which ensures maximum dissemination and a wider impact of our publications.

The book as a whole is distributed by MDPI under the terms and conditions of the Creative Commons license CC BY-NC-ND.

Contents

About the Special Issue Editor ix

Jessica S. Gubbels
Environmental Influences on Dietary Intake of Children and Adolescents
Reprinted from: *Nutrients* 2020, 12, 922, doi:10.3390/nu12040922 1

Edward Leigh Gibson, Odysseas Androutsos, Luis Moreno, Paloma Flores-Barrantes, Piotr Socha, Violeta Iotova, Greet Cardon, Ilse De Bourdeaudhuij, Berthold Koletzko, Simona Skripkauskaite, Yannis Manios and on behalf of the Toybox-study Group
Influences of Parental Snacking-Related Attitudes, Behaviours and Nutritional Knowledge on Young Children's Healthy and Unhealthy Snacking: The ToyBox Study
Reprinted from: *Nutrients* 2020, 12, 432, doi:10.3390/nu12020432 7

Wendy Van Lippevelde, Leentje Vervoort, Jolien Vangeel and Lien Goossens
Can Parenting Practices Moderate the Relationship between Reward Sensitivity and Adolescents' Consumption of Snacks and Sugar-Sweetened Beverages?
Reprinted from: *Nutrients* 2020, 12, 178, doi:10.3390/nu12010178 25

Yukako Tani, Takeo Fujiwara, Satomi Doi and Aya Isumi
Home Cooking and Child Obesity in Japan: Results from the A-CHILD Study
Reprinted from: *Nutrients* 2019, 11, 2859, doi:10.3390/nu11122859 51

Fiona Lavelle, Tony Benson, Lynsey Hollywood, Dawn Surgenor, Amanda McCloat, Elaine Mooney, Martin Caraher and Moira Dean
Modern Transference of Domestic Cooking Skills
Reprinted from: *Nutrients* 2019, 11, 870, doi:10.3390/nu11040870 61

Sacha Verjans-Janssen, Dave Van Kann, Stef Kremers, Steven Vos, Maria Jansen and Sanne Gerards
A Cross-Sectional Study on the Relationship between the Family Nutrition Climate and Children's Nutrition Behavior
Reprinted from: *Nutrients* 2019, 11, 2344, doi:10.3390/nu11102344 75

Liisa Korkalo, Kaija Nissinen, Essi Skaffari, Henna Vepsäläinen, Reetta Lehto, Riikka Kaukonen, Leena Koivusilta, Nina Sajaniemi, Eva Roos and Maijaliisa Erkkola
The Contribution of Preschool Meals to the Diet of Finnish Preschoolers
Reprinted from: *Nutrients* 2019, 11, 1531, doi:10.3390/nu11071531 89

Reetta Lehto, Carola Ray, Liisa Korkalo, Henna Vepsäläinen, Kaija Nissinen, Leena Koivusilta, Eva Roos and Maijaliisa Erkkola
Fruit, Vegetable, and Fibre Intake among Finnish Preschoolers in Relation to Preschool-Level Facilitators and Barriers to Healthy Nutrition
Reprinted from: *Nutrients* 2019, 11, 1458, doi:10.3390/nu11071458 105

Sara E. Benjamin-Neelon, Amelie A. Hecht, Thomas Burgoine and Jean Adams
Perceived Barriers to Fruit and Vegetable Gardens in Early Years Settings in England: Results from a Cross-Sectional Survey of Nurseries
Reprinted from: *Nutrients* 2019, 11, 2925, doi:10.3390/nu11122925 119

Claie E. Holley, Carolynne Mason and Emma Haycraft
Opportunities and Challenges Arising from Holiday Clubs Tackling Children's Hunger in the
UK: Pilot Club Leader Perspectives
Reprinted from: *Nutrients* **2019**, *11*, 1237, doi:10.3390/nu11061237 . . . . **131**

Nina Bartelink, Patricia van Assema, Stef Kremers, Hans Savelberg, Dorus Gevers and
Maria Jansen
Unravelling the Effects of the Healthy Primary School of the Future: For Whom and Where Is
It Effective?
Reprinted from: *Nutrients* **2019**, *11*, 2119, doi:10.3390/nu11092119 . . . . **143**

Anna Kiss, József Popp, Judit Oláh and Zoltán Lakner
The Reform of School Catering in Hungary: Anatomy of a Health-Education Attempt
Reprinted from: *Nutrients* **2019**, *11*, 716, doi:10.3390/nu11040716 . . . . **159**

Almudena Garrido-Fernández, Francisca María García-Padilla, José Luis Sánchez-Ramos,
Juan Gómez-Salgado, Gabriel H. Travé-González and Elena Sosa-Cordobés
Food Consumed by High School Students during the School Day
Reprinted from: *Nutrients* **2020**, *12*, 485, doi:10.3390/nu12020485 . . . . **179**

Roel C.J. Hermans, Koen Smit, Nina van den Broek, Irma J. Evenhuis and Lydian Veldhuis
Adolescents' Food Purchasing Patterns in the School Food Environment: Examining the Role
of Perceived Relationship Support and Maternal Monitoring
Reprinted from: *Nutrients* **2020**, *12*, 733, doi:10.3390/nu12030733 . . . . **197**

Rubén Trigueros, Luis A. Mínguez, Jerónimo J. González-Bernal, Maha Jahouh,
Raul Soto-Camara and José M. Aguilar-Parra
Influence of Teaching Style on Physical Education Adolescents' Motivation and
Health-Related Lifestyle
Reprinted from: *Nutrients* **2019**, *11*, 2594, doi:10.3390/nu11112594 . . . . **211**

Rubén Trigueros, Luis A. Mínguez, Jerónimo J. González-Bernal, José M. Aguilar-Parra,
Raúl Soto-Cámara, Joaquín F. Álvarez and Patricia Rocamora
Physical Education Classes as a Precursor to the Mediterranean Diet and the Practice of
Physical Activity
Reprinted from: *Nutrients* **2020**, *12*, 239, doi:10.3390/nu12010239 . . . . **225**

Julia Díez, Alba Cebrecos, Alba Rapela, Luisa N. Borrell, Usama Bilal and Manuel Franco
Socioeconomic Inequalities in the Retail Food Environment around Schools in a Southern
European Context
Reprinted from: *Nutrients* **2019**, *11*, 1511, doi:10.3390/nu11071511 . . . . **237**

Jaapna Dhillon, L. Karina Diaz Rios, Kaitlyn J. Aldaz, Natalie De La Cruz, Emily Vu,
Syed Asad Asghar, Quintin Kuse and Rudy M. Ortiz
We Don't Have a Lot of Healthy Options: Food Environment Perceptions of First-Year, Minority
College Students Attending a Food Desert Campus
Reprinted from: *Nutrients* **2019**, *11*, 816, doi:10.3390/nu11040816 . . . . **251**

Charlene Elliott
Tracking Kids' Food: Comparing the Nutritional Value and Marketing Appeals of
Child-Targeted Supermarket Products Over Time
Reprinted from: *Nutrients* **2019**, *11*, 1850, doi:10.3390/nu11081850 . . . . **267**

Christine D. Czoli, Elise Pauzé and Monique Potvin Kent
Exposure to Food and Beverage Advertising on Television among Canadian Adolescents,
2011 to 2016
Reprinted from: *Nutrients* **2020**, *12*, 428, doi:10.3390/nu12020428 . . . . **283**

About the Special Issue Editor

Jessica Sophia Gubbels (PhD). Dr. Jessica Gubbels is an associate professor at the Department of Health Promotion within Maastricht University, the Netherlands. Her research mainly focuses on the (environmental) determinants of health behavior of young children and their families. Most of her projects focus on the influence of parents and childcare. She has a special interest in the interaction between determinants of health behavior. In addition to her research in the European context, she supervises several PhD-projects in developing countries, including Sudan, Lebanon, and Uganda. She also teaches within various programs, including the bachelor programs of Health Sciences, Psychology, and European Public Health, as well as the master program in Health Education and Promotion. She is a frequent keynote speaker at national and international conferences for both practice and research, and is a member of specialist committees of the Dutch Health Council. She has received various prestigious fellowships and grants.

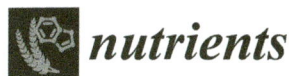

Editorial

Environmental Influences on Dietary Intake of Children and Adolescents

Jessica S. Gubbels

Department of Health Promotion, NUTRIM School of Nutrition and Translational Research in Metabolism, Maastricht University, NL-6200 MD, Maastricht, The Netherlands; jessica.gubbels@maastrichtuniversity.nl

Received: 17 March 2020; Accepted: 19 March 2020; Published: 27 March 2020

Introduction

Childhood is a crucial period for establishing lifelong healthy nutritional habits [1]. The environment can have an important influence on these habits [2]. According to the ANGELO framework [3], the environment can be operationalized through distinguishing between four environmental types: The physical environment (what is available), the social environment (what are the attitudes/beliefs of important others), the political environment (what are the rules), and the economic environment (what are the costs) [3]. The studies described in the current special issue cover these various types of environmental influences within different settings, including home and school, on children and adolescents' dietary intake.

Several studies in the special issue focused on environmental influences in the home setting. Parents play an important role in forming their children's dietary habits and are important gatekeepers for children's behavior [4,5]. Gibson and colleagues [6] examined parental influences on snacking in preschoolers in a large cross-European sample. Parents' own snacking behavior and rules about snacking were significantly associated with the intake of their children, but parents' educational level and nutritional knowledge were also important predictors. Interestingly, the parental influences were different for healthy and unhealthy snacking [6]. In an older sample, Van Lippevelde and colleagues [7] showed that health-promoting parenting practices were associated with reduced sugar sweetened beverage intake and increased healthy snack intake, while health-reducing practices were associated with increased unhealthy snack intake. Van Lippevelde and colleagues [7] also examined whether the parenting practices moderated the positive relationship between adolescents' reward sensitivity and unhealthy dietary intake, but this was not the case. Interestingly, they did find indications of such an interaction when using the parent-reported instead of the adolescent-reported parenting practices as a moderator [7]. This stresses the importance of carefully considering our methodology to assess environmental influences, also taking the child's perspective of the environment into account [8]. In addition, Hermans and colleagues [9] showed that parental influence on adolescents' dietary intake even reaches beyond the home setting: Support from mothers was positively associated with adolescents bringing healthy products to school, and negatively associated with their purchase of sweet snacks in and around school [9].

Tani, Fujiwara, Doi, and Isumi [10] examined the association between home cooking and childhood obesity in a large sample of primary school children in Japan. Children living in households with a low frequency of home cooking were more than twice as likely to be obese as those in a household with high cooking frequency were. This association was partially mediated by children's diet (vegetable, breakfast, and snack intake), suggesting that home cooking is associated with healthy intake, which, in turn, decreases the risk for obesity [10]. Home cooking and family meals are important indicators of family functioning [11], and can thus be regarded an important target for future obesity prevention interventions. Transference of cooking skills from parents to their children could be a key aspect in increasing home cooking. Lavelle and colleagues [12] examined such transference of cooking skills in a qualitative study among Irish mothers. Although mothers expressed a desire for teaching their children to cook, various barriers to actually involving children in cooking were identified. These barriers included children's lack of interest in cooking, clingy behavior and messiness in the kitchen, and pickiness with regard to food. This points out that parents may need some help in dealing with practical barriers to involving their children in the kitchen, as well to motivate their children to actually get involved [12].

In addition to parental influences, increasing attention is being paid to the influence of the broader family system on children's dietary intake [13]. In the current special issue, Verjans-Janssen and colleagues [14] examined the associations between the Family Nutrition Climate—i.e., the family's shared perceptions and cognitions regarding healthy nutrition [15]—and dietary intake of primary school children. Several subscales, as well as the total Family Nutrition Scale, were positively associated with healthy intake behaviors, including increased fruit, vegetable, and water intake, and decreased soft drink and sweets intake [14]. This underlines the importance of the family-level influences in addition to parental influences.

Furthermore, parents often share responsibility for caring for their child with (pre)schools and childcare facilities. Whereas the majority of young children in OECD (Organisation for Economic Co-operation and Development)-countries attend some form of preschool or organized childcare [16], almost all older children and adolescents attend some type of education [17]. In the current special issue, various papers addressed the influence of care and educational facilities.

With regards the youngest children, Korkalo and colleagues [18] showed that preschool meals contribute to over half of weekday energy intake in young Finnish children. This shows the important influence preschools can have on children's diets. Preschool meals were relatively healthy, being high in fibers, fish, unsaturated fats, and several vitamins, and low in added sugar. However, fruit consumption at preschool was low and salt intake was relatively high [18]. These findings point out the specific intake behaviors that need to be addressed in future interventions. In another study from Finland, Lehto and colleagues [19] examined the association of various facilitators and barriers at preschool, with children's fruit, vegetable, and fiber intake in those preschools. One of the main predictors of healthy intake was the presence of food policies [19]. Policies are crucial for the longer-term maintenance of potential intervention effects [20], preventing that established environmental changes slowly dilute and eventually diminish over time. Surprisingly, the study of Lehto et al. [19] did not find any influence of center cooking facilities, resources, or staff education on children's intake, which might imply that a lack of resources and facilities does not necessarily hinder healthy dietary intake. Benjamin Neelon and colleagues [21] also examined barriers to the implementation of intervention in childcare settings, though specifically for fruit and vegetable gardens. Fruit and vegetable garden projects have been previously shown to increase children's intake of fruit and vegetables (e.g., [22], but to date few interventions in Early Care and Education settings have included gardening [23]). Benjamin Neelon and colleagues [21] showed that although the majority (81%) of the English childcare settings was interested in implementing gardens, various practical barriers hindered actual implementation, including lack of space, expertise and time. This is in line with the findings of Holley and colleagues [24], who identified various barriers and challenges for free food provision at holiday clubs to tackle children's hunger. Although reported effects did not only include tackling of hunger, but also creating positive food experiences and promoting social interactions and positive behavior in general, the reported challenges, including resources constraints, hindered implementation [24]. This indicates that a tailored approach is necessary when implementing intervention approaches, taking into account intermediaries' needs and barriers, as well as their strengths [25].

Moving on to primary schools, Bartelink and colleagues examined effects of an integrated intervention on children's diet and physical activity in a large quasi-experimental study in the Netherlands [26]. They found the intervention to have favorable effects on children's diet and physical activity. However, the effects on diet were only present when the full intervention was implemented: Schools that skipped the free healthy lunch that was part of the intervention only found effects on physical activity. In addition, the intervention showed less favorable effects on younger children and children with a low socioeconomic status (SES). These findings of Bartelink and colleagues [26] are in line with an ecological systems view of environmental influences on behavior [27–29], which states that environmental influences on diet are context-specific (like children's SES in the study by Bartelink et al.) as well as person-specific (in line with the diminished effects depending on children's age in the study). Hence, determinants of behavior cannot be viewed in isolation. They influence each other, and it is their combined influence that determines behavior [30]. This stresses the importance of a broad, integrative approach in interventions. The findings of Kiss and colleagues [31] underline this. In their analysis of the reform of the school catering system in Hungary, they showed that changed regulations (i.e., the political environment) are not necessarily translated into action. All involved sectors need to be on board, and interaction and dialogue between stakeholders needs to be facilitated. Furthermore, they stressed that there is no universal solution fitting all settings and all children [31], in line with the different effects depending on contextual and person-related factors reported by Bartelink et al. [26].

Diet is also a concern within secondary schools. Garrido-Fernández and colleagues [32] showed that adolescents were more likely to consume unhealthy snacks when they attended a school with a cafeteria. Hence, while school cafeteria might have large potential to improve children's diet and prevent overweight [33], this potential is often not utilized in practice [32]. In addition to the physical environment at secondary schools, the social environment is also very important. Trigueros and colleagues [34,35] showed that teaching style during Physical Education (PE) classes was associated with Portuguese adolescents' motivation, which, in turn, was related to their diet and physical activity. Their findings support the Self Determination Theory [36]: Satisfaction of the basic human psychological needs (autonomy, competence, and relatedness) was crucial for the adolescent's motivation toward PE classes. Students that were highly motivated consumed more healthy foods and less unhealthy foods and were more active. As such, Trigueros et al. [34,35] provide us with insight into some of the cognitive factors that precede behavioral decisions regarding dietary intake and how the environment can support these cognitive processes. The results can therefore be used by interventions addressing PE classes and teaching styles.

Moving from the school setting to the surrounding neighborhood environment, Díez and colleagues [37] examined socioeconomic inequalities in the food environment around schools in Spain. They showed that 95% of the schools were surrounded by unhealthy food retailers within a short range, with a median of 17 unhealthy food outlets per school. A worrying addition to this was that unhealthy food retailers were both closer and higher in number for schools in low-SES neighborhoods [37], indicating that children from a lower SES background are growing up in a less healthy food environment. Dhillon and colleagues [38] painted an equally problematic picture regarding the food environment of college students living on a food-desert campus in the United States. Performing a qualitative focus group study, they showed that there was a lack of adequate, acceptable, affordable, and accessible food within students' environment. Healthy foods, such as fruit, were too expensive and often not available at campus, and it was very difficult to get food from outside the campus area [38]. Based on the studies of Díez [37] and Dhillon [38], we can conclude that both the overwhelming offer of unhealthy foods and the lack of healthy foods around educational facilities are very problematic.

Within food outlets, the study by Elliott [39] showed that 88% of Canadian child-targeted products was not suitable for marketing to children. Interestingly, the percentage of children's products that was unsuitable was stable between 2009 and 2017. At both time points, over 70% of children's food products was too high in sugar. However, a very large increase in nutrition claims was visible in the observed time period. Also, the use of several marketing techniques aimed at children (e.g., the use of cartoon images and child fonts) increased, while the use of other approaches decreased (e.g., the use of games on the package). The study by Elliott [39] showed the significant pressure to eat unhealthy foods that is exerted by marketing. In line with this, the findings of Czoli et al. [40] showed that although overall exposure to food advertisements among Canadian children decreased, advertisements were dominated by fast food and sugary drinks. More strict regulation of marketing directed at children and adolescent is therefore urgently needed, which should be directed at the different settings and media that youngsters encounter.

In conclusion, the papers in the current issue underline the importance of the environment in influencing children's and adolescents' dietary intake across different settings and types of environments. In addition, the papers identified some crucial barriers and facilitators for the implementation of environmental changes to enable a healthy diet for young children. The special issue therefore provides some important directions for both future research and practice.

Funding: This research received no external funding.

Conflicts of Interest: The authors declare no conflict of interest.

References

1. Craigie, A.M.; Lake, A.A.; Kelly, S.A.; Adamson, A.J.; Mathers, J.C. Tracking of obesity-related behaviours from childhood to adulthood: A systematic review. *Maturitas* **2011**, *70*, 266–284. [CrossRef]
2. Brug, J.; Kremers, S.P.; Lenthe, F.; Ball, K.; Crawford, D. Environmental determinants of healthy eating: In need of theory and evidence. *Proc. Nutr. Soc.* **2008**, *67*, 307–316. [CrossRef]
3. Swinburn, B.; Egger, G.; Raza, F. Dissecting obesogenic environments: The development and application of a framework for identifying and prioritizing environmental interventions for obesity. *Prev. Med.* **1999**, *29 Pt 1*, 563–570. [CrossRef]
4. Larsen, J.K.; Hermans, R.C.J.; Sleddens, E.F.C.; Engels, R.C.; Fisher, J.O.; Kremers, S.P.J. How parental dietary behavior and food parenting practices affect children's dietary behavior. Interacting sources of influence? *Appetite* **2015**, *89*, 246–257. [CrossRef]
5. Scaglioni, S.; Arrizza, C.; Vecchi, F.; Tedeschi, S. Determinants of children's eating behavior. *Am. J. Clin. Nutr.* **2011**, *84* (Suppl. 6), 2006S–2011S. [CrossRef]
6. Gibson, E.L.; Androutsos, O.; Moreno, L.; Flores-Barrantes, P.; Socha, P.; Iotova, V.; Cardon, G.; de Bourdeaudhuij, I.; Koletzko, B.; Skripkauskaite, S.; et al. Influences of parental snacking-related attitudes, behaviours and nutritional knowledge on young children's healthy and unhealthy snacking: The ToyBox Study. *Nutrients* **2020**, *12*, 432. [CrossRef]
7. Van Lippenvelde, W.; Vervoort, L.; Vangeel, L.; Goossens, L. Can parenting practices moderate the relationship between reward sensitivity and adolescents' consumption of snacks and sugar-sweetened beverages? *Nutrients* **2020**, *12*, 178. [CrossRef]
8. Taylor, A.; Wilson, C.; Slater, A.; Mohr, P. Parent- and child-reported parenting. Associations with child weight-related outcomes. *Appetite* **2011**, *57*, 700–706. [CrossRef]
9. Hermans, R.C.J.; Smit, K.; Van den Broek, N.; Evenhuis, I.J.; Veldhuis, L. Adolescents' food purchasing patterns in the school food environment: Examining the role of perceived relationship support and maternal monitoring. *Nutrients* **2020**, *12*, 733. [CrossRef]
10. Tani, Y.; Fujiwara, T.; Doi, S.; Isumi, A. Home cooking and child obesity in Japan: Results from the A-CHILD study. *Nutrients* **2019**, *11*, 2859. [CrossRef]
11. Walton, K.; Horton, N.J.; Rifas-Shiman, S.L.; Field, A.E.; Austin, B.; Haycraft, E.; Breen, A.; Haines, J. Exploring the role of family functioning in the association between frequence of family dinners and dietary intake among adolescents and young adults. *JAMA Netwo. Open* **2018**, *1*, e185217. [CrossRef]
12. Lavelle, F.; Benson, T.; Hollywood, L.; Surgenor, D.; McCloat, A.; Mooney, E.; Breen, A.; Haines, J. Modern transference of domestic cooking skills. *Nutrients* **2019**, *11*, 870. [CrossRef]
13. Niermann, C.Y.N.; Gerards, S.M.P.L.; Kremers, S.P.J. Conceptualizing family influences on children's energy balance-related behaviors: Levels of Interacting Family Environmental Subsystems (The LIFES Framework). *Int. J. Environ. Res. Public Health* **2018**, *15*, 2714. [CrossRef]
14. Verjans-Janssen, S.; Van Kann, D.; Kremers, S.; Vos, S.; Jansen, M.; Gerards, S. A cross-sectional study on the relationship between the Family Nutrition Climate and children's nutrition behavior. *Nutrients* **2019**, *11*, 2344. [CrossRef]
15. Niermann, C.Y.N.; Krapf, F.; Renner, B.; Reiner, M.; Woll, A. Familiy health climate scale (FHC-scale): Development and validation. *Int. J. Behav. Nutr. Phys. Act.* **2014**, *11*, 30. [CrossRef]

16. OECD Social Policy Division—DIrectorate of Employment LaSA. *PF3.2: Enrolment in Childcare and Pre-School*; OECD: Paris, France, 2019.
17. OECD Social Policy Division—Directorate of Employment LaSA. *Educational Attainment by Gender*; OECD: Paris, France, 2019.
18. Korkalo, L.; Nissinen, K.; Skaffari, E.; Vepsäläinen, H.; Lehto, R.; Kaukonen, R.; Koivusilta, L.; Sajaniemi, N.; Roos, E.; Erkkola, M.; et al. The contribution of preschool meals to the diet of Finnish Preschoolers. *Nutrients* **2019**, *11*, 1531. [CrossRef]
19. Lehto, R.; Ray, C.; Korkalo, L.; Vepsäläinen, H.; Nissinen, K.; Koivusilta, L.; Roos, E.; Erkkola, M. Fruit, vegetable, and fibre intake among Finnish preschoolers in Relation to preschool-level facilitators and barriers to healthy nutrition. *Nutrients* **2019**, *11*, 1458. [CrossRef]
20. Glasgow, R.E.; Vogt, T.M.; Boles, S.M. Evaluating the public health impact of health promotion interventions: The RE-AIM framework. *Am. J. Public Health* **1999**, *89*, 1322–1327. [CrossRef]
21. Benjamin Neelon, S.E.; Hecht, A.A.; Burgoine, T.; Adams, J. Perceived barriers to fruit and vegetable gardens in early year settings in England: Results from a cross-sectional survey of nurseries. *Nutrients* **2019**, *11*, 2925. [CrossRef]
22. Evans, A.; Ranjit, N.; Rutledge, R.; Medina, J.; Jennings, R.; Smiley, A.; Stigler, M.; Hoelscher, D. Exposure to multiple components of a garden-based intervention for middle school students increases fruit and vegetable consumption. *Health Promot. Pract.* **2012**, *13*, 608–616. [CrossRef]
23. Hodder, R.K.; Stacey, F.G.; O'Brien, K.M.; Wyse, R.J.; Clinton-McHarg, T.; Tzelepsis, F.; Bartlem, K.M.; Sutherland, R.; James, E.L.; Barnes, C.; et al. Interventions for increasing fruit and vegetables consumption in children aged five years and under. *Cochrane Database Syst. Rev.* **2018**, *1*, Cd008552.
24. Holley, C.; Mason, C.; Haycraft, E. Opportunities and challenges arising from holday clubs tackling children's hunger in the UK: Pilot club leader perspectives. *Nutrients* **2019**, *11*, 1237. [CrossRef]
25. Wiltsey Stirman, S.; Kimberly, J.; Cook, N.; Calloway, A.; Castro, F.; Charns, M. The sustainability of new programs and innovations: A review of the empirical literature and recommendations for future research. *Implement. Sci.* **2012**, *7*, 17. [CrossRef]
26. Bartelink, N.; Van Assema, P.; Kremers, S.; Savelberg, H.; Gevers, D.; Jansen, M. Unravelling the effects of the healthy primary school of the future: For whom and where is it effective? *Nutrients* **2019**, *11*, 2119. [CrossRef]
27. Gubbels, J.S.; Van Kann, D.H.; de Vries, N.K.; Thijs, C.; Kremers, S.P. The next step in health behavior research: The need for ecological moderation analyses—An application to diet and physical activity at childcare. *Int. J. Behav. Nutr. Phys. Act.* **2014**, *11*, 52. [CrossRef]
28. Spence, J.C.; Lee, R.E. Toward a comprehensive model of physical activity. *Psychol. Sport Exerc.* **2003**, *4*, 7–24. [CrossRef]
29. Friedman, S.L.; Wachs, T.D. *Measuring Environment across the Life Span: Emerging Methods and Concepts*; American Psychological Association: Washington, DC, USA, 1999.
30. Kremers, S.P. Theory and practice in the study of influences on energy balance-related behaviors. *Patient Educ. Couns.* **2010**, *79*, 291–298. [CrossRef]
31. Kiss, A.; Popp, J.; Oláh, J.; Lakner, Z. The reform of school catering in Hungary: Anatomy of a health-education attempt. *Nutrients* **2019**, *11*, 716. [CrossRef]
32. Garrido-Fernández, A.; García-Padilla, F.M.; Sánchez-Ramos, J.L.; Gómez-Saldago, J.; Travé-González, G.H.; Sosa-Cordobés, E. Food consumed by high school students during the school day. *Nutrients* **2020**, *12*, 485. [CrossRef]
33. Driessen, C.E.; Cameron, A.J.; Thornton, L.E.; Lai, S.K.; Barnett, L.M. Effect of changes to the school food environment on eating behaviours and/or body weight in children: A systematic review. *Pediatric Obes. Obes. Manag.* **2014**, *15*, 968–982. [CrossRef]
34. Trigueros, R.; Mínguez, L.A.; González-Bernal, J.J.; Jahouh, M.; Soto-Camara, R.; Aguilar-Parra, J.M. Influence of teaching style on physical education adolescents' motivation and health-related lifestyle. *Nutrients* **2019**, *11*, 2594. [CrossRef]
35. Trigueros, R.; Mínguez, L.A.; González-Bernal, J.J.; Aguilar-Parra, J.M.; Soto-Camara, R.; Álvarez, J.F.; Rocamora, P. Physical Education classes as a precursor or the Mediterranean diet and the practice of physical activity. *Nutrients* **2020**, *12*, 239. [CrossRef]
36. Deci, E.L.; Ryan, R.M. Optimizing students' motivation in the era of testing and pressure: A Self-Determination Theory perspective. In *Building Autonomous Learners*; Springer: Singapore, 2016.

37. Diez, J.; Cebrecos, A.; Rapela, A.; Borrell, L.N.; Bilal, U.; Franco, M. Socioeconomic inequalitites in the retail food environment around schools in a Southern European context. *Nutrients* **2019**, *11*, 1511. [CrossRef]
38. Dhillon, J.; Diaz Rios, L.K.; Aldaz, K.J.; De La Cruz, N.; Vu, E.; Asad Asghar, S.; Kuse, Q.; Ortiz, R.M. We don't have a lot of healthy options: Food environment perceptions of first-year, minority college students attending a food desert campus. *Nutrients* **2019**, *11*, 816. [CrossRef]
39. Elliott, C. Tracking kids' food: Comparing the nutritional value and marketing appeals of child-targeted supermaket products over time. *Nutrients* **2019**, *11*, 1850. [CrossRef]
40. Czoli, C.D.; Pauzé, E.; Potvin Kent, M. Exposure to food and beverage advertising on television among Canadian Adolescents, 2011 to 2016. *Nutrients* **2020**, *12*, 428. [CrossRef]

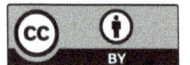

© 2020 by the author. Licensee MDPI, Basel, Switzerland. This article is an open access article distributed under the terms and conditions of the Creative Commons Attribution (CC BY) license (http://creativecommons.org/licenses/by/4.0/).

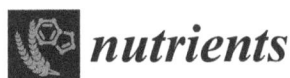

Article

Influences of Parental Snacking-Related Attitudes, Behaviours and Nutritional Knowledge on Young Children's Healthy and Unhealthy Snacking: The ToyBox Study

Edward Leigh Gibson [1,*], Odysseas Androutsos [2], Luis Moreno [3,4,5], Paloma Flores-Barrantes [3,4,5], Piotr Socha [6], Violeta Iotova [7], Greet Cardon [8], Ilse De Bourdeaudhuij [8], Berthold Koletzko [9], Simona Skripkauskaite [1], Yannis Manios [10] and on behalf of the Toybox-study Group [†]

1. Department of Psychology, University of Roehampton, London SW15 4JD, UK; s.skripkauskaite@bangor.ac.uk
2. Department of Nutrition and Dietetics, School of Physical Education, Sport Science and Dietetics, University of Thessaly, 42132 Trikala, Greece; oandroutsos@uth.gr
3. GENUD (Growth, Exercise, NUtrition and Development) Research Group, Faculty of Health Sciences, University of Zaragoza, Edificio del SAI, C/Pedro Cerbuna s/n, 50009 Saragossa, Spain; lmoreno@unizar.es (L.M.); pfloresbarrantes@gmail.com (P.F.-B.)
4. Instituto Agroalimentario de Aragón (IA2), 50013 Saragossa, Spain
5. Fundación Instituto de Investigación Sanitaria Aragón (IIS Aragón), 50009 Saragossa, Spain
6. The Children's Memorial Health Institute, 04-730 Warsaw, Poland; p.socha@ipczd.pl
7. Department of Pediatrics, Medical University of Varna, 9002 Varna, Bulgaria; violeta.iotova@mu-varna.bg
8. Department of Movement and Sports Sciences, Ghent University, 9000 Ghent, Belgium; greet.cardon@ugent.be (G.C.); Ilse.Debourdeaudhuij@UGent.be (I.D.B.)
9. Dr von Hauner Children's Hospital, LMU-Ludwig-Maximilians-University at Munich, D-80337 Munich, Germany; Berthold.Koletzko@med.uni-muenchen.de
10. Department of Nutrition and Dietetics, School of Health Science and Education, Harokopio University, 17671 Athens, Greece; manios.toybox@hua.gr
* Correspondence: l.gibson@roehampton.ac.uk
† Membership of ToyBox-study group is provided in the Acknowledgments.

Received: 29 December 2019; Accepted: 4 February 2020; Published: 7 February 2020

Abstract: This study investigated parental influences on preschool children's healthy and unhealthy snacking in relation to child obesity in a large cross-sectional multinational sample. Parents and 3–5 year-old child dyads (n = 5185) in a kindergarten-based study provided extensive sociodemographic, dietary practice and food intake data. Parental feeding practices that were derived from questionnaires were examined for associations with child healthy and unhealthy snacking in adjusted multilevel models, including child estimated energy expenditure, parental education, and nutritional knowledge. Parental healthy and unhealthy snacking was respectively associated with their children's snacking (both $p < 0.0001$). Making healthy snacks available to their children was specifically associated with greater child healthy snack intake ($p < 0.0001$). Conversely, practices that were related to unhealthy snacking, i.e., being permissive about unhealthy snacking and acceding to child demands for unhealthy snacks, were associated with greater consumption of unhealthy snacks by children, but also less intake of healthy snacks (all $p < 0.0001$). Parents having more education and greater nutritional knowledge of snack food recommendations had children who ate more healthy snacks (all $p < 0.0001$) and fewer unhealthy snacks ($p = 0.002$, $p < 0.0001$, respectively). In the adjusted models, child obesity was not related to healthy or unhealthy snack intake in these young children. The findings support interventions that address parental practices and distinguish between healthy and unhealthy snacking to influence young children's dietary patterns.

Keywords: child obesity; snacking; preschool children; nutrition; parents; feeding practices; Europe

1. Introduction

Trends in childhood obesity are a concern in many countries, with evidence for increasing prevalence of obesity, even in preschool children [1]. Numerous interventions have been attempted, addressing eating, drinking, and activity energy-balance related behaviours, primarily in school-aged children, but with mixed success [2–4]. In younger children, family environment, and particularly parental feeding practices, are strong predictors of both children's diet [5] and adiposity [6], and so successful interventions should include these aspects.

Snacking is an important energy-balance related dietary behaviour in children: young children have proportionately the highest nutritional and energetic requirements of any stage of the lifespan [7]; thus, frequent eating, including snacking between meals, is typical, easily reinforced, and avoids acute nutritional deficits that might otherwise limit physical and psychological development [8,9]. Therefore, snacking can substantially contribute to daily energy intake; for example, one recent comparison of four national nutritional surveys of 4–13-year-old children found that snacking provided up to one-third of energy intake [10]. Furthermore, there is concern that children's choice of snacks are often particularly high in sugar and fat [11,12]. Therefore, it is important to distinguish between snacking on foods with a healthy nutrient profile (e.g., fruit and vegetables, unsweetened dairy) from those with unhealthy profiles (e.g., those high in fat, sugar, and/or salt, but low in essential nutrients), and to understand their determinants [8].

The strong influence of parental eating behaviour and feeding practices on children's diet is well established [6,13]. However, there is less understanding of parental influences, specifically on children's snacking behaviours [14,15], i.e., energy consumption between meals, particularly in relation to how different healthy or unhealthy snacking habits, might contribute to children's risk of obesity [16]. A recent systematic review of 47 studies on parenting practices that included information on children's snacking found that 39 of these studies concerned parenting practices not specifically related to snacking [17]. Furthermore, the most consistent significant associations were that parental restriction of food was related to higher levels of child snacking, which suggests reactive rather than proactive parenting [17]. This reactive parenting appears to be a common response [18], with such parental food restriction also being positively associated with child obesity [19]. By contrast, there is a paucity of evidence for beneficial effects of proactive parenting, such as modelling, on children's snacking *per se*, although the shared family environment is known to explain most of the variance in snack preferences in preschool children [17,20].

Baseline data from the ToyBox-study (www.toybox-study.eu), a six-country kindergarten-based, family-involved intervention to improve energy-balance related behaviours in preschool children [21], provided the opportunity to examine cross-sectional relationships between parental feeding practices and their children's snacking, in a large and diverse international, yet thoroughly observed, sample. ToyBox-study surveyed parents from six European countries in detail about their attitudes to snacking, their practices in feeding their children, and their own and their children's frequencies of healthy and unhealthy snacking. At the time, these data were collected, there had been little research into relations between parental practices and young children's snacking behaviours, with the exception of the development of the Toddler Snack Food Feeding Questionnaire [22]. Moreover, that study only examined associations between parental practices and unhealthy snacking, and found little association with child obesity. More recently, Davison et al. [15] conducted a qualitative study while using semi-structured interviews of caregivers' snack feeding practices for preschool children. They proposed four dimensions: autonomy support (praise/ support/modelling of healthy snacking/child-centered provision); structure (planning/ routine/availability/monitoring); coercive control (snacks to manage behaviour/unilateral decisions/restriction/pressure); and, permissiveness (no rules/disinterest/emotion-based feeding). By comparison, a quantitative cluster analysis of a

21-item 'Comprehensive Snack Parenting Questionnaire' [23] reported four-dimensional clusters of parental practices: "high covert control and rewarding", "low covert control and non-rewarding", "high involvement and supportive", and "low involvement and indulgent". Parents practising "high involvement and supportive" feeding had children who tended to eat energy-dense snacks least often.

The ToyBox-study questionnaires completed by parents included various items that were related to snacking practices, and in relation to parental nutritional knowledge. Our interest was primarily in examining supra-country patterns for both healthy and unhealthy snacking using hierarchical modelling to control for country differences, although some differences in unhealthy snacking between countries have been reported for the ToyBox-study [24]. Thus, as in the above studies, the present study focused on examining the dimensional structure of responses (grouping of item response variation) on items that were related to parental feeding practices, as being behaviourally and psychometrically more meaningful than examining associations with individual questionnaire items. Therefore, we applied multilevel modelling to determine the independent influences of these parents' feeding practices, their own snacking, and the parents' nutritional knowledge in relation to snacks, on both healthy and unhealthy snacking by their children.

2. Materials and Methods

2.1. Study Design

The Toybox-study was an intervention with a cluster randomized design, having two phases of data collection, at the baseline and at post-intervention (2012–2013). A detailed description of the ToyBox-study design is provided elsewhere [25]. The present study considers the baseline data only. The missing data were not replaced. The ToyBox-study adhered to the Declaration of Helsinki and the conventions of the Council of Europe on human rights and biomedicine. All the countries (Belgium, Bulgaria, Germany, Greece, Poland, and Spain) obtained ethical clearance from the relevant ethical committees and local authorities; all the parents/caregivers provided a signed consent form before being enrolled in the study.

2.2. Participants

Parents or primary caregivers (97% mothers) and their children attending kindergarten while aged 3.5–5.5 years old were recruited to the ToyBox-study, a European Commission-funded large-scale kindergarten-based, family-involved intervention in preschool children, and their families from six European countries: Belgium, Bulgaria, Germany, Greece, Poland, and Spain.

The study sample was composed of preschool children and their families, who were approached via kindergartens that were recruited from three socioeconomic levels of municipalities within each country. All the data presented in the present study were obtained between May and June 2012, while using standard methods and equipment that were applied by trained researchers. Initially, 10,632 parents/caregivers of preschoolers from six European countries provided written informed consent to participate in the ToyBox cross-sectional study. Of these, 8117 parents/caregivers (76.3%) filled in the CORE Questionnaire, and 7244 parents/caregivers (68.1%) filled in the Food Frequency Questionnaire [24]. Demographic information is not available on those parents who failed to participate in questionnaire completion.

Family, sociodemographic, and behavioural data were self-reported by parents and caregivers via the CORE-questionnaire (CORE-Q), including their years of education, weight and height, and their child's sex, and details regarding parental feeding practices and attitudes, which were derived from extensive focus group research and shown to be reliable [26]. Parents also completed a highly structured food frequency questionnaire concerning their child's diet (Child FFQ); this has been validated in a subsample from the ToyBox-study, with moderate to good validity, including for snack foods, such as biscuits [27]. As this study specifically concerns the influence of parental feeding practices, to improve the validity of any associations between the feeding practices and/or obesity of the primary carer and that of the child, we only analysed parent/guardian-child dyads, where the primary carer who completed the questionnaires was also the person who usually cooked for the child and fed the child, as determined by the responses to relevant questions on the CORE-Q. The questionnaires can be found online (www.toybox-study.eu) and detailed information on the development, test-retest reliability, and validity has been described elsewhere [26,28,29].

2.3. Predictor Variables

2.3.1. Derivation of Scales for Parental Attitudes and Practices Regarding Snacking

At the time this study was designed, behavioural models specifically characterising parental feeding practices in relation to child snacking were not available, although three questionnaires have been recently developed in this area [22,23,30]. Nevertheless, as parental practices were of interest in the ToyBox-Study, the CORE-Q contained relevant questions. Although the large multinational sample and intervention design did not allow for a standard psychometric validation, we were interested in examining the possible dimensional structure of the set of questions on this topic, and so applied psychometric analyses to determine this. Thus, suitable items were selected from the CORE-Q based on representing specific beliefs, attitudes, and practices of the parents in regard to their child's snacking behaviour. This section of the questionnaire was headed "Please read the following statements and tick the boxes most appropriate to your situation for morning, afternoon and evening snacks (responses on a five-point Likert scale, from 1 = "strongly disagree" to 5 = "strongly agree"). An initial item analysis was carried out, and after examination of the correlation matrix, some items were excluded as being too similar to others: the remaining 12 items had acceptable distributions, with skewness ranging from 0.05 to −1.06, means ranging from 2.12 to 4.18 (on a 1–5 scale), and the smallest SD = 0.78. Therefore, Principal Components Analysis (PCA) was used to assess these items for potential contribution to unique scales with Promax non-orthogonal rotation. The pattern matrix (Table 1) suggested four factor components (2–4 items per factor with loadings above 0.40). These are labelled as follows: component 1 (3 items) = 'Healthy snack provision'; component 2 (2 items) = 'Permissive healthy snacking'; component 3 (3 items) = 'Unhealthy snacks child responsive'; and, component 4 (4 items) = 'Permissive unhealthy snacking'. Thus, the scale scores were generated from the means of the respective items, having reverse-scored items 9 and 12 (Table 1) for the component 4 scale. These four derived variables were normally distributed. For scales consisting of 2–4 items only, within-scale reliability is likely to be limited [31], but the interest here is in dimensionality derived from the PCA [32]; nevertheless, Guttman's λ_2 values [33] were computed, as follows: healthy snack provision $\lambda_2 = 0.60$; permissive healthy snacking $\lambda_2 = 0.73$; unhealthy snacks child responsive $\lambda_2 = 0.51$; and, permissive unhealthy snacking $\lambda_2 = 0.49$.

Table 1. Pattern matrix from PCA with Promax rotation[a] of parent/carer attitudes and practices from CORE-questionnaire (CORE-Q) item responses related to child snacking.

CORE-Q Items	Component			
	1	2	3	4
1. I make dairy snacks regularly available for my child	**0.812**			
2. I make cereals/bread snacks regularly available for my child	**0.727**	0.136	0.141	
3. I make fruit or vegetables snacks regularly available for my child	**0.625**		−0.276	
4. My child is allowed to eat dairy or cereals/bread as snacks without asking	0.141	**0.849**		
5. My child is allowed to eat fruits or vegetables as snacks without asking		**0.838**		
6. If I prohibit my child to eat a sweet or salty snack, I find it difficult to stick to my rules if he/she starts nagging	−0.119	0.106	**0.733**	
7. I find it difficult to restrain myself from eating sweet or salty snacks because of the presence of my child	0.168	−0.169	**0.686**	
8. I give sweet or salty snacks to my child as a reward or to comfort him/her	−0.126		**0.663**	
9. My child is allowed to eat sweet or salty snacks only at certain occasions i.e., birthdays	0.228		0.177	**−0.726**
10. I make sweet or salty snacks regularly available for my child	0.145		0.153	**0.707**
11. I think eating sweet or salty snacks is not bad for my child	0.135	−0.276		**0.603**
12. My child is not allowed to snack while watching TV		−0.324		**−0.454**

Note: Extraction Method: PCA. [a] Rotation Method: Promax with Kaiser Normalization. Rotation converged in 6 iterations. Item loadings in bold indicate those used for that scale.

2.3.2. Parent/Carer Nutritional Knowledge for Snacks

Questions that were related to parental nutritional knowledge were embedded in the CORE-Q. We used these to develop a measure of nutritional knowledge in relation to snack foods, by establishing a scoring system that was based on expert consensus. Our scoring system incorporated recommendations for both healthy and unhealthy snack foods, and quantified disparity from those recommendations, which allowed for a more nuanced and varied scale scoring than previously derived from this questionnaire [34]: moreover, our method is similar to one that has previously been shown to result in more general nutritional knowledge scores being predictive of children's eating behaviour [35]. A summary measure of parents' understanding of recommended healthy snacking patterns was derived from responses to a question "What do you think is an acceptable consumption of the following food items for 4–6 year-old children?" for each of 10 possible food categories. There were eight possible responses: never; on certain occasions i.e., birthdays; 1 or less times per week; 2–4 times per week; 5–6 times per week; 1–2 times per day; 3–4 times per day; and, 5 or more times per day. The food categories were: sweets/candies/chocolate; biscuits/cookies/cakes/muffins; crisps and other similar salty snacks; fruit and vegetables; pizza, cheese pies/meat pies; milk (plain); yogurt (plain); milk (flavoured); yogurt (flavoured); and, cheese.

The present study interpreted recommendations for snack food consumption based upon the dietary recommendations of the Belgian Health Council, the World Health Organization, and the advice for school food standards for England [36], combined with data on habitual dietary intake in the Belgian population [37] since food-based dietary guidelines (FBDG) for preschool children only exist on a national basis. These FBDG are very similar to dietary guidelines in other countries [38], which makes these guidelines applicable for a European population of preschoolers [39].

On this basis, expert consensus was achieved (Toybox-study Group) on what frequencies of consumption would be recommended for each of these categories, for four to six year-old children, as shown in Table 2, with the exception of cheese for which no consensus was reached. For each category, recommendations encompassed two or three possible frequency responses. Subsequently, responses were recoded to indicate the closeness to the recommendations by giving a maximum score to responses equal to the recommendations, and then one point was subtracted for each frequency level by which the responses differed from recommendations. The maxima were set at either six or seven, depending on whether recommended frequencies spanned two or three levels, so that the minimum possible score for any category was one. For example, if a caregiver indicated that they believed that salty snacks were recommended to be eaten '1 or less times per week', i.e., one level above the nearest recommended frequency, they would be scored as $6 - 1 = 5$ for that response.

Table 2. Description of recommendations for frequency consumption of different snack food categories for preschool children.

Snack Food Category	Recommended Frequency of Consumption
sweets/candies/chocolate	Never to 1 or less times per week
biscuits/cookies/cakes/muffins	Never to 'on certain occasions'
crisps and other similar salty snacks	Never to 'on certain occasions'
fruit and vegetables	3–4 times to 5 or more times per day
pizza, cheese pies/meat pies	'On certain occasions' to '1 or less times per week'
milk (plain)	1–2 to 3–4 times per day
Yogurt (plain)	1–2 to 3–4 times per day
milk (flavoured)	Never to 1 or less times per week
yogurt (flavoured)	Never to 1 or less times per week

Note: Based on national guidelines and expert consensus from the ToyBox-study Group (see text for references).

These individual snack category knowledge scores were summed to provide an overall snack nutritional knowledge score. As this score was negatively skewed, the variable was reversed, then natural log transformed, and then unreversed to maintain the original score direction. This final transformed variable was normally distributed.

2.3.3. Parent/Carer Snack Modelling Behaviour

From the CORE-Q, the principal parental modelling variables were derived from parents' reports of frequency of consuming various snack foods, from a question asking "How often do you consume the following items as a snack (in between your main meals)?". The foods listed were: Nuts/peanuts; Cakes/muffins; Wholemeal Bread; Biscuits/cookies; Crisps and other similar salty snacks; Crackers, breadsticks; Chocolate; Sweets/candies; Cheese; Cheese pies/meat pies; Yogurt/fresh cheeses; Pizza; Fresh fruits; and, Vegetables.

Frequency categories were: never; 1 or less times per week; 2–4 times per week; 5–6 times per week; 1–2 times per day; 3–4 times per day; and, 5 or more times per day. The frequencies were recoded to times per day using mid-point frequencies as follows: 0; 0.143; 0.429; 0.786; 1.5; 3.5; and, 5.

These were used to form a total frequency per day of consuming healthy or unhealthy snack foods, by summing two groups of snack food categories, as follows: 'healthy snacks': nuts, wholemeal bread, yogurt, fruits, vegetables; 'unhealthy snacks': cakes, biscuits, salty snacks, chocolate, sweets, pies, and pizza. These variables were positively skewed and so were transformed by natural logarithm. The transformed variables were normally distributed.

A general parent snacking frequency variable was derived from questions asking "How often do you usually have something to eat as snack between the meals during weekdays, for morning, afternoon and evening snack", with frequency responses ranging from "never" (scored 0), then "On 1 day" up to "on 5 days". The same questions were asked about weekends but responses included "never", "On 1 day" and "On 2 days". The responses were summed to provide a score of overall frequencies of snacking per week. This variable was normally distributed (range 0 to 21, which is the full possible range).

2.4. Anthropometry

Two consecutive measurements of children's weight to the nearest 100 g while using electronic scales (types SECA 861 and SECA 813; Seca, Hamburg, Germany) and height to the nearest 0.1 cm using a portable stadiometer (types SECA 225 and SECA 214; Seca) were taken. For anthropometric measurements, the children were measured in light clothing without shoes, and were asked to stand still in an erect position. Body mass index (BMI; weight, kg/(height, m)^2) z-scores (zBMI) were calculated with use of the LMS method and children were categorized as normal weight or overweight/obese [40]. Parental age, height, and weight were obtained by self-report on the CORE-Q. Parental BMI was positively skewed and so was transformed to a non-skewed distribution by natural logarithm prior to parametric statistical analyses.

Resting energy expenditure (REE) for the children (3–10 years old) was calculated while using the Schofield equation, including both height and weight, as recommended for such populations [41]. This enabled energy needs to be controlled for when, for example, relating child zBMI to snack intake variables.

2.5. Dependent Variables

2.5.1. Child snack Intakes from Child Food Frequency Questionnaire

Two variables were derived from the Child FFQ: first, daily intakes were estimated from the product of the frequency of consumption per day and the standard portion size for that food, as specified on the questionnaire. The intakes of likely snack foods were then grouped into 'healthy' and 'unhealthy' lists, as follows: Healthy snack foods: Plain yogurt; cheese; fresh fruit; raw vegetables; unsweetened cereals; wholemeal bread and similar bakery products. Unhealthy snack foods: chocolate; cakes; biscuits; pastries; sweet spreads; salty snacks; and, sugar-based desserts.

Intakes within each group were summed to provide child healthy and unhealthy snack intake variables. The child unhealthy snack intake variable was positively skewed and so was transformed by a natural logarithm. The transformed variable was normally distributed.

2.5.2. Child Snacking Tendencies

An overall estimate of frequency of child snacking behaviour was derived from the question "How often does your child eat something in between meals?", with the response frequencies ranging from "never or less than once a month" to "every day". The responses were recoded into child snacking frequency per week. However, this variable was somewhat bipolar distributed; therefore, the variable was recoded to form a dichotomous categorical variable, where those children reported to snack either 5–6 days a week or every day were classified as 'snacking most days' (60.6%), and the remaining children were classified as 'not snacking most days' (36.9%; 2.5% missing).

2.6. Alpha Level Adjustment

Alpha level for statistical significance was set at 0.01 due to the large sample size and large number of tests examined.

2.7. Data Analysis

Simple correlations were tested with Pearson's r and partial correlations (r_p), with variables being transformed to normalise if needed. For adjusted models, multilevel modelling was employed to predict child snack intake, using nlme package [42] in R [43], as this acknowledges the hierarchical structure of the data and it is robust against missing values [44]. Two hierarchical models were built, modelling healthy and unhealthy child snack intake. For both models, a two-level hierarchical structure was utilized (i.e., country/child). To be precise, each child with information on child anthropometry, parental attitudes, knowledge, modelling behaviour, and educational status as predictors was nested within the country information. Allowing for intercepts to vary across countries significantly improved the model fit for predicting child healthy snack intake ($\chi^2(1) = 275.43$, $p < 0.001$), and child unhealthy snack intake ($\chi^2(1) = 60.20$, $p < 0.001$), thus justifying the use of multilevel analyses.

For each analysis, adding predictor variables one by one and comparing the current model with the previous one, to develop a final model, created multiple models with fixed effects. Chi-square (χ^2) test of change in log-likelihood with full maximum-likelihood estimation (ML) was used to compare a model fit of different models [45]. The list of relevant predictor variables for each model was decided prior to the analyses and no predictors were excluded from the model due to lack of significance in order to evaluate whether and how much each hypothesised variable predicted the relevant outcome. Once fixed effects were modelled, the existence of random effects was also evaluated.

3. Results

3.1. Participants

From the original sample of 7076 parent-child dyads, 5185 were available for analyses, which included parents reporting involvement in cooking for and feeding their child. Of this sample, 97% of participating parent/caregivers were mothers, 2.4% were fathers, the remaining 0.6% being step-parents or classified as other; the parent/caregiver is referred to here as 'parent'. There were 2685 (51.8%) boys and 2500 (48.2%) girls. Table 3 provides descriptive data for the parents and children.

Table 3. Descriptive statistics for participant characteristics.

	N	Mean	SD	Min.	Max.
Child Age (years)	5183	4.75	0.43	3.50	5.49
Parent/Carer Age (years)	5158	35.60	4.82	21	66
Parent BMI	5080	23.49	4.14	15.23	60.24
Child zBMI	5000	0.22	1.03	−5.87	4.01
Child healthy snack intake (g/d)	5156	256.1	139.7	0.0	842.9
Child unhealthy snack intake (g/d)	5149	57.3	42.4	0.0	374.6
Child resting energy expenditure (kcal/d)	5000	883.65	61.66	701.06	1276.50

3.2. Differences in Child zBMI and Snack Consumption by Country

Child zBMI significantly varied across the six countries (Table 4: one-way ANOVA, country effect, $F(5, 4994) = 18.1$, $p < 0.001$), with the most marked difference being that zBMI for Greece was higher than all other countries.

Table 4. Differences by country in child zBMI and measures of healthy and unhealthy snack consumption, and the ratio of healthy to unhealthy snack intake. Data are expressed as means (95% CIs).

Country	N Range [1]	Child zBMI	Snacks Per Week	Healthy Snack Intake [2] (g/d)	Unhealthy Snack Intake [2] (g/d)	Healthy: Unhealthy Snack Ratio [3]
Belgium	692–700	0.22 [a] (0.15–0.29)	6.11 [a] (5.99–6.23)	219.5 [a] (209.3–229.6)	67.1 [a] (63.9–70.3)	4.24 [a] (3.97–4.51)
Bulgaria	580–606	0.24 [a] (0.16–0.32)	5.13 [bc] (4.95–5.30)	328.9 [b] (318.0–339.8)	64.2 [b] (60.7–67.6)	10.26 [b] (8.56–11.96)
Germany	871–948	0.06 [b] (−0.01–0.12)	5.43 [b] (5.30–5.56)	279.7 [c] (270.7–288.7)	50.4 [bc] (47.6–53.3)	8.38 [bc] (7.43–9.33)
Greece	1258–1306	0.43 [c] (0.37–0.49)	5.43 [b] (5.31–5.55)	248.3 [d] (240.8–255.8)	56.9 [c] (54.5–59.3)	8.60 [bc] (7.60–9.59)
Poland	1055–1065	0.10 [ab] (0.04–0.16)	4.81 [c] (4.69–4.95)	248.2 [d] (240.1–256.2)	55.4 [c] (52.9–58.0)	8.64 [bc] (7.47–9.81)
Spain	517–535	0.21 [ab] (0.12–0.30)	2.00 [d] (1.79–2.20)	209.6 [a] (198.0–221.2)	53.8 [ac] (50.2–57.5)	6.58 [ac] (5.69–7.48)

[1] Sample sizes varied slightly for complete data for each measure within countries. [2] Estimated marginal means adjusted for child resting energy expenditure as a significant covariate. For unhealthy snack intake, analyses were performed on Ln-transformed data. [3] Healthy snack intake divided by unhealthy snack intake, excluding zero values for either variable; a higher number represents a healthier snacking profile. [abcd] Differing superscript letters within each column indicate significant differences between countries (Bonferroni multiple comparisons).

For frequency of snacks per week, Belgium showed the highest, whereas Spain showed the lowest frequency when compared to the other countries (Table 4: one-way ANOVA, country effect, $F(5, 5052) = 271.2$, $p < 0.001$; REE was not a significant covariate for snacking frequency in ANCOVA).

Healthy and unhealthy snack intakes also varied by country but contrasted with differences in snacking frequency. For healthy snack intake, Belgium and Spain showed the lowest intakes, and Bulgaria the highest (Table 4: adjusted for child REE, ANCOVA country effect, $F(5, 4965) = 63.9$, $p < 0.001$; REE covariate, $F(1, 4965) = 33.4$, $p < 0.001$). For unhealthy snack intake, Belgium was notably higher than all other countries (ANCOVA on Ln-transformed data adjusted for REE, country effect, $F(5, 4957) = 20.9$, $p < 0.001$; REE covariate, $F(1, 4965) = 4.01$, $p < 0.05$). We also report the ratio of healthy to unhealthy snack intake, since this provides an indicator of the healthiness of snacking behaviour, independent of overall snack intake: this again varied across countries, with Belgium having the least healthy profile (lowest ratio) as compared to other countries, although not significantly different from the next lowest, Spain (Table 4: one-way ANOVA, country effect, $F(5, 5091) = 11.2$, $p < 0.001$).

3.3. Is Parental Snacking Behaviour Associated with Child Healthy and Unhealthy Snacking?

The overall estimate of parent's weekly snacking frequency was unrelated to child healthy snack intake, but it was associated with greater child unhealthy snack intake (Table 5). Parents' healthy snacking frequency was associated with greater child healthy, but not unhealthy, snack intake. Conversely, parents' unhealthy snacking frequency was associated with greater unhealthy, but not healthy, child snack intake.

Table 5. Correlations (Pearson's r) between parent snacking practices and child snacking behaviour.

Parental Predictor Variables	Child Healthy Snack Intake [a]	Child Unhealthy Snack Intake [b]
Parent healthy snacks/day	0.204 **	−0.014
Parent unhealthy snacks/day	−0.009	0.255 **
Parent snacks/week	0.008	0.121 **
Healthy snack provision	0.115 **	0.018
Permissive healthy snacking	0.075 **	0.006
Unhealthy snacks child responsive	−0.150 *	0.157 **
Permissive unhealthy snacking	−0.136 **	0.249 **
Knowledge of snack recommendations	0.166 **	−0.210 **

* $p < 0.01$, ** $p < 0.001$ for significant Pearson's r correlation (2-tailed). Significance also indicated in bold. [a] N ranges from 5088 to 5122; [b] N ranges from 5081 to 5115.

Furthermore, children who snacked on most days of the week had parents who snacked more often ($n = 3193$, mean [SD] = 11.04 [5.52] times per week) than did children who did not snack on most days of the week ($n = 1798$, mean [SD] = 8.37 [5.29] times per week), $t(3861.3) = 16.89$ $p < 0.001$; adjusted for unequal variances, Levene's $F = 6.80$, $p = 0.009$).

3.4. Are Parental Attitudes and Practices Concerning Snacking Associated with Child Healthy and Unhealthy Snack Intakes?

Providing healthy snacks, and being permissive about allowing healthy snacking were both associated with greater child healthy snack intake, but not with child unhealthy snack intake. Conversely, allowing for unhealthy snacking was strongly associated with greater child unhealthy snack intake, but negatively related to healthy snack intake (Table 5). Similarly, responding to child demands for unhealthy snacks was associated with higher unhealthy snack consumption and less healthy snack consumption by their children.

Greater parent/caregiver understanding of recommendations for snack food consumption for young children was associated with more child healthy snack intake and less child unhealthy snack intake. Moreover, parents with more years of education also had greater knowledge regarding snack recommendations (Pearson's $r(5030) = 0.126$, $p < 0.001$).

These associations, although cross-sectional, suggest that parental snacking behaviour and practices may be influencing both child healthy and unhealthy snack consumption.

3.5. Associations between Snacking Behaviours and Child Obesity

In zero-order correlations, child zBMI was positively associated with children's reported intake of healthy snacks ($r(4972) = 0.051$, $p < 0.001$), but unrelated to unhealthy snack intake ($r(4964) = 0.007$, $p = 0.612$). More parental years of education was associated with higher child healthy snack intake ($r(5050) = 0.081$, $p < 0.001$) and lower unhealthy snack intake ($r(5042) = −0.042$, $p = 0.003$), and with lower child zBMI ($r(4895) = −0.071$, $p < 0.001$).

However, because zBMI is strongly related to REE ($r(5000) = 0.667$, $p < 0.001$), which in turn could drive snack intake, partial correlations were used to control for any influence of REE. zBMI was no longer associated with either healthy ($r_p(4953) = −0.005$, $p = 0.699$) or unhealthy ($r_p(4953) = 0.000$, $p = 0.994$) snack intake with these adjusted partial correlations.

In line with this lack of relationship between zBMI and child snacking, only one significant relationship for snacking attitudes and practices of parents was seen with child zBMI among these partial correlations: children with higher zBMI had parents who tended to report being less permissive regarding healthy snacking by their child ($r_p(4819) = -0.060$, $p < 0.001$). Knowledge of snack recommendations was weakly positively related to zBMI in these adjusted analyses ($r_p = 0.029$, $p = 0.041$), although not significantly at $p < 0.01$. Neither permissiveness nor responsiveness for unhealthy snacking, nor provisioning for healthy snacking, were related to zBMI in these partial correlations (respectively, $r_p = 0.011, 0.001, 0.008$).

3.6. Hierarchical Multilevel Modelling of Predictors of Child Snack Intake

Hierarchical linear regression, or multilevel modelling is the more powerful method for testing for adjusted associations in these hierarchical data. These models adjust for any potentially significant variance due to differences between kindergartens or countries; in this case, the best model used two levels, child nested in country. Tables 6 and 7 present these regression results for predictors of child healthy and unhealthy snack intake, respectively.

Table 6. Hierarchical linear regression statistics for predictors of child healthy snack intake.

Predictor	B (SE)	t(4700)	Predictive p Value
Child zBMI	1.43 (2.48)	0.58	0.565
Resting energy expenditure	0.18 (0.04)	4.24	<0.0001
Parent unhealthy snack intake	3.30 (1.32)	2.50	0.013
Parent healthy snack intake	5.23 (0.59)	8.84	<0.0001
Parent snacking frequency	0.82 (0.37)	2.25	0.025
Knowledge of recommendations	32.99 (4.05)	8.14	<0.0001
Unhealthy snack permissiveness	−17.43 (3.17)	5.50	<0.0001
Unhealthy snack responsiveness	−16.21 (2.64)	6.15	<0.0001
Healthy snack permissiveness	−0.83 (1.97)	0.42	0.675
Healthy snack provision	28.50 (3.06)	9.33	<0.0001
Parent/carer education level	7.42 (1.70)	4.35	<0.0001

Note: The multilevel model accounts for variance at the levels of child (1) and country (2). Child zBMI was a significant fit in the model (Log Likelihood Ratio = 18.30, $p < 0.0001$) but not a significant multilevel predictor of child healthy snack intake. Sex and SES were not related to the dependent variable in this model. Strongest predictors shown in bold.

Table 7. Hierarchical linear regression statistics for predictors of child unhealthy snack intake.

Predictor	B (SE)	t(4693)	Predictive p Value
Child zBMI	−0.62 (0.77)	0.80	0.423
Resting energy expenditure	0.03 (0.02)	2.55	0.011
Parent unhealthy snack intake	4.90 (0.41)	11.83	<0.0001
Parent healthy snack intake	0.10 (0.18)	0.53	0.593
Parent snacking frequency	0.15 (0.11)	1.34	0.180
Knowledge of recommendations	−10.91 (1.26)	8.64	<0.0001
Unhealthy snack permissiveness	8.65 (0.98)	8.85	<0.0001
Unhealthy snack responsiveness	4.90 (0.82)	5.98	<0.0001
Healthy snack permissiveness	1.54 (0.61)	2.53	0.012
Healthy snack provision	0.89 (0.94)	0.95	0.341
Parent/carer education level	−1.64 (0.53)	3.10	0.002

Note: The multilevel model accounts for variance at the levels of child (1) and country (2). Sex and SES were not related to the dependent variable. Strongest predictors shown in bold.

In addition to REE, which was a strong predictor, child healthy snack intake was independently associated with having parents who had more years of education, had better knowledge of snack recommendations, ate more healthy snacks, provided more healthy snacks to their children, and were more restrictive of unhealthy snack consumption (Table 6). Child zBMI was unrelated to healthy snack intake.

In contrast, for child unhealthy snack intake, REE was relatively weakly positively related, implying mainly non-regulatory (e.g., hedonic) drivers to eat such snacks (Table 7). Children who ate more unhealthy snacks had parent/carers who ate more unhealthy snacks, were less restrictive of their children eating such snacks, had fewer years of education, and were less knowledgeable about snack recommendations. Child unhealthy snack intake was also unrelated to parents' healthy snacking, implying a specific association to the class of snack.

4. Discussion

This study has applied some novel behavioural measures of parental attitudes, as well as their own snacking behaviour, to both healthy and unhealthy child snacking behaviour, in a cross-sectional analysis of a large and well-measured sample of 3.5–5.5 year-old children. The findings contribute to the limited existing literature on this topic [30], and they provide some useful and novel understandings of the differential influences of parental behaviour on healthy and unhealthy snacking by their children, and implications for obesity risk in young children.

There was clear evidence that parental habitual snacking was associated with, and likely influenced, their child's snacking: thus, for the specific parental snack frequency variables, parental healthy and unhealthy snack intake predicted respective child healthy and unhealthy snack intake, but not vice-versa. Furthermore, children who snacked on most days had parents who reported snacking more frequently than did the parents of children who did not snack on most days. These associations could reflect the child acquiring snacking habits through parental modelling of snacking, although other mechanisms could be involved, including exposure and opportunity via snack availability in the home. Our data do not allow for us to distinguish these possibilities for certain, although the parent/carer was specifically the main feeder of their child here, parent/carer snack intake was predictive of child snack intake independently of a measure of snack provision, and parental modelling has been shown to promote both snacking [46,47] and fruit and vegetable consumption [35,48,49].

The parental feeding strategies for young children are known to result in differential effects on the healthiness of their children's diets [50,51]. Here, being permissive about their child's snacking promoted only unhealthy snack intake, whereas children's healthy snack intake was higher in parents who were specifically less permissive of, or less responsive to, unhealthy snacking. It is possible that the more hedonically attractive, and energy-dense, nature of unhealthy snacks makes them more amenable to such parental strategies or simple modelling effects than might be the case for healthier snacks, at least in young children [52,53]. A key variable that was not directly assessed here might be expressed preference as opposed to just intake, as in another study maternal food preferences were an important predictor of children's intake of healthy foods but not unhealthy foods [53]. Nevertheless, in this study, healthy snack provision did appear to promote specifically healthy snack intake, independent of parental intake, nutritional knowledge, or education. It should also be noted that these results are independent of country differences, as this level was controlled for in the multilevel modelling. Nevertheless, we replicated the earlier report from ToyBox-study data that Belgium children appear to most frequently snack [24], and extend this to show that their snacking profile was the least healthy of the six countries. Presumably, the country differences in snacking reflect a combination of cultural, economic, environmental, and food availability influences.

To summarise, beyond potential modelling effects from eating snacks (to the extent to which this happened in the child's presence), our findings from the measures representing parental snack feeding practices were also significantly associated with the children's healthy and unhealthy snack consumption. On the positive side, parents' practices of making healthy snacks available to their children was associated with greater child healthy snack intake, but it did not relate to unhealthy snack intake. Conversely, parental practices that are related to unhealthy snacking, i.e., being permissive about unhealthy snacking including making them available, and being responsive or acceding to child demands for unhealthy snacks, was associated with the greater consumption of unhealthy snacks by children, but also less intake of healthy snacks. This suggests that when unhealthy snacking is encouraged, their intake displaces healthy snacks from children's diet, although the reverse might not be the case.

In addition to these parental practices regarding their children's snacking, parents having greater nutritional knowledge of snack food recommendations had children who ate more healthy snacks and fewer unhealthy snacks. This measure was a strong predictor of child healthy vs. unhealthy snacking, independent of education level: thus, this finding supports the use of nutritional education for parents as an aspect of interventions addressing children's diets and obesity risk [34]. The weak tendency for higher child zBMI to be associated with greater parental nutritional knowledge was an unexpected finding: if not a chance result, it could perhaps indicate some reverse causality, i.e., greater interest in dietary recommendations among parents with more overweight children.

The associations between parental snacking practices and their children's snacking shows that such parenting techniques are significant influences on healthy and unhealthy snacking in these young children: thus, practitioners should educate parents regarding the importance of their own behaviours, as well as instilling knowledge of snack food group recommendations, whilst being aware that less educated parents are particularly at risk of unhealthy parental practices [54,55]. Furthermore, such advice is supported by evidence that interventions, such as the ToyBox-study, can improve relevant parental snacking practices and rule-setting, as well as nutritional knowledge of parents [34]. However, there was little support here for associations between child snacking and child obesity, which is in agreement with a previous analysis of associations between unhealthy snacking and baseline BMI in these children, although soft drink consumption, which was not examined here, was found to be positively related to BMI [56]. One reason might be that this age range is approaching the age (5–6 years old) at which BMI typically reaches a minimum ('adiposity rebound'), thus limiting the variance in BMI, before rising again through to adulthood. The limited associations between either child snacking or parental snacking practices and child obesity are also consistent with other studies of parental and child snacking behaviours and obesity in similar aged young children [22,30]. Still, children starting the adiposity rebound at a younger age are much more likely to be obese in adulthood [57], so preschool child overweight or obesity is still a concern; furthermore, child obesity dramatically increases during early school years, and unhealthy energy-dense snacking is likely to be a contributory factor [12]. Moreover, we did find evidence that parents who were less permissive in encouraging healthy snacking had children with higher zBMI; this might indicate that healthy snacks, which are generally lower in energy density than unhealthy snacks, could help displace unhealthy snacks and so reduce the children's overall energy intake.

With this in mind, particularly from a research perspective, an innovation in this study was to include REE as a predictor alongside BMI, in an attempt to separate the impact that greater energy needs *per se* might have on snack intake from other behavioural characteristics that may be inherently linked to being a heavier child. For instance, snacking, especially as defined by eating energy-dense food between meals, has been considered to be an expression of 'eating in the absence of hunger', which has been associated with an increased adiposity in young children [8,58], perhaps due to weaker appetite regulation in more overweight children [59], which in turn could result from parental use of controlling feeding practices [60]. However, the inclusion of REE in the regression analyses resulted in REE, but not zBMI being a significant predictor of both healthy and unhealthy snack intake in our fully adjusted multilevel models. It should also be noted that, despite zBMI being greater in Greece than the other intervention countries, as was previously observed [61], our hierarchical analyses controlled for such country-level variation. Furthermore, although sex differences in the associations between fruit and vegetable intake and child obesity have been reported for this ToyBox-Study cohort (albeit a smaller sample) [56], we did not find an effect of sex on healthy or unhealthy child snack intake in our multilevel models, including REE. Therefore, investigators should consider controlling for differences in physiological energy requirements that vary with body mass, age, and sex when examining relationships between children's snack intake, obesity and potential behavioural risk factors; then, for example, any associations between snacking-related behaviours and child obesity would not be confounded by greater energy needs in more overweight or at least heavier, older, or faster-growing children.

This study is limited by the self-report nature of the behavioural variables, and the development of new measures without full psychometric validation. A further limitation of our observations is that the effect sizes were generally moderate to very small, and the associations cross-sectional: thus, it must be acknowledged that other factors, some of which may covary with snacking, which have not been addressed here, could play more important roles in linking parental and child behaviour to child obesity risk [62,63]. It is also possible that unhealthy snacking has not yet had time to influence the development of obesity in these young children; however, we only examined cross-sectional relationships at baseline in order to benefit from the largest sample size.

One factor not measured here that could disrupt simple associations between overweight and obesity, healthy or unhealthy snacking, parental practices, and indeed fruit and vegetable intake, is the children's fussy eating tendencies, since fussy eaters will tend to avoid snacking on healthy foods, yet also tend to be thinner [64,65]. In fact, parents often struggle to find successful strategies for promoting healthy eating in picky/fussy children [66]. Moreover, it is likely that associations between energy-dense snack consumption and obesity will increase with age of the child [56,58].

5. Conclusions

Child obesity was unrelated to their (healthy or unhealthy) snack intake, in adjusted models that included energy requirements, parental education, and feeding practices, perhaps reflecting the young age of the children and the greater importance of parental influences. Clear independent predictors of both healthy and unhealthy snacking included knowledge of dietary recommendations for snack foods (negative for unhealthy snacking), parent/carer education, and parent/carer snack intake. Unhealthy snacking can lead to dietary habits that are harmful to health, irrespective of obesity, and these findings could help to support interventions for improving children's nutritional status, as well as the dissemination of healthy dietary practices to parents of young children.

Author Contributions: Study conceptualisation, E.L.G., G.C., I.D.B., B.K., Y.M. and O.A.; Methodology, E.L.G., L.M., P.F.-B., P.S., V.I., G.C., I.D.B., B.K., Y.M. and O.A.; Formal Analysis, E.L.G. and S.S.; Investigation and data collection, all authors; Data Curation, E.L.G., L.M., S.S., Y.M. and O.A.; Writing—Original Draft Preparation, E.L.G., V.I., G.C., I.D.B., B.K., and O.A.; Writing—Review & Editing, E.L.G., L.M., P.F.-B., V.I., G.C., I.D.B., B.K., S.S., Y.M. and O.A.; Visualization, E.L.G.; Supervision, Y.M. and O.A.; Project Administration, Y.M. and O.A.; Resources, Y.M., I.D.B., B.K., L.M., V.I. and P.S.; Funding Acquisition, Y.M., I.D.B., B.K., L.M., V.I., and P.S. All authors revised the manuscript for important intellectual content, read and approved the final manuscript. All authors have read and agreed to the published version of the manuscript.

Funding: The ToyBox study was funded by the Seventh Framework Programme (CORDIS FP7) of the European Commission under grant agreement no. 245200. The content of this article reflects only the authors' views and the European Community is not liable for any use that may be made of the information contained therein. Funding from this grant is not available to cover APC fees.

Acknowledgments: The authors would like to thank the members of the ToyBox study group: Coordinator: Y.M.; Project manager: O.A.; Steering Committee: Y.M., B.K., I.D.B., Mai Chin A Paw, L.M., Carolyn Summerbell, Tim Lobstein, Lieven Annemans, Goof Buijs; External Advisors: John Reilly, Boyd Swinburn, Dianne Ward; Harokopio University (Greece): Y.M., O.A., Eva Grammatikaki, Christina Katsarou, Eftychia Apostolidou, Anastasia Livaniou, Eirini Efstathopoulou, Paraskevi- Eirini Siatitsa, Angeliki Giannopoulou, Effie Argyri, Konstantina Maragkopoulou, Athanasios Douligeris, Roula Koutsi; Ludwig Maximilians Universitaet Muenchen (Germany): B.K., Kristin Duvinage, Sabine Ibrügger, Angelika Strauß, Birgit Herbert, Julia Birnbaum, Annette Payr, Christine Geyer; Ghent University (Belgium): Department of Movement and Sports Sciences: I.D.B., Greet Cardon, Marieke De Craemer, Ellen De Decker; Department of Public Health: Lieven Annemans, Stefaan De Henauw, Lea Maes, Carine Vereecken, Jo Van Assche, Lore Pil; VU University Medical Center EMGO Institute for Health and Care Research (The Netherlands): EMGO Institute for Health and Care Research: Mai Chin A Paw, Saskia te Velde; University of Zaragoza (Spain): L.M., Theodora Mouratidou, Juan Fernandez, Maribel Mesana, Pilar De Miguel-Etayo, Esther M. González-Gil, Luis Gracia-Marco, Beatriz Oves, Paloma Flores Barran; Oslo and Akershus University College of Applied Sciences (Norway): Agneta Yngve, Susanna Kugelberg, Christel Lynch, Annhild Mosdøl, Bente B. Nilsen; University of Durham (UK): Carolyn Summerbell, Helen Moore, Wayne Douthwaite, Catherine Nixon; State Institute of Early Childhood Research (Germany): Susanne Kreichauf, Andreas Wildgruber; Children's Memorial Health Institute (Poland): Piotr Socha, Zbigniew Kulaga, Kamila Zych, Magdalena Góźdź, Beata Gurzkowska, Katarzyna Szott; Medical University of Varna (Bulgaria): Violeta Iotova, Mina Lateva, Natalya Usheva, Sonya

Galcheva, Vanya Marinova, Zhaneta Radkova, Nevyana Feschieva; International Association for the Study of Obesity (UK): Tim Lobstein, Andrea Aikenhead; CBO B.V. (the Netherlands): Goof Buijs, Annemiek Dorgelo, Aviva Nethe, Jan Jansen; AOK-Verlag (Germany): Otto Gmeiner, Jutta Retterath, Julia Wildeis, Axel Günthersberger; Roehampton University (UK): Leigh Gibson; University of Luxembourg (Luxembourg): Claus Voegele.

Conflicts of Interest: The authors declare no conflict of interest.

References

1. World Health Organisation. *Report of the Commission on Ending Childhood Obesity*; World Health Organisation: Geneva, Switzerland, 2016.
2. Colquitt, J.L.; Loveman, E.; O'Malley, C.; Azevedo, L.B.; Mead, E.; Al-Khudairy, L.; Ells, L.J.; Metzendorf, M.I.; Rees, K. Diet, physical activity, and behavioural interventions for the treatment of overweight or obesity in preschool children up to the age of 6 years. *Cochrane Database Syst. Rev.* **2016**, *3*. [CrossRef] [PubMed]
3. Gibson, E.L.; Kreichauf, S.; Wildgruber, A.; Vogele, C.; Summerbell, C.D.; Nixon, C.; Moore, H.; Douthwaite, W.; Manios, Y.; ToyBox-Study Group. A narrative review of psychological and educational strategies applied to young children's eating behaviours aimed at reducing obesity risk. *Obes. Rev.* **2012**, *13* (Suppl. 1), 85–95. [CrossRef] [PubMed]
4. Waters, E.; de Silva-Sanigorski, A.; Hall, B.J.; Brown, T.; Campbell, K.J.; Gao, Y.; Armstrong, R.; Prosser, L.; Summerbell, C.D. Interventions for preventing obesity in children. *Cochrane Database Syst. Rev.* **2011**. [CrossRef] [PubMed]
5. Savage, J.S.; Fisher, J.O.; Birch, L.L. Parental influence on eating behavior: Conception to adolescence. *J. Law Med. Ethics* **2007**, *35*, 22–34. [CrossRef]
6. Birch, L.L.; Ventura, A.K. Preventing childhood obesity: What works? *Int. J. Obes.* **2009**, *33*, S74–S81. [CrossRef]
7. Wang, Z. High ratio of resting energy expenditure to body mass in childhood and adolescence: A mechanistic model. *Am. J. Hum. Biol.* **2012**, *24*, 460–467. [CrossRef]
8. Bellisle, F. Meals and snacking, diet quality and energy balance. *Physiol. Behav.* **2014**, *134*, 38–43. [CrossRef]
9. Gibson, E.L.; Wardle, J. Energy density predicts preferences for fruit and vegetables in 4-year-old children. *Appetite* **2003**, *41*, 97–98. [CrossRef]
10. Wang, D.; van der Horst, K.; Jacquier, E.F.; Afeiche, M.C.; Eldridge, A.L. Snacking patterns in children: A comparison between Australia, China, Mexico, and the US. *Nutrients* **2018**, *10*. [CrossRef]
11. Dunford, E.K.; Popkin, B.M. 37 year snacking trends for US children 1977–2014. *Pediatr. Obes.* **2018**, *13*, 247–255. [CrossRef]
12. Public Health England. PHE Launches Change4Life Campaign around Children's Snacking. Available online: https://www.gov.uk/government/news/phe-launches-change4life-campaign-around-childrens-snacking (accessed on 9 March 2018).
13. Yee, A.Z.; Lwin, M.O.; Ho, S.S. The influence of parental practices on child promotive and preventive food consumption behaviors: A systematic review and meta-analysis. *Int. J. Behav. Nutr. Phys. Act.* **2017**, *14*, 47. [CrossRef] [PubMed]
14. Corsini, N.; Kettler, L.; Danthiir, V.; Wilson, C. Parental feeding practices to manage snack food intake: Associations with energy intake regulation in young children. *Appetite* **2018**, *123*, 233–240. [CrossRef] [PubMed]
15. Davison, K.K.; Blake, C.E.; Blaine, R.E.; Younginer, N.A.; Orloski, A.; Hamtil, H.A.; Ganter, C.; Bruton, Y.P.; Vaughn, A.E.; Fisher, J.O. Parenting around child snacking: Development of a theoretically-guided, empirically informed conceptual model. *Int. J. Behav. Nutr. Phys. Act.* **2015**, *12*, 109. [CrossRef] [PubMed]
16. Kral, T.V.E.; Chittams, J.; Moore, R.H. Relationship between food insecurity, child weight status, and parent-reported child eating and snacking behaviors. *J. Spec. Pediatr. Nurs.* **2017**, *22*. [CrossRef] [PubMed]
17. Blaine, R.E.; Kachurak, A.; Davison, K.K.; Klabunde, R.; Fisher, J.O. Food parenting and child snacking: A systematic review. *Int. J. Behav. Nutr. Phys. Act.* **2017**, *14*, 146. [CrossRef]
18. Webber, L.; Cooke, L.; Hill, C.; Wardle, J. Child adiposity and maternal feeding practices: A longitudinal analysis. *Am. J. Clin. Nutr.* **2011**, *92*, 1423–1428. [CrossRef]

19. Webber, L.; Hill, C.; Cooke, L.; Carnell, S.; Wardle, J. Associations between child weight and maternal feeding styles are mediated by maternal perceptions and concerns. *Eur. J. Clin. Nutr.* **2010**, *64*, 259–265. [CrossRef]
20. Fildes, A.; van Jaarsveld, C.H.; Llewellyn, C.H.; Fisher, A.; Cooke, L.; Wardle, J. Nature and nurture in children's food preferences. *Am. J. Clin. Nutr.* **2014**, *99*, 911–917. [CrossRef]
21. Manios, Y.; Grammatikaki, E.; Androutsos, O.; Chinapaw, M.J.; Gibson, E.L.; Buijs, G.; Iotova, V.; Socha, P.; Annemans, L.; Wildgruber, A.; et al. A systematic approach for the development of a kindergarten-based intervention for the prevention of obesity in preschool age children: The ToyBox-study. *Obes. Rev.* **2012**, *13* (Suppl. 1), 3–12. [CrossRef]
22. Corsini, N.; Wilson, C.; Kettler, L.; Danthiir, V. Development and preliminary validation of the Toddler Snack Food Feeding Questionnaire. *Appetite* **2010**, *54*, 570–578. [CrossRef]
23. Gevers, D.W.M.; Kremers, S.P.J.; de Vries, N.K.; van Assema, P. The Comprehensive Snack Parenting Questionnaire (CSPQ): Development and test-retest reliability. *Int. J. Environ. Res. Public Health* **2018**, *15*, 862. [CrossRef] [PubMed]
24. De Craemer, M.; Lateva, M.; Iotova, V.; De Decker, E.; Verloigne, M.; De Bourdeaudhuij, I.; Androutsos, O.; Socha, P.; Kulaga, Z.; Moreno, L.; et al. Differences in energy balance-related behaviours in European preschool children: The ToyBox-study. *PLoS ONE* **2015**, *10*, e0118303. [CrossRef] [PubMed]
25. Manios, Y.; Androutsos, O.; Katsarou, C.; Iotova, V.; Socha, P.; Geyer, C.; Moreno, L.; Koletzko, B.; De Bourdeaudhuij, I.; ToyBox-study Group. Designing and implementing a kindergarten-based, family-involved intervention to prevent obesity in early childhood: The ToyBox-study. *Obes. Rev.* **2014**, *15* (Suppl. 3), 5–13. [CrossRef] [PubMed]
26. Gonzalez-Gil, E.M.; Mouratidou, T.; Cardon, G.; Androutsos, O.; De Bourdeaudhuij, I.; Gozdz, M.; Usheva, N.; Birnbaum, J.; Manios, Y.; Moreno, L.A.; et al. Reliability of primary caregivers reports on lifestyle behaviours of European pre-school children: The ToyBox-study. *Obes. Rev.* **2014**, *15* (Suppl. 3), 61–66. [CrossRef] [PubMed]
27. Mouratidou, T.; Mesana Graffe, M.I.; Huybrechts, I.; De Decker, E.; De Craemer, M.; Androutsos, O.; Manios, Y.; Galcheva, S.; Lateva, M.; Gurzkowska, B.; et al. Reproducibility and relative validity of a semiquantitative food frequency questionnaire in European preschoolers: The ToyBox study. *Nutrition* **2019**, *65*, 60–67. [CrossRef] [PubMed]
28. Huybrechts, I.; De Backer, G.; De Bacquer, D.; Maes, L.; De Henauw, S. Relative validity and reproducibility of a food-frequency questionnaire for estimating food intakes among Flemish preschoolers. *Int. J. Environ. Res. Public Health* **2009**, *6*, 382–399. [CrossRef]
29. Mouratidou, T.; Miguel, M.L.; Androutsos, O.; Manios, Y.; De Bourdeaudhuij, I.; Cardon, G.; Kulaga, Z.; Socha, P.; Galcheva, S.; Iotova, V.; et al. Tools, harmonization and standardization procedures of the impact and outcome evaluation indices obtained during a kindergarten-based, family-involved intervention to prevent obesity in early childhood: The ToyBox-study. *Obes. Rev.* **2014**, *15* (Suppl. 3), 53–60. [CrossRef]
30. Davison, K.K.; Blake, C.E.; Kachurak, A.; Lumeng, J.C.; Coffman, D.L.; Miller, A.L.; Hughes, S.O.; Power, T.G.; Vaughn, A.F.; Blaine, R.E.; et al. Development and preliminary validation of the Parenting around SNAcking Questionnaire (P-SNAQ). *Appetite* **2018**, *125*, 323–332. [CrossRef]
31. Rammstedt, B.; Beierlein, C. Can't We Make It Any Shorter? The limits of personality assessment and ways to overcome them. *J. Individ. Differ.* **2014**, *35*, 212–220. [CrossRef]
32. Sijtsma, K. On the Use, the Misuse, and the Very Limited Usefulness of Cronbach's Alpha. *Psychometrika* **2009**, *74*, 107–120. [CrossRef]
33. Guttman, L. A basis for analyzing test-retest reliability. *Psychometrika* **1945**, *10*, 255–282. [CrossRef] [PubMed]
34. Lambrinou, C.P.; van Stralen, M.M.; Androutsos, O.; Cardon, G.; De Craemer, M.; Iotova, V.; Socha, P.; Koletzko, B.; Moreno, L.A.; Manios, Y. Mediators of the effectiveness of a kindergarten-based, family-involved intervention on pre-schoolers' snacking behaviour: The ToyBox-study. *Public Health Nutr.* **2019**, *22*, 157–163. [CrossRef] [PubMed]
35. Gibson, E.L.; Wardle, J.; Watts, C.J. Fruit and vegetable consumption, nutritional knowledge and beliefs in mothers and children. *Appetite* **1998**, *31*, 205–228. [CrossRef] [PubMed]
36. Department for Education, England. Standards for school food in England. Available online: https://www.gov.uk/government/publications/standards-for-school-food-in-england (accessed on 12 December 2017).

37. De Keyzer, W.; Lin, Y.; Vereecken, C.; Maes, L.; Van Oyen, H.; Vanhauwaert, E.; De Backer, G.; De Henauw, S.; Huybrechts, I. Dietary sources of energy and macronutrient intakes among Flemish preschoolers. *Arch. Public Health* **2011**, *69*, 5. [CrossRef]
38. European Food Information Council. Food-based dietary guidelines in Europe. Available online: http://www.eufic.org/en/healthy-living/article/food-based-dietary-guidelines-in-europe (accessed on 16 March 2018).
39. Nutrition Information Centre, Belgium. De Actieve Voedingsdriehoek Voor Kleuters. Available online: http://www.123aantafel.be/03/03btabel2.html (accessed on 28 February 2018).
40. Cole, T.J.; Lobstein, T. Extended international (IOTF) body mass index cut-offs for thinness, overweight and obesity. *Pediatr. Obes.* **2012**, *7*, 284–294. [CrossRef]
41. Rodriguez, G.; Moreno, L.A.; Sarria, A.; Fleta, J.; Bueno, M. Resting energy expenditure in children and adolescents: Agreement between calorimetry and prediction equations. *Clin. Nutr.* **2002**, *21*, 255–260. [CrossRef]
42. Pinheiro, J.; Bates, D.; DebRoy, S.; Sarkar, D.; Team, R.C. Nlme: Linear and nonlinear mixed effects models. Available online: https://CRAN.R-project.org/package=nlme (accessed on 17 July 2018).
43. R Development Core Team. *R: A language and environment for statistical computing*; R Foundation for Statistical Computing: Vienna, Austria, 2015; Available online: http://www.R-project.org (accessed on 2 April 2018).
44. Baayen, R.H.; Davidson, D.J.; Bates, D.M. Mixed-effects modeling with crossed random effects for subjects and items. *J. Memory Lang.* **2008**, *59*, 390–412. [CrossRef]
45. Field, A.P.; Miles, J.; Field, Z. *Discovering Statistics Using R.*; SAGE Publications Ltd.: London, UK, 2012; p. 992.
46. Brown, R.; Ogden, J. Children's eating attitudes and behaviour: A study of the modelling and control theories of parental influence. *Health Educ. Res.* **2004**, *19*, 261–271. [CrossRef]
47. Dickens, E.; Ogden, J. The role of parental control and modelling in predicting a child's diet and relationship with food after they leave home a prospective study. *Appetite* **2014**, *76*, 23–29. [CrossRef]
48. Cooke, L.J.; Wardle, J.; Gibson, E.L.; Sapochnik, M.; Sheiham, A.; Lawson, M. Demographic, familial and trait predictors of fruit and vegetable consumption by pre-school children. *Public Health Nutr.* **2004**, *7*, 295–302. [CrossRef]
49. Draxten, M.; Fulkerson, J.A.; Friend, S.; Flattum, C.F.; Schow, R. Parental role modeling of fruits and vegetables at meals and snacks is associated with children's adequate consumption. *Appetite* **2014**, *78*, 1–7. [CrossRef] [PubMed]
50. Kristiansen, A.L.; Bjelland, M.; Himberg-Sundet, A.; Lien, N.; Andersen, L.F. Associations between sociocultural home environmental factors and vegetable consumption among Norwegian 3-5-year olds: BRA-study. *Appetite* **2017**, *117*, 310–320. [CrossRef]
51. Russell, C.G.; Haszard, J.J.; Taylor, R.W.; Heath, A.-L.M.; Taylor, B.; Campbell, K.J. Parental feeding practices associated with children's eating and weight: What are parents of toddlers and preschool children doing? *Appetite* **2018**, *128*, 120–128. [CrossRef] [PubMed]
52. Beets, M.W.; Tilley, F.; Kyryliuk, R.; Weaver, R.G.; Moore, J.B.; Turner-McGrievy, G. Children select unhealthy choices when given a choice among snack offerings. *J. Acad. Nutr. Diet.* **2014**, *114*, 1440–1446. [CrossRef] [PubMed]
53. Johnson, L.; van Jaarsveld, C.H.; Wardle, J. Individual and family environment correlates differ for consumption of core and non-core foods in children. *Br. J. Nutr.* **2011**, *105*, 950–959. [CrossRef]
54. Fisher, J.O.; Wright, G.; Herman, A.N.; Malhotra, K.; Serrano, E.L.; Foster, G.D.; Whitaker, R.C. Snacks are not food. Low-income, urban mothers' perceptions of feeding snacks to their preschool-aged children. *Appetite* **2015**, *84*, 61–67. [CrossRef]
55. Miguel-Berges, M.L.; Zachari, K.; Santaliestra-Pasias, A.M.; Mouratidou, T.; Androutsos, O.; Iotova, V.; Galcheva, S.; De Craemer, M.; Cardon, G.; Koletzko, B.; et al. Clustering of energy balance-related behaviours and parental education in European preschool children: The ToyBox study. *Br. J. Nutr.* **2017**, *118*, 1089–1096. [CrossRef]
56. Cardon, G.; De Bourdeaudhuij, I.; Iotova, V.; Latomme, J.; Socha, P.; Koletzko, B.; Moreno, L.; Manios, Y.; Androutsos, O.; De Craemer, M.; et al. Health related behaviours in normal weight and overweight preschoolers of a large pan-European sample: The ToyBox-Study. *PLoS ONE* **2016**, *11*, e0150580. [CrossRef]

57. Whitaker, R.C.; Pepe, M.S.; Wright, J.A.; Seidel, K.D.; Dietz, W.H. Early adiposity rebound and the risk of adult obesity. *Pediatrics* **1998**, *101*, e5. [CrossRef]
58. Hill, C.; Llewellyn, C.H.; Saxton, J.; Webber, L.; Semmler, C.; Carnell, S.; van Jaarsveld, C.H.M.; Boniface, D.; Wardle, J. Adiposity and 'eating in the absence of hunger' in children. *Int. J. Obes.* **2008**, *32*, 1499–1505. [CrossRef]
59. Carnell, S.; Benson, L.; Gibson, E.L.; Mais, L.A.; Warkentin, S. Caloric compensation in preschool children: Relationships with body mass and differences by food category. *Appetite* **2017**, *116*, 82–89. [CrossRef] [PubMed]
60. Birch, L.L.; Fisher, J.O.; Davison, K.K. Learning to overeat: Maternal use of restrictive feeding practices promotes girls' eating in the absence of hunger. *Am. J. Clin. Nutr.* **2003**, *78*, 215–220. [CrossRef] [PubMed]
61. Manios, Y.; Androutsos, O.; Katsarou, C.; Vampouli, E.A.; Kulaga, Z.; Gurzkowska, B.; Iotova, V.; Usheva, N.; Cardon, G.; Koletzko, B.; et al. Prevalence and sociodemographic correlates of overweight and obesity in a large Pan-European cohort of preschool children and their families: The ToyBox study. *Nutrition* **2018**, *55*, 192–198. [CrossRef] [PubMed]
62. Llewellyn, C.; Wardle, J. Behavioral susceptibility to obesity: Gene-environment interplay in the development of weight. *Physiol. Behav.* **2015**, *152*, 494–501. [CrossRef] [PubMed]
63. Carnell, S.; Wardle, J. Appetite and adiposity in children: Evidence for a behavioral susceptibility theory of obesity. *Am. J. Clin. Nutr.* **2008**, *88*, 22–29. [CrossRef]
64. Dubois, L.; Farmer, A.P.; Girard, M.; Peterson, K. Preschool children's eating behaviours are related to dietary adequacy and body weight. *Eur. J. Clin. Nutr.* **2007**, *61*, 846–855. [CrossRef]
65. Gibson, E.L.; Cooke, L. Understanding food fussiness and its implications for food choice, health, weight and interventions in young children: The impact of Professor Jane Wardle. *Curr. Obes. Rep.* **2017**, *6*, 46–56. [CrossRef]
66. Russell, C.G.; Worsley, A.; Campbell, K.J. Strategies used by parents to influence their children's food preferences. *Appetite* **2015**, *90*, 123–130. [CrossRef]

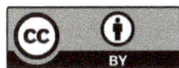 © 2020 by the authors. Licensee MDPI, Basel, Switzerland. This article is an open access article distributed under the terms and conditions of the Creative Commons Attribution (CC BY) license (http://creativecommons.org/licenses/by/4.0/).

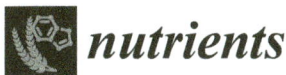

Article

Can Parenting Practices Moderate the Relationship between Reward Sensitivity and Adolescents' Consumption of Snacks and Sugar-Sweetened Beverages?

Wendy Van Lippevelde [1,2,*], Leentje Vervoort [3], Jolien Vangeel [4] and Lien Goossens [3]

1. Department of Marketing, Innovation and Organisation, Ghent University, 9000 Ghent, Belgium
2. Department of Nutrition and Public Health, University of Agder, 4604 Kristiansand, Norway
3. Department of Developmental, Personality and Social Psychology, Ghent University, 9000 Ghent, Belgium; Leentje.Vervoort@ugent.be (L.V.); Lien.Goossens@ugent.be (L.G.)
4. Department of Business studies and Business Administration, Karel De Grote University College, 2000 Antwerp, Belgium; Jolien.Vangeel@kdg.be
* Correspondence: Wendy.VanLippevelde@ugent.be; Tel.: +32-486-155780

Received: 5 November 2019; Accepted: 18 December 2019; Published: 8 January 2020

Abstract: Background: Reward sensitivity has been associated with adolescents' intake of unhealthy snacks and sugar-sweetened beverages. However, so far, there are no studies published describing the impact of parenting practices on this relationship. The present study will, therefore, investigate whether food parenting practices can moderate the association between reward sensitivity and diet intakes. Method: A cross-sectional research study was conducted among 14- to 16-year old Flemish adolescents (n = 867, age 14.7 ± 0.8 y, 48.1% boys) and a subset of their parents (n = 131), collecting data on daily intakes, reward sensitivity, and food parenting practices. Linear regression was used to assess the moderation effect of parenting practices (both adolescent- and parent-reported) on the relationship between reward sensitivity, and diet using SPSS 25.0. Results: In the main analysis (adolescent-reported), no significant moderation effects were found for parenting practices on the relationship between reward sensitivity and diet. However, the sensitivity analysis (parent-reported) showed a moderation effect for health-reducing parenting practices on the association between reward sensitivity and unhealthy snack intake (β = 0.297, 95% CI = 0.062, 0.531, p = 0.01). Conclusion: Given the difference in the effect of parenting practices between the adolescent- and parent-reported data, our inconclusive findings warrant more research in larger adolescent-parent dyad samples.

Keywords: adolescent; reward sensitivity; parents; nutrition; environment; snacks; sugar-sweetened beverages

1. Introduction

Adolescents' eating pattern is characterized by a high intake of energy-dense snacks and sugar-sweetened beverages (SSBs) [1,2]. Research demonstrates that over-consumption of these unhealthy snacks and SSBs is predictive of obesity and other health problems [3–5]. In the current obesogenic environment, there is an abundance of palatable foods and sugar-sweetened drinks [6,7]. Therefore, it is important to increase our knowledge on which factors explain adolescents' increased intake of unhealthy snacks and SSBs.

At the individual level, some adolescents seem to be more vulnerable to increase their food intake when they are faced with highly palatable (or reinforcing) foods like energy-dense snacks or SSBs [8]. More specifically, recent research seems to indicate that high levels of the temperamental trait of reward sensitivity may increase youngsters' vulnerability to over-consumption of palatable foods and SSBs [8].

Reward sensitivity can be defined as the proneness to detect signals of reward in the environment and to experience positive effects in rewarding situations [9,10]. More specifically, it can be seen as the reflection of interindividual differences in the sensitivity of the behavioral activation system (BAS-system). An individual with a strongly reactive approach system (i.e., a sensitive behavioral activation system), will be highly sensitive to reward or to cues that signal reward [11]. Previous studies related higher levels of reward sensitivity to an increased experience of food cravings, more emotional eating, and an increased risk of being overweight in children and adults [9,12,13]. However, the study by De Cock and colleagues [8] was the first to demonstrate that adolescents' self-reported reward sensitivity was positively associated with daily unhealthy snack intake and the intake of SSBs (especially in girls).

Importantly, adolescents' food choices may not only be explained by individual characteristics but also by environmental factors [14]. Decades of research have shown that the home environment plays an important role in shaping children's eating habits [15–18]. In general, parenting practices refer to the behaviors or actions (intentional or unintentional) performed by parents for child-rearing purposes that influence their child's attitudes, behaviors, or beliefs [15]. Specific practices that are used within the context of feeding are called food parenting practices. Such practices may be of more or less controlling nature. Controlling practices are regarded as attempts by parents to regulate or influence the child's eating behavior by pressuring the child to eat certain foods or to empty his plate and by restricting the intake of energy-dense food [16]. Previous research shows that the use of controlling food parenting practices such as pressure to eat and restriction are related to more negative eating and weight-related outcomes because they disrupt children's innate self-regulation mechanisms [17]. Therefore, these parenting practices can be considered health-reducing. For example, Birch and colleagues [17] found that maternal restriction of the child's food intake at five years predicted more eating in the absence of hunger when the child was between seven and nine years old, especially in overweight children. Less controlling practices like monitoring, encouragement, as well as modeling of healthy eating behavior and making healthy food available at home are considered more adaptive and health-promoting since they appear to be associated with more positive eating- and weight-related outcomes. For example, parental encouragement and modeling of healthy eating have been associated with healthy eating in children [15,16,18].

Past research often focuses on how food parenting practices influence dietary intake in toddlers and elementary school-aged children, and to date, far less studies have been carried out in samples of adolescents. Although adolescence is a developmental period that is characterized by an increased strive for autonomy, at the same time, adolescent boys and girls are still dependent on their parents, and the quality of the parent-child relationship remains important for determining food intake [19]. In adolescent samples, some European studies examined the association between more general parenting styles, such as authoritative, authoritarian, indulgent and neglectful parenting, and consumption behavior [20,21]. Regarding the role of more specific food parenting practices, Loth and colleagues [22] found in their population-based study in the US that the use of controlling food-related parenting practices such as pressure to eat and the restriction is related to adolescents' weight status. In a recent study, it was also demonstrated that more use of controlling parenting practices, where rules and limits are put forward to avoid junk food and SSBs, seems associated with more consumption of junk foods and SSBs in the US adolescents [23]. As it is the case in younger children, some studies in adolescent samples also concluded that having family meals on a regular basis, and modeling and encouragement of healthful eating by parents are more health-promoting as they are associated with less fast food consumption and more healthy eating in their adolescents [24,25]. However, more research is needed to unravel whether and how food parenting practices are implicated in determining adolescents' eating behavior in this challenging developmental period.

In recent developmental models such as the goodness of fit model [26], it is generally assumed that the interaction between a children's and adolescents' temperament and its environment is one of the core mechanisms leading to (mal)adaptive behavior. When the environment is able to recognize and accommodate a child's and adolescent's temperament, development is more likely to be prosperous than when there is no compatibility between a child's and adolescent's temperament and the environment in which it grows up. In line with this view, unhealthy eating and drinking behavior (such as increased intake of energy-dense snacks and SSBs) in adolescents may be seen as a result of the interaction between adolescents' level of reward sensitivity and their parents' use of certain food parenting practices. Therefore, in the present study, we aim to investigate whether food parenting practices moderate the negative impact of reward sensitivity on the intake of snacks and SSBs in adolescents. More specifically, we hypothesize that health-promoting (i.e., availability of healthy products) parenting practices attenuate this relationship, whereas health-reducing (i.e., coercive control) parenting practices strengthen this negative relationship.

2. Materials and Methods

2.1. Study Procedure

The present study was a secondary data analysis on data from the REWARD project (http://www.rewardstudy.be). The overall aim of this project was to provide evidence for a new public health framework to improve the eating patterns of children and adolescents by focusing on individual differences in reward sensitivity. Data were collected between September and December 2013 in a representative sample of adolescents recruited in the third and fourth grades of 20 secondary schools in Flanders (Belgium). Additionally, parents of the participating adolescents were also invited to fill out the parent questionnaire (one parent per adolescent). Parents' passive consent and adolescents' active consent were obtained prior to participation of the adolescents, and parents' active consent was given for their own participation. Of the 1210 selected adolescents, 6% were absent or not allowed to participate, and 3% returned a questionnaire of unsatisfactory quality (defined as more than 33% of the questions not completed or straight-lining responses) for further use. More detailed information on the study procedure and used materials can be found elsewhere [8,27]. The study protocol was approved by the Ethics Committee of the Ghent University Hospital and performed in accordance with the ethical standards laid down in Belgian national laws and the Declaration of Helsinki.

2.2. Measures

The adolescent questionnaire assessed socio-demographics, reward sensitivity, perceived parenting practices, and snack and sugar-sweetened beverage intake. The parent questionnaire also assessed socio-demographics and applied parenting practices.

2.3. Adolescents' Intake of Sugar-Sweetened Beverages (SSB) and (Un)Healthy Snacks

Snack food and sugar-sweetened beverage (SSB) consumption was assessed using a Food Frequency Questionnaire (FFQ) for adolescents [27], based on the validated diet quality index for children [28]. The six categories used were: 0 = never or seldom; 1 = 1–3 days/month; 2 = 1 days/week; 3 = 2–4 days/week; 4 = 5–6 days/week; 5 = every day. These categories were recoded into the frequency of consumption per week: 0 = never or seldom; 0.5 = 1–3 days/month; 1 = 1 days/week; 3 = 2–4 days/week; 5.5 = 5–6 days/week; 7 = every day [28]. The FFQ probes for the consumption of snacks and beverages within a reference period of one month. The 28 snack items were: chocolate and pralines, candy bars, candy, dry cookies, other cookies such as chocolate cookies, breakfast rolls, pastries, breakfast cereals, unsweetened yogurt, sweetened yogurt, pudding, mousses, ice-cream, popsicles, dried fruit, fruit, raw vegetables, nuts and seeds, sandwiches with sweet or savory spread, cheese or meat cubes, crisps and similar products, other savory snacks such as breadsticks, sausage/cheese rolls, and pizza, other fried snacks such as spring rolls and cheese croquettes, French fries, kebab, hamburgers, and pasta cups. Included sugar-sweetened beverage items were energy drinks, sports drinks, soft drinks. Snacks were classified as either healthy or unhealthy using the UK Ofcom nutrient profiling model [29]. Following this scoring system, the FFQ snack items chocolate and pralines, candy bars, candy, dry cookies, other cookies such as chocolate cookies, breakfast rolls, pastries, breakfast cereals, pudding, mousses, ice-cream, popsicles, cheese or meat cubes, crisps and similar products, other savory snacks such as bread sticks, sausage/cheese rolls and pizza, other fried snacks such as spring rolls and cheese croquettes, French fries, hamburgers were considered to be unhealthy (20) and the other FFQ snack items healthy (8). Depending on the item, 4–6 portion-size categories (in g or mL) were provided together with a list of common standard measures as examples of the quantity of consumption for the most frequently consumed food items by adolescents within that category, as reported in the European HELENA study [8]. The average (in g or mL) of the portion ranges and the lowest/highest category ±0.67 was used to calculate the quantity of the consumption. For instance, for candy the following portion sizes were given 9 g or less (i.e., 6 g), 10–34 g (i.e., 22 g), 35–59 g (i.e., 47 g), 60–84 g (i.e., 72 g), 85–109 g (i.e., 97 g), and 110 g or more (i.e., 183.3 g), together with the following examples of portions—one small bag of M&M's = 45 g and one wine gum = 4 g. The daily intake of each FFQ item was obtained by multiplying the frequency of consumption per week with the quantity of consumption (g or mL) divided by 7. The overall daily intakes per item were then summed to obtain the daily intakes of unhealthy snacks (g), healthy snacks (g), and SSBs (mL). Zero imputation (i.e., assumption of no consumption) was used for food items that were left blank. We had complete cases for 87% of the snack items, 8.2% had a missing for one item, and less than five percent had more than one missing for the snack items. For the SSBs, less than two percent had one or more missing items for the SSB items.

2.4. Adolescents' Reward Sensitivity

Reward Sensitivity (RS) was indexed by the BAS-scale of a Dutch age-downward version one of Carver and White's BIS/BAS scale [30]. Thirteen items are scored on a four-point scale (1 = not at all true, 2 = somewhat not true, 3 = somewhat true, 4 = all true), and summed to obtain Total RS scores. Psychometrics of this Dutch version of the BIS/BAS-scales are evaluated in Dutch and Flemish children and adolescents aged 8–18 years [30,31], evidencing that the total scale is a valid measurement of RS in children and adolescents with higher scores indicating more RS (range 13–52). The internal consistency of the total scale in the present sample was very good (Cronbach's α = 0.82).

2.5. Health-Promoting and Health-Reducing Food-Parenting Practices Perceived by Adolescents and Parents

The food parenting practices were assessed separately in both adolescents (adolescent-reported) and their parents (parent-reported) by 21 items (using five-point Likert scales) from the adolescent and parent version of the Child Feeding Questionnaire [32] and the Comprehensive Feeding Practices Questionnaire [33]. Both questionnaires have been tested for their validity and reliability. Measured constructs were modeling (three items), monitoring (seven items), encouragement (five items), availability (two items), restriction (one item), and pressure to eat (three items). The items of the first four constructs were combined—based on both theoretical and empirical grounds—into the overall construct "health-promoting parenting practices". The items of the latter two constructs were combined—based on theory and empirical grounds—into the overall construct "health-reducing parenting practices".

2.6. Potential Confounders

The following a-priori defined covariables were considered as potential confounders due to a known association with diet [34]). Adolescents' age, gender, family situation (traditional = the two parents living together versus non-traditional), education type (general versus vocational; technical versus vocational), and parents' age, gender, and socio-economic status (based on education of mother and father), and meal patterns (daily breakfast, lunch, and dinner versus not daily breakfast, lunch, and dinner) were assessed via self-reported questionnaires.

2.7. Statistical Analyses

2.7.1. Main Analysis

Descriptive statistics were produced (see Table 1). Analyses were conducted on complete cases, and therefore only included participants who had valid measures for reward sensitivity, covariables, parenting practices, and diet outcomes. To investigate the moderation effects of both health-promoting and health-reducing parental practices on the association between reward sensitivity and SSB and (un)healthy snack intake in adolescents, a set of hierarchical linear regression models were conducted using SPSS version 25.0. First, an unadjusted model without the interaction term BAS total*parenting practices (model 1); second, an unadjusted model with the interaction term BAS total*parenting practices (model 2); third, a model adjusting for adolescents' age (continuous), gender (dichotomous), family situation (dichotomous), and education type (two dummies were created) (model 3); and finally a model that included the covariables adjusted for in model 3 plus additional adjustment for breakfast, lunch, and dinner habits (model 4).

Table 1. Participant characteristics* in those eligible and included and those eligible but excluded due to missing data on at least one independent or co-variable.

	Eligible & Included $n = 867$ Mean ± SD or %	Eligible but Missing data on Independent or Co-Variables $n = 237$ Mean ± SD or %	p-Value
Baseline Characteristics			
Age	14.7 ± 0.8	14.8 ± 0.9	0.2
Boys	48.1	58.2	<0.001
Family type			
Traditional	70.9	70.5	0.9
Other	29.1	29.5	
School type			
General	48.9	35.9	
Technical	34.4	32.5	<0.001
Vocational	16.7	31.6	
Independent Variables			
BAS total (1–52)	31.9 ± 6.4	30.6 ± 6.8	0.02
Health-promoting parenting practices (1–5)	3.11 ± 0.65	3.06 ± 0.65	0.3
Health-reducing parenting practices (1–5)	2.91 ± 0.81	2.89 ± 0.73	0.7
Dietary Outcomes			
Daily intake of sugar–sweetened beverages [in mL]	361.8 ± 398	427.4 ± 512.5	0.07
Daily intake of healthy snacks [in g]	182.7 ± 216.2	168.8 ± 277.2	0.4
Daily intake of unhealthy snacks [in g]	256.4 ± 287.3	280.6 ± 361.8	0.4

BAS total (Behavioral Activation System) is an indicator of Reward sensitivity, SD = standard deviation, g = grams, mL = milliliter.

2.7.2. Sensitivity Analysis

Sensitivity analyses were performed to evaluate the robustness of the findings (see Appendix A, Tables A1–A6) by rerunning the analyses first including all cases, regardless of missing values; second with ≥3 SD outlier exclusion for the dietary intake variables, and third using the (health-promoting and health-reducing) parenting practices reported by the parents. Generally, findings were similar under these conditions and therefore will not be commented on further, apart from the significant moderation effect in the parent sample.

3. Results

3.1. Description of Sample

One-thousand one-hundred and four adolescents (and 158 parents) completed the questionnaires. The complete-cases analysis sample was comprised of 867 adolescents (and 131 parents). Table 1 presents characteristics of the adolescent sample. The mean age of the participants was 14.7; there were slightly fewer boys (48.1%). Most adolescents came from traditional families, and most participating adolescents were in general education. The participating parents had a mean age of 44.7 ± 3.7, were mostly mothers (81.7%), and from higher SES families (76.3%). Mean health-promoting and health-reducing parenting practices were respectively 3.6 ± 0.4 and 2.7 ± 0.7.

3.2. Moderation Effect of Health-Promoting and Health-Reducing Parenting Practices

Tables 2 and 3 show the associations between reward sensitivity, the (adolescent-reported) parenting practices, and covariables, and the included dietary measures (i.e., daily intake of SSB, healthy and unhealthy snacks). Despite several significant main associations between reward sensitivity and parenting practices and SSB, healthy and unhealthy snack consumption (also reported in [27]), no significant moderation effects were found for health-promoting or health-reducing parenting practices on the relationship between reward sensitivity and the diet measures.

Table 2. Associations between reward sensitivity and adolescents' intake of sugar-sweetened beverages, healthy and unhealthy snacks, and the moderating role of (adolescent-reported) health-promoting parenting practices ($n = 867$).

	Model 1		Model 2		Model 3		Model 4	
	B (95% CI)	p-Value	B (95% CI)	p-Value	B (95% CI)	p-Value	B (95% CI)	p-Value
Outcome: Sugar-sweetened beverages	Adjusted R^2 = 0.046		Adjusted R^2 = 0.046		Adjusted R^2 = 0.122		Adjusted R^2 = 0.125	
BAS total	0.103 (0.038, 0.168)	0.002	0.109 (0.043, 0.175)	0.001	0.97 (0.033, 0.162)	0.003	0.096 (0.031, 0.160)	0.004
Health-promoting parenting practices	−0.200 (−0.266, −0.135)	<0.001	−0.204 (−0.270, −0.139)	<0.001	−0.152 (−0.217, −0.087)	<0.001	−0.144 (−0.210, −0.079)	<0.001
BAS total * Health-promoting parenting practices			0.032 (−0.029, 0.094)	0.3	0.021 (−0.038, 0.080)	0.5	0.023 (−0.037, 0.082)	0.5
Age					0.006 (−0.073, 0.086)	0.9	−0.003 (−0.083, 0.077)	0.9
Gender [Ref: boy]					−0.432 (−0.558, −0.305)	<0.001	−0.452 (−0.580, −0.323)	<0.001
Family type [Ref: not traditional]					−0.067 (−0.207, 0.073)	0.3	−0.050 (−0.190, 0.091)	0.5
School type General [Ref: Vocational]					−0.427 (−0.617, −0.238)	<0.001	−0.409 (−0.600, −0.218)	<0.001
School type Technical [Ref: Vocational]					−0.171 (−0.362, 0.021)	0.08	−0.167 (−0.359, 0.024)	0.09
Breakfast [Ref: Not daily]							−0.158 (−0.294, −0.023)	0.2
Lunch [Ref: Not daily]							−0.022 (−0.179, 0.136)	0.8
Dinner [Ref: Not daily]							0.087 (−0.127, 0.301)	0.4
Outcome: Healthy Snack intake	Adjusted R^2 = 0.018		Adjusted R^2 = 0.017		Adjusted R^2 = 0.021		Adjusted R^2 = 0.020	
BAS total #	0.070 (0.004, 0.136)	0.04	0.069 (0.002, 0.136)	0.04	0.067 (0.000, 0.135)	0.05	0.067 (−0.001, 0.136)	0.05
health-promoting parenting practices	0.120 (0.054, 0.186)	<0.001	0.121 (0.054, 0.187)	<0.001	0.111 (0.043, 0.180)	0.001	0.107 (0.038, 0.176)	0.003
BAS total * health-promoting parenting practices			−0.005 (−0.067, 0.058)	0.9	−0.002 (−0.064, 0.061)	1.0	−0.001 (−0.064, 0.062)	1.0
Age					−0.001 (−0.085, 0.082)	1.0	0.002 (−0.082, 0.087)	1.0
Gender [Ref: boy]					0.118 (−0.015, 0.252)	0.08	0.126 (−0.010, 0.262)	0.07
Family type [Ref: not traditional]					−0.029 (−0.177, 0.119)	0.7	−0.034 (−0.183, 0.114)	0.6
School type General [Ref: Vocational]					0.080 (−0.120, 0.280)	0.4	0.071 (−0.131, 0.273)	0.5
School type Technical [Ref: Vocational]					−0.083 (−0.285, 0.119)	0.4	−0.084 (−0.287, 0.119)	0.4
Breakfast [Ref: Not daily]							0.082 (−0.061, 0.226)	0.3
Lunch [Ref: Not daily]							−0.043 (−0.209, 0.124)	0.6
Dinner [Ref: Not daily]							−0.002 (−0.229, 0.225)	1.0
Outcome: Unhealthy Snack intake	Adjusted R^2 = 0.017		Adjusted R^2 = 0.017		Adjusted R^2 = 0.021		Adjusted R^2 = 0.020	
BAS total	0.147 (0.081, 0.213)	<0.001	0.069 (0.085, 0.220)	<0.001	0.146 (0.079, 0.213)	<0.001	0.143 (0.076, 0.210)	<0.001

Table 2. Cont.

	Model 1		Model 2		Model 3		Model 4	
	B (95% CI)	p-Value	B (95% CI)	p-Value	B (95% CI)	p-Value	B (95% CI)	p-Value
Health-promoting parenting practices	−0.056 (−0.122, 0.010)	0.1	−0.060 (−0.126, 0.007)	0.08	−0.030 (0.097, 0.037)	0.4	−0.029 (−0.097, 0.038)	0.4
BAS total * Health-promoting parenting practices			0.030 (−0.032, 0.092)	0.3	0.025 (−0.036, 0.086)	0.4	0.024 (−0.037, 0.086)	0.4
Age					−0.002 (−0.084, 0.080)	1.0	−0.005 (−0.088, 0.078)	0.9
Gender [Ref: boy]					−0.328 (−0.459, −0.196)	<0.001	−0.335 (−0.468, −0.201)	<0.001
Family type [Ref: not traditional]					0.097 (−0.048, 0.242)	0.2	0.098 (−0.048, 0.244)	0.2
School type General [Ref: Vocational]					−0.292 (−0.488, −0.095)	0.004	−0.280 (−0.478, −0.081)	0.006
School type Technical [Ref: Vocational]					−0.167 (−0.365, 0.031)	0.1	−0.160 (−0.359, 0.039)	0.1
Breakfast [Ref: Not daily]							0.011 (−0.130, 0.152)	0.8
Lunch [Ref: Not daily]							−0.041 (−0.205, 0.123)	0.6
Dinner [Ref: Not daily]							−0.097 (−0.320, 0.125)	0.4

* Results in the table are for complete cases (n = 867) with unstandardized B values; Model 1 includes the main independent variables (BAS total, Health-promoting parenting practices); Model 2 includes the main independent variables (BAS total, Health-promoting parenting practices) and the interaction; Model 3 includes adjustments for age, gender, family type (traditional versus other), and school type (general, technical, vocational); Model 4 includes model 3 adjustments plus additional adjustments for breakfast, lunch, and dinner patterns. [#] BAS total (Behavioral Activation System) is an indicator of Reward sensitivity.

Table 3. Associations between reward sensitivity and adolescents' intake of sugar-sweetened beverages, healthy and unhealthy snacks, and the moderating role of (adolescent-reported) health-reducing parenting practices (n = 867).

	Model 1		Model 2		Model 3		Model 4	
	B (95% CI)	p-Value	B (95% CI)	p-Value	B (95% CI)	p-Value	B (95% CI)	p-Value
Outcome: Sugar-sweetened beverages	Adjusted R² = 0.006		Adjusted R² = 0.005		Adjusted R² = 0.100		Adjusted R² = 0.106	
BAS total [#]	0.092 (0.025, 0.160)	0.007	0.092 (0.025, 0.160)	0.007	0.080 (0.015, 0.145)	0.02	0.079 (0.014, 0.144)	0.02
Health-reducing parenting practices	−0.011 (−0.078, 0.056)	0.8	−0.011 (−0.079, 0.056)	0.7	0.001 (−0.064, 0.066)	1.0	−0.005 (−0.070, 0.060)	0.9
BAS total * Health-reducing parenting practices			0.006 (−0.056, 0.067)	0.9	−0.001 (−0.060, 0.058)	1.0	0.001 (−0.058, 0.059)	1.0
Age					0.016 (−0.065, 0.096)	0.7	0.003 (−0.078, 0.084)	0.9
Gender [Ref: boy]					−0.453 (−0.581, −0.325)	<0.001	−0.476 (−0.605, −0.346)	<0.001
Family type [Ref: not traditional]					−0.093 (−0.234, 0.049)	0.2	−0.072 (−0.214, 0.070)	0.3
School type General [Ref: Vocational]					−0.509 (−0.697, −0.320)	<0.001	−0.480 (−0.670, −0.289)	<0.001
School type Technical [Ref: Vocational]					−0.238 (−0.429, −0.046)	0.02	−0.227 (−0.419, −0.036)	0.02

Table 3. Cont.

	Model 1		Model 2		Model 3		Model 4	
	B (95% CI)	p-Value	B (95% CI)	p-Value	B (95% CI)	p-Value	B (95% CI)	p-Value
Breakfast [Ref: Not daily]							−0.191 (−0.328, −0.055)	0.006
Lunch [Ref: Not daily]							−0.007 (−0.166, 0.153)	0.9
Dinner [Ref: Not daily]							0.068 (−0.149, 0.285)	0.5
Outcome: Healthy Snack intake	Adjusted R^2 = 0.004		Adjusted R^2 = 0.005		Adjusted R^2 = 0.012		Adjusted R^2 = 0.011	
BAS total	0.079 (0.011, 0.146)	0.02	0.078 (0.010, 0.145)	0.02	0.078 (0.010, 0.146)	0.03	0.077 (0.009, 0.146)	0.03
health-reducing parenting practices	−0.007 (−0.74, 0.061)	0.8	−0.003 (−0.071, 0.064)	0.9	−0.005 (−0.073, 0.063)	0.9	−0.002 (−0.070, 0.067)	1.0
BAS total * health-reducing parenting practices			−0.043 (−0.105, 0.018)	0.2	−0.044 (−0.105, 0.018)	0.2	−0.044 (−0.106, 0.017)	0.2
Age					−0.012 (−0.096, 0.073)	0.8	−0.006 (−0.091, 0.080)	0.9
Gender [Ref: boy]					0.134 (0.000, 0.269)	0.05	0.144 (0.008, 0.280)	0.04
Family type [Ref: not traditional]					−0.018 (−0.166, 0.131)	0.8	−0.026 (−0.175, 0.123)	0.7
School type General [Ref: Vocational]					0.134 (−0.063, 0.332)	0.2	0.118 (−0.082, 0.318)	0.2
School type Technical [Ref: Vocational]					−0.038 (−0.239, 0.162)	0.7	−0.044 (−0.245, 0.158)	0.7
Breakfast [Ref: Not daily]							0.108 (−0.036, 0.251)	0.1
Lunch [Ref: Not daily]							−0.050 (−0.218, 0.117)	0.6
Dinner [Ref: Not daily]							0.009 (−0.219, 0.237)	0.9
Outcome: Unhealthy Snack intake	Adjusted R^2 = 0.024		Adjusted R^2 = 0.027		Adjusted R^2 = 0.067		Adjusted R^2 = 0.064	
BAS total	0.131 (0.064, 0.198)	<0.001	0.130 (0.063, 0.196)	<0.001	0.123 (0.056, 0.189)	<0.001	0.121 (0.055, 0.188)	<0.001
Health-reducing parenting practices	0.074 (0.007, 0.141)	0.03	0.079 (0.012, 0.146)	0.02	0.089 (0.023, 0.155)	0.008	0.086 (0.020, 0.153)	0.01
BAS total * Health-reducing parenting practices			−0.059 (−0.120, 0.002)	0.06	−0.060 (−0.120, −0.001)	0.05	−0.060 (−0.120, 0.0000)	0.05
Age					0.007 (−0.075, 0.089)	0.9	0.005 (−0.078, 0.088)	0.9
Gender [Ref: boy]					−0.346 (−0.476, −0.215)	<0.001	−0.349 (−0.481, −0.216)	<0.001
Family type [Ref: not traditional]					0.080 (−0.064, 0.224)	0.3	0.079 (−0.066, 0.225)	0.3
School type General [Ref: Vocational]					−0.305 (−0.497, −0.113)	0.002	−0.298 (−0.493, −0.103)	0.003
School type Technical [Ref: Vocational]					−0.192 (−0.387, 0.003)	0.05	−0.187 (−0.383, 0.009)	0.06
Breakfast [Ref: Not daily]							0.017 (−0.123, 0.157)	0.8
Lunch [Ref: Not daily]							−0.023 (−0.186, 0.140)	0.8
Dinner [Ref: Not daily]							−0.077 (−0.299, 0.145)	0.5

* Results in the table are for complete cases (n = 867) with unstandardized B values; Model 1 includes the main independent variables (BAS total, health-reducing parenting practices); Model 2 includes the main independent variables (BAS total, health-promoting parenting practices) and the interaction term; Model 3 includes adjustments for age, gender, family type (traditional versus other), and school type (general, technical, vocational); Model 4 includes model 3 adjustments plus additional adjustment for breakfast, lunch, and dinner patterns. # BAS total (Behavioral Activation System) is an indicator of Reward sensitivity.

In the sensitivity analyses, we did find a moderation effect for parent-reported health-reducing parenting practices on the relationship between reward sensitivity and unhealthy snack intake. Figure 1 presents this interaction effect and shows a more unhealthy snack intake when using more health-reducing parenting practices compared to a lower intake of unhealthy snacks when using less health-reducing parenting practices among highly reward sensitive adolescents. Figure 1 shows no difference between the use of health-reducing parenting practices among adolescents with lower reward sensitivity.

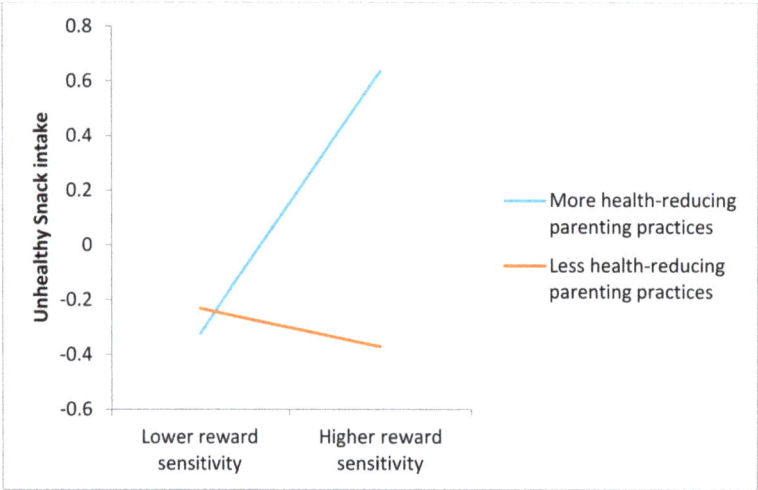

Figure 1. The moderation effect of Reward Sensitivity and Health-reducing parenting practices on the intake of unhealthy snacks.

4. Discussion

The present study investigated whether the influence of reward sensitivity, a known determinant of snack and SSB intake in adolescents [8], might be affected by either health-promoting or health-reducing food parenting practices. Following the goodness-of-fit [26] model, suggesting that the interaction between an adolescent's temperament and its environment is one of the core mechanisms leading to a (mal)adaptive behavior, we assumed that the association between reward sensitivity and unhealthy eating and drinking behavior might be attenuated by health-promoting parenting practices while being enhanced by health-reducing parenting practices. Although the data reported by the adolescents partly supported the role of both reward sensitivity and parenting practices separately, they did not provide evidence for their interactive role in unhealthy and healthy snack intake and SSB consumption in adolescents. Based on the analysis of the complete case, data suggested that higher reward sensitivity was associated with a higher intake of healthy and unhealthy snacks and higher consumption of SSB. This finding is in line with previous research where it was found that higher levels of reward sensitivity were associated with eating- and weight-related outcomes such as the increased experience of food cravings, more emotional eating, and an increased risk for being overweight in children and adults [9,12,13].

However, when diet outliers were removed, these effects were no longer significant. In contrast, the effects of parenting practices were more robust and survived all sensitivity analyses. Increased use of health-promoting parenting practices was associated with reduced SSB consumption and increased healthy snack intake, while increased use of health-reducing parenting practices was associated with increased unhealthy snack intake. These results are in line with previous studies [22,23] and seem to demonstrate that according to the adolescents themselves, parental variables (in this case, parenting practices) still play an important role in explaining adolescents' eating and drinking behavior. Although these results are only cross-sectional, they do seem to indicate that during the developmental stage of adolescence, where increased autonomy is required, working with parents to address their adolescents' eating behavior may still be an effective intervention strategy.

Parent-reported data on parenting practices; however, did provide evidence for their interactive role with reward sensitivity in explaining adolescents' unhealthy snack intake. More specifically, results demonstrate that health-reducing parenting practices strengthen the association between adolescents' reward sensitivity and unhealthy snack intake. In other words, in line with the assumptions of the goodness of fit model [26], unhealthy eating behavior may be explained by a 'poorness of fit' between adolescent's vulnerable temperament and their parents' food-related parenting practices. The other two outcomes, SSB consumption, and healthy snack intake, were not determined by parenting practices (either alone or in interaction with reward sensitivity).

The present study has several strengths. First of all, the divergence of the results obtained through adolescent and parent report point to the relevance of multi-informant assessment. Although considered best practice in developmental psychopathology research [35], this approach is less often used in nutrition research. However, both parents and adolescents might experience, and thus, report on a certain concept (like parenting) differently, which might at the one sight create measurement error but, on the other side, open up a broader view on its role in determining behavior. Previous studies, including both child- and parent-report in investigating parental influence, showed stronger associations with child eating behavior for the child perception than parent perception [36]. In the present study, we were able to collect both parents- and adolescent-reported data on food parenting practices in a small subsample of our participants, giving a first impression on its role in snack and SSB intake in adolescents. The results based on parent-report; however, need replication. Future research might aim to collect data in a large and representative sample of adolescent-parent dyads. In order to get a more comprehensive view of how parents influence their adolescents' eating behavior, other methodologies are required. For example, observational methods can provide information about the verbal and non-verbal context of behavioral dynamics during mealtimes, e.g., [37].

A large sample is necessary to have enough power to detect small effects. We assumed that the effect sizes of the determinants under study would be small because eating behavior has multiple determinants that act together on different levels [1,14]. Therefore, we collected data in a large sample. In order to be able to generalize our results to the Flemish population of adolescents between 14 and 16 years, we ensured that our sample was representative. In addition to its multi-informant assessment of parenting practices and its large and representative sample, another strength of the present study is its use of validated instruments to assess reward sensitivity [30] and snack and SSB intake [27].

Some limitations have to be noted, as well. First, parenting practices were assessed through a purpose-built questionnaire, using a selection of relevant items borrowed from several instruments on food parenting practices, being the Child Feeding Questionnaire [32], and the Comprehensive Feeding Practices Questionnaire [33]. Future research might benefit from using the validated instruments themselves. Moreover, as argued by other researchers, different concepts are often used to study food parenting practices, and future research should strive for more consensus on how to operationalize and measure different practices [38]. Next, only a limited subsample of parents reported on their parenting practices, which call into question the representativeness of this subsample in comparison to the entire sample and the population. Furthermore, because of the cross-sectional nature of the present study, no conclusions can be drawn regarding the direction of the associations and causality. In order to examine whether reward sensitivity, parenting practices, and their interaction predict unhealthy snacking and the intake of SSB, longitudinal and experimental designs are needed. Moreover, future research may investigate whether other environmental factors interact with reward sensitivity to explain adolescent's intake of snacks and SSB [11]. For example, previous research found evidence for the role of peer consumption and the school environment in explaining adolescents' snack and soft drink consumption [39]. Studying how individual (intrapersonal) characteristics interact with different environmental factors may result in a more comprehensive explanation of adolescents' eating/snacking behavior and may lead to more tailored intervention efforts that target factors at multiple levels of influence.

To conclude, the present study investigated whether health-promoting or health-reducing food parenting practices could impact the relationship between reward sensitivity and dietary intake in adolescents. The main analysis on the adolescent-reported data did not show any moderating effect of food parenting practices. This finding indicates that, although reward sensitivity and parenting practices were uniquely associated with dietary intake, they do not seem to interact based on adolescent-reported data. Other—for example, observational—measures and multiple informants are needed to investigate further whether and how parenting practices impact the relation between temperamental traits and adolescents' dietary intake. Especially since the sensitivity analysis using the small sample of parent-reported data showed an interactive role with reward sensitivity in explaining adolescents' unhealthy snack intake. This finding indicates that health-reducing parenting practices seemed to strengthen the association between adolescents' reward sensitivity and unhealthy snack intake. Nevertheless, more longitudinal and intervention research in larger samples of adolescent-parent dyads is necessary to further investigate the impact of both health-promoting and health-reducing parenting practices on the relationship between reward sensitivity and diet intakes of adolescents.

Author Contributions: W.V.L., L.V., L.G. were involved in the study conceptualization. W.V.L., J.V. collected the data. W.V.L., L.V. conducted the analyses. W.V.L., L.V., L.G. were involved in the interpretation of the analyses. W.V.L., L.V., L.G. drafted the manuscript. All authors contributed to the interpretation of the results and provided feedback on the drafts before submission. All authors have read and agreed to the published version of the manuscript.

Acknowledgments: This study was supported by the agency for Innovation by Science and Technology (IWT) of Flanders (Belgium) (grant number SBO120054). The sponsor was not involved in the study design, collection, analysis, or interpretation of the data. The first and corresponding author had access to all data at all times and had the final responsibility to submit the manuscript for publication.

Conflicts of Interest: The authors declare that there were no conflicts of interest.

Appendix A

Sensitivity Analyses

Table A1. Associations between reward sensitivity and adolescents' intake of sugar-sweetened beverages, healthy and unhealthy snacks, and the moderating role of (adolescent-reported) health-promoting parenting practices for all cases ($n = 1104$).

Outcomes	Model 1		Model 2		Model 3		Model 4	
	B (95% CI)	p-Value	B (95% CI)	p-Value	B (95% CI)	p-Value	B (95% CI)	p-Value
Outcome: Sugar-Sweetened Beverages	Adjusted R^2 = 0.041		Adjusted R^2 = 0.040		Adjusted R^2 = 0.122		Adjusted R^2 = 0.124	
BAS total [#]	0.118 (0.057, 0.179)	<0.001	0.121 (0.059, 0.182)	<0.001	0.114 (0.054, 0.173)	<0.001	0.112 (0.052, 0.172)	<0.001
Health-promoting parenting practices	−0.179 (−0.241, −0.118)	<0.001	−0.180 (−0.243, −0.118)	<0.001	−0.132 (−0.193, −0.070)	<0.001	−0.126 (−0.187, −0.064)	<0.001
BAS total * Health-promoting parenting practices			0.015 (−0.043, 0.073)	0.6	0.002 (−0.054, 0.057)	0.9	0.003 (−0.052, 0.059)	0.9
Age					−0.016 (−0.090, 0.058)	0.7	−0.025 (−0.099, 0.050)	0.5
Gender [Ref: boy]					−0.447 (−0.566, −0.327)	<0.001	−0.468 (−0.590, −0.347)	<0.001
Family type [Ref: not traditional]					−0.106 (−0.238, 0.026)	0.1	−0.089 (−0.222, 0.044)	0.2
School type General [Ref: Vocational]					−0.443 (−0.615, −0.271)	<0.001	−0.421 (−0.595, −0.248)	<0.001
School type Technical [Ref: Vocational]					−0.158 (−0.332, 0.016)	0.08	−0.151 (−0.325, 0.023)	0.09
Breakfast [Ref: Not daily]							−0.133 (−0.261, −0.006)	0.04
Lunch [Ref: Not daily]							−0.042 (−0.192, 0.107)	0.6
Dinner [Ref: Not daily]							0.050 (−0.149, 0.248)	0.6
Outcome: Healthy Snack intake	Adjusted R^2 = 0.016		Adjusted R^2 = 0.015		Adjusted R^2 = 0.021		Adjusted R^2 = 0.021	
BAS total	0.045 (−0.021, 0.112)	0.2	0.046 (−0.022, 0.114)	0.2	0.039 (−0.029, 0.107)	0.3	0.040 (−0.028, 0.108)	0.3
Health-promoting parenting practices	0.134 (0.066, 0.202)	<0.001	0.134 (0.066, 0.202)	<0.001	0.138 (0.069, 0.208)	<0.001	0.131 (0.060, 0.201)	<0.001
BAS total * Health-promoting parenting practices			0.003 (−0.061, 0.066)	0.9	0.004 (−0.059, 0.068)	0.9	0.005 (−0.058, 0.069)	0.9
Age					−0.011 (−0.095, 0.073)	0.8	−0.003 (−0.088, 0.081)	0.9
Gender [Ref: boy]					0.103 (−0.034, 0.239)	0.1	0.118 (−0.020, 0.257)	0.09
Family type [Ref: not traditional]					−0.037 (−0.188, 0.113)	0.6	−0.047 (−0.198, 0.105)	0.5
School type General [Ref: Vocational]					−0.067 (−0.263, 0.129)	0.5	−0.087 (−0.285, 0.111)	0.4
School type Technical [Ref: Vocational]					−0.234 (−0.432, −0.036)	0.02	−0.239 (−0.438, −0.041)	0.02

Table A1. Cont.

Outcomes	Model 1		Model 2		Model 3		Model 4	
	B (95% CI)	p-Value	B (95% CI)	p-Value	B (95% CI)	p-Value	B (95% CI)	p-Value
Breakfast [Ref: Not daily]							0.136 (−0.009, 0.282)	0.07
Lunch [Ref: Not daily]							−0.049 (−0.219, 0.122)	0.6
Dinner [Ref: Not daily]							0.031 (−0.195, 0.257)	0.8
Outcome: Unhealthy Snack Intake	Adjusted R^2 = 0.014		Adjusted R^2 = 0.013		Adjusted R^2 = 0.053		Adjusted R^2 = 0.051	
BAS total	0.125 (0.061, 0.188)	<0.001	0.129 (0.065, 0.194)	<0.001	0.124 (0.060, 0.188)	<0.001	0.123 (0.059, 0.187)	<0.001
Health-promoting parenting practices	−0.039 (−0.104, 0.026)	0.2	−0.041 (−0.105, 0.024)	0.2	−0.009 (−0.075, 0.056)	0.8	−0.012 (−0.078, 0.054)	0.7
BAS total * Health-promoting parenting practices			0.027 (−0.034, 0.087)	0.4	0.020 (−0.040, 0.079)	0.5	0.019 (−0.040, 0.079)	0.5
Age					−0.020 (−0.099, 0.059)	0.6	−0.018 (−0.097, 0.062)	0.7
Gender [Ref: boy]					−0.348 (−0.476, −0.220)	<0.001	−0.344 (−0.474, −0.214)	<0.001
Family type [Ref: not traditional]					0.057 (−0.084, 0.199)	0.4	0.052 (−0.090, 0.195)	0.5
School type General [Ref: Vocational]					−0.350 (−0.534, −0.165)	<0.001	−0.354 (−0.541, −0.168)	<0.001
School type Technical [Ref: Vocational]					−0.217 (−0.403, −0.031)	0.02	−0.217 (−0.404, −0.031)	0.02
Breakfast [Ref: Not daily]							0.067 (−0.070, 0.203)	0.3
Lunch [Ref: Not daily]							−0.025 (−0.186, 0.135)	0.8
Dinner [Ref: Not daily]							−0.054 (−0.267, 0.159)	0.6

* Results in the table are for all cases (n = 1104) with unstandardized B values; Model 1 includes the main independent variables (BAS total, Health-promoting parenting practices); Model 2 includes the main independent variables (BAS total, Health-promoting parenting practices) and the interaction; Model 3 includes adjustments for age, gender, family type (traditional versus other), and school type (general, technical, vocational); Model 4 includes model 3 adjustments plus additional adjustment for breakfast, lunch, and dinner patterns. # BAS total (Behavioral Activation System) is an indicator of Reward sensitivity.

Table A2. Associations between reward sensitivity and adolescents' intake of sugar-sweetened beverages, healthy and unhealthy snacks, and the moderating role of (adolescent-reported) Health-reducing parenting practices for all cases (n = 1104).

Outcomes	Model 1		Model 2		Model 3		Model 4	
	B (95% CI)	p-Value	B (95% CI)	p-Value	B (95% CI)	p-Value	B (95% CI)	p-Value
Outcome: Sugar-Sweetened Beverages	Adjusted R² = 0.009		Adjusted R² = 0.008		Adjusted R² = 0.107		Adjusted R² = 0.110	
BAS total #	0.102 (0.039, 0.165)	0.002	0.102 (0.039, 0.165)	0.001	0.095 (0.035, 0.156)	0.002	0.095 (0.035, 0.155)	0.002
Health-reducing parenting practices	0.007 (−0.057, 0.072)	0.8	0.007 (−0.058, 0.071)	0.8	0.022 (−0.040, 0.084)	0.5	0.016 (−0.046, 0.078)	0.6
BAS total * Health-reducing parenting practices			0.008 (−0.050, 0.066)	0.8	−0.004 (−0.059, 0.051)	0.9	−0.002 (−0.058, 0.053)	0.9
Age					−0.002 (−0.078, 0.073)	1.0	−0.013 (−0.089, 0.063)	0.7
Gender [Ref: boy]					−0.463 (−0.584, −0.342)	<0.001	−0.486 (−0.609, −0.364)	<0.001

Table A2. Cont.

Outcomes	Model 1		Model 2		Model 3		Model 4	
	B (95% CI)	p-Value	B (95% CI)	p-Value	B (95% CI)	p-Value	B (95% CI)	p-Value
Family type [Ref: not traditional]					−0.130 (−0.264, 0.003)	0.06	−0.110 (−0.245, 0.024)	0.1
School type General [Ref: Vocational]					−0.517 (−0.689, −0.344)	<0.001	−0.488 (−0.663, −0.314)	<0.001
School type Technical [Ref: Vocational]					−0.224 (−0.399, −0.049)	0.01	−0.214 (−0.389, −0.038)	0.02
Breakfast [Ref: Not daily]							−0.157 (−0.286, −0.029)	0.02
Lunch [Ref: Not daily]							−0.028 (−0.180, 0.123)	0.7
Dinner [Ref: Not daily]							0.034 (−0.167, 0.235)	0.7
Outcome: Healthy Snack Intake	Adjusted R^2 = 0.001		Adjusted R^2 = 0.001		Adjusted R^2 = 0.007		Adjusted R^2 = 0.009	
BAS total	0.061 (−0.007, 0.129)	0.08	0.062 (−0.006, 0.130)	0.07	0.058 (−0.010, 0.126)	0.1	0.057 (−0.011, 0.126)	0.1
Health-reducing parenting practices	−0.026 (−0.096, 0.043)	0.5	−0.028 (−0.098, 0.041)	0.4	−0.031 (−0.101, 0.039)	0.4	−0.025 (−0.096, 0.045)	0.5
BAS total * Health-reducing parenting practices			0.031 (−0.031, 0.094)	0.3	0.030 (−0.033, 0.092)	0.4	0.029 (−0.034, 0.092)	0.4
Age					−0.025 (−0.111, 0.061)	0.6	−0.015 (−0.102, 0.071)	0.7
Gender [Ref: boy]					0.120 (−0.018, 0.258)	0.09	0.138 (−0.002, 0.278)	0.05
Family type [Ref: not traditional]					0.001 (−0.150, 0.153)	1.0	−0.012 (−0.165, 0.140)	0.9
School type General [Ref: Vocational]					−0.007 (−0.203, 0.189)	0.9	−0.035 (−0.233, 0.164)	0.7
School type Technical [Ref: Vocational]					−0.181 (−0.380, 0.018)	0.08	−0.191 (−0.391, 0.008)	0.06
Breakfast [Ref: Not daily]							0.158 (0.012, 0.304)	0.04
Lunch [Ref: Not daily]							−0.057 (−0.229, 0.115)	0.5
Dinner [Ref: Not daily]							0.049 (−0.179, 0.278)	0.7
Outcome: Unhealthy Snack Intake	Adjusted R^2 = 0.015		Adjusted R^2 = 0.014		Adjusted R^2 = 0.058		Adjusted R^2 = 0.056	
BAS total	0.111 (0.046, 0.175)	0.001	0.111 (0.046, 0.176)	0.001	0.106 (0.043, 0.170)	0.001	0.106 (0.042, 0.170)	0.001
Health-reducing parenting practices	0.062 (−0.004, 0.128)	0.07	0.061 (−0.005, 0.128)	0.07	0.072 (0.007, 0.137)	0.03	0.073 (0.007, 0.139)	0.03
BAS total * Health-reducing parenting practices			0.006 (−0.053, 0.066)	0.8	0.001 (−0.057, 0.060)	1.0	0.001 (−0.058, 0.059)	1.0
Age					−0.011 (−0.091, 0.069)	0.8	−0.008 (−0.088, 0.073)	0.9
Gender [Ref: boy]					−0.362 (−0.490, −0.234)	<0.001	−0.355 (−0.485, −0.225)	<0.001
Family type [Ref: not traditional]					0.056 (−0.085, 0.197)	0.4	0.049 (−0.094, 0.191)	0.5
School type General [Ref: Vocational]					−0.365 (−0.547, −0.182)	<0.001	−0.373 (−0.558, −0.188)	<0.001
School type Technical [Ref: Vocational]					−0.240 (−0.425, −0.055)	0.01	−0.242 (−0.428, −0.057)	0.01
Breakfast [Ref: Not daily]							0.069 (−0.067, 0.206)	0.3
Lunch [Ref: Not daily]							−0.012 (−0.172, 0.149)	0.9
Dinner [Ref: Not daily]							−0.034 (−0.247, 0.179)	0.8

* Results in the table are for all cases (n = 1104) with unstandardized B values; Model 1 includes the main independent variables (BAS total, Health-reducing parenting practices); Model 2 includes the main independent variables (BAS total, Health-promoting parenting practices) and the interaction term; Model 3 includes adjustments for age, gender, family type (traditional versus other), and school type (general, technical, vocational); Model 4 includes model 3 adjustments plus additional adjustment for breakfast, lunch, and dinner patterns. # BAS total (Behavioral Activation System) is an indicator of Reward sensitivity.

Table A3. Associations between reward sensitivity and adolescents' intake of sugar-sweetened beverages, healthy and unhealthy snacks, and the moderating role of (adolescent-reported) Health-promoting parenting practices for complete cases, excluding diet outliers ($n = 560$).

Outcomes	Model 1		Model 2		Model 3		Model 4	
	B (95% CI)	p-Value	B (95% CI)	p-Value	B (95% CI)	p-Value	B (95% CI)	p-Value
Outcome: Sugar-sweetened beverages	Adjusted R^2 = 0.006		Adjusted R^2 = 0.011		Adjusted R^2 = 0.043		Adjusted R^2 = 0.048	
BAS total [#]	0.019 (−0.029, 0.066)	0.4	0.021 (−0.026, 0.068)	0.4	0.021 (−0.025, 0.068)	0.4	0.020 (−0.027, 0.066)	0.4
Health-promoting parenting practices	−0.056 (−0.105, −0.006)	0.03	−0.055 (−0.105, −0.006)	0.03	−0.039 (−0.090, 0.011)	0.1	−0.031 (−0.082, 0.054)	0.2
BAS total * Health-promoting parenting practices			0.051 (0.001, 0.101)	0.04	0.045 (−0.005, 0.094)	0.8	0.046 (−0.003, 0.095)	0.07
Age					0.006 (−0.051, 0.064)	<0.001	−0.004 (−0.062, 0.054)	0.9
Gender [Ref: boy]					−0.192 (−0.282, −0.101)	0.3	−0.205 (−0.297, −0.114)	<0.001
Family type [Ref: not traditional]					−0.058 (−0.159, 0.042)	0.5	−0.043 (−0.145, 0.058)	0.4
School type General [Ref: Vocational]					−0.047 (−0.198, 0.104)	0.7	−0.035 (−0.187, 0.118)	0.7
School type Technical [Ref: Vocational]							0.038 (−0.116, 0.192)	0.6
Breakfast [Ref: Not daily]							−0.114 (−0.212, −0.017)	0.02
Lunch [Ref: Not daily]							−0.031 (−0.143, 0.081)	0.6
Dinner [Ref: Not daily]							0.053 (−0.111, 0.216)	0.5
Outcome: Healthy Snack intake	Adjusted R^2 = 0.013		Adjusted R^2 = 0.012		Adjusted R^2 = 0.047		Adjusted R^2 = 0.044	
BAS total	0.004 (−0.046, 0.055)	0.9	0.003 (−0.047, 0.054)	0.9	0.008 (−0.042, 0.057)	0.8	0.008 (−0.042, 0.058)	0.7
Health-promoting parenting practices	0.082 (0.029, 0.135)	0.002	0.082 (0.029, 0.134)	0.002	0.050 (−0.004, 0.104)	0.07	0.052 (−0.003, 0.106)	0.06
BAS total * Health-promoting parenting practices			−0.018 (−0.071, 0.035)	0.5	−0.009 (−0.062, 0.043)	0.7	−0.009 (−0.061, 0.044)	0.8
Age					−0.025 (−0.086, 0.036)	0.4	−0.028 (−0.090, 0.034)	0.4
Gender [Ref: boy]					0.139 (0.043, 0.236)	0.005	0.138 (0.040, 0.235)	0.006
Family type [Ref: not traditional]					0.052 (−0.055, 0.160)	0.3	0.060 (−0.049, 0.168)	0.3
School type General [Ref: Vocational]					0.249 (0.088, 0.410)	0.002	0.245 (0.082, 0.409)	0.003
School type Technical [Ref: Vocational]					0.128 (−0.036, 0.292)	0.1	0.126 (−0.039, 0.291)	0.1
Breakfast [Ref: Not daily]							−0.045 (−0.150, 0.059)	0.4
Lunch [Ref: Not daily]							−0.007 (−0.127, 0.113)	0.9
Dinner [Ref: Not daily]							0.081 (−0.094, 0.256)	0.4
Outcome: Unhealthy Snack intake	Adjusted R^2 = 0.001		Adjusted R^2 < 0.001		Adjusted R^2 = 0.027		Adjusted R^2 = 0.029	
BAS total	0.030 (−0.006, 0.065)	0.1	0.030 (−0.005, 0.066)	0.1	0.033 (−0.003, 0.068)	0.07	0.035 (0.000, 0.071)	0.05
Health-promoting parenting practices	−0.009 (−0.046, 0.028)	0.6	−0.009 (−0.046, 0.028)	0.6	−0.012 (−0.050, 0.026)	0.5	−0.013 (−0.052, 0.025)	0.5
BAS total * Health-promoting parenting practices			0.011 (−0.026, 0.049)	0.6	0.006 (−0.031, 0.044)	0.7	0.007 (−0.030, 0.045)	0.7
Age					0.003 (−0.041, 0.047)	0.9	0.004 (−0.040, 0.048)	0.9
Gender [Ref: boy]					−0.132 (−0.200, −0.063)	<0.001	−0.127 (−0.196, −0.058)	<0.001

Table A3. Cont.

Outcomes	Model 1		Model 2		Model 3		Model 4	
	B (95% CI)	p-Value	B (95% CI)	p-Value	B (95% CI)	p-Value	B (95% CI)	p-Value
Family type [Ref: not traditional]							0.073 (−0.004, 0.150)	0.06
School type General [Ref: Vocational]							0.033 (−0.082, 0.149)	0.6
School type Technical [Ref: Vocational]							0.066 (−0.051, 0.183)	0.3
Breakfast [Ref: Not daily]					0.068 (−0.008, 0.145)	0.08	−0.017 (−0.091, 0.056)	0.6
Lunch [Ref: Not daily]					0.048 (−0.067, 0.162)	0.4	0.004 (−0.081, 0.089)	0.9
Dinner [Ref: Not daily]					0.073 (−0.044, 0.189)	0.2	0.124 (0.000, 0.248)	0.05

* Results in the table are for complete cases but excluding outliers for diet >3 SD ($n = 560$); Model 1 includes the main independent variables (BAS total, Health-promoting parenting practices); Model 2 includes the main independent variables (BAS total, Health-promoting parenting practices) and the interaction; Model 3 includes adjustments for age, gender, family type (traditional versus other), and school type (general, technical, vocational); Model 4 includes model 3 adjustments plus additional adjustment for breakfast, lunch, and dinner patterns. # BAS total (Behavioral Activation System) is an indicator of Reward sensitivity.

Table A4. Associations between reward sensitivity and adolescents' intake of sugar-sweetened beverages, healthy and unhealthy snacks, and the moderating role of (adolescent-reported) Health-reducing parenting practices for complete cases excluding diet outliers ($n = 560$).

Outcomes	Model 1		Model 2		Model 3		Model 4	
	B (95% CI)	p-Value	B (95% CI)	p-Value	B (95% CI)	p-Value	B (95% CI)	p-Value
Outcome: Sugar-Sweetened Beverages	Adjusted $R^2 = 0.002$		Adjusted $R^2 < 0.001$		Adjusted $R^2 = 0.041$		Adjusted $R^2 = 0.047$	
BAS total [#]	0.006 (−0.042, 0.054)	0.8	0.007 (−0.041, 0.055)	0.8	0.007 (−0.041, 0.054)	0.8	0.006 (−0.041, 0.054)	0.8
Health-reducing parenting practices	0.038 (−0.008, 0.085)	0.1	0.038 (−0.010, 0.085)	0.1	0.047 (0.000, 0.054)	0.05	0.045 (−0.002, 0.092)	0.06
BAS total * Health-reducing parenting practices			−0.014 (−0.059, 0.032)	0.6	−0.013 (−0.058, 0.032)	0.6	−0.011 (−0.056, 0.034)	0.6
Age					0.017 (−0.041, 0.075)	0.6	0.007 (−0.052, 0.065)	0.8
Gender [Ref: boy]					−0.205 (−0.296, −0.115)	<0.001	−0.217 (−0.309, −0.126)	<0.001
Family type [Ref: not traditional]					−0.064 (−0.165, 0.036)	0.2	−0.048 (−0.149, 0.054)	0.4
School type General [Ref: Vocational]					−0.071 (−0.219, 0.076)	0.3	−0.054 (−0.204, 0.096)	0.5
School type Technical [Ref: Vocational]					0.015 (−0.138, 0.167)	0.9	0.025 (−0.128, 0.178)	0.7
Breakfast [Ref: Not daily]							−0.119 (−0.216, −0.023)	0.02
Lunch [Ref: Not daily]							−0.017 (−0.129, 0.096)	0.8
Dinner [Ref: Not daily]							0.059 (−0.105, 0.223)	0.5
Outcome: Healthy Snack Intake	Adjusted $R^2 < 0.001$		Adjusted $R^2 < 0.001$		Adjusted $R^2 = 0.047$		Adjusted $R^2 = 0.044$	
BAS total	0.019 (−0.033, 0.070)	0.5	0.019 (−0.032, 0.071)	0.5	0.022 (−0.028, 0.072)	0.4	0.022 (−0.028, 0.073)	0.4
Health-reducing parenting practices	−0.037 (−0.087, 0.014)	0.2	−0.038 (−0.088, 0.013)	0.1	−0.046 (−0.095, 0.004)	0.07	−0.045 (−0.095, 0.005)	0.08
BAS total * Health-reducing parenting practices			−0.017 (−0.066, 0.032)	0.5	−0.015 (−0.063, 0.033)	0.5	−0.015 (−0.063, 0.033)	0.5
Age					−0.033 (−0.094, 0.029)	0.3	−0.034 (−0.097, 0.028)	0.3
Gender [Ref: boy]					0.152 (0.056, 0.249)	0.002	0.151 (0.053, 0.249)	0.003
Family type [Ref: not traditional]					0.059 (−0.048, 0.166)	0.3	0.066 (−0.042, 0.175)	0.2

Table A4. Cont.

Outcomes	Model 1		Model 2		Model 3		Model 4	
	B (95% CI)	p-Value	B (95% CI)	p-Value	B (95% CI)	p-Value	B (95% CI)	p-Value
School type General [Ref: Vocational]					0.276 (0.119, 0.433)	0.001	0.272 (0.112, 0.433)	0.001
School type Technical [Ref: Vocational]					0.148 (−0.014, 0.310)	0.07	0.146 (−0.017, 0.309)	0.08
Breakfast [Ref: Not daily]							−0.032 (−0.135, 0.072)	0.5
Lunch [Ref: Not daily]							−0.020 (−0.141, 0.100)	0.7
Dinner [Ref: Not daily]							0.078 (−0.097, 0.254)	0.4
Outcome: Unhealthy Snack Intake	Adjusted R² = 0.010		Adjusted R² = 0.013		Adjusted R² = 0.041		Adjusted R² = 0.045	
BAS total	0.021 (−0.015, 0.057)	0.2	0.022 (−0.014, 0.058)	0.2	0.023 (−0.013, 0.058)	0.2	0.025 (−0.011, 0.061)	0.2
Health-reducing parenting practices	0.041 (0.006, 0.076)	0.02	0.039 (0.004, 0.074)	0.03	0.045 (0.010, 0.080)	0.01	0.050 (0.015, 0.085)	0.01
BAS total * Health-reducing parenting practices			−0.027 (−0.061, 0.007)	0.1	−0.022 (−0.055, 0.012)	0.2	−0.023 (−0.057, 0.011)	0.2
Age					0.009 (−0.034, 0.053)	0.7	0.011 (−0.033, 0.055)	0.6
Gender [Ref: boy]					−0.140 (−0.208, −0.071)	<0.001	−0.134 (−0.202, −0.065)	<0.001
Family type [Ref: not traditional]					0.063 (−0.013, 0.138)	0.1	0.066 (−0.010, 0.143)	0.09
School type General [Ref: Vocational]					0.043 (−0.068, 0.153)	0.5	0.025 (−0.088, 0.137)	0.7
School type Technical [Ref: Vocational]					0.066 (−0.048, 0.181)	0.3	0.058 (−0.057, 0.172)	0.3
Breakfast [Ref: Not daily]							−0.017 (−0.090, 0.055)	0.6
Lunch [Ref: Not daily]							0.017 (−0.068, 0.101)	0.7
Dinner [Ref: Not daily]							0.139 (0.015, 0.262)	0.03

* Results in the table are for complete cases but excluding outliers for diet >3 SD (n = 560); Model 1 includes the main independent variables (BAS total, Health-reducing parenting practices); Model 2 includes the main independent variables (BAS total, Health-promoting parenting practices) and the interaction term; Model 3 includes adjustments for age, gender, family type (traditional versus other), and school type (general, technical, vocational); Model 4 includes model 3 adjustments plus additional adjustment for breakfast, lunch, and dinner patterns. # BAS total (Behavioral Activation System) is an indicator of Reward sensitivity.

Table A5. Associations between reward sensitivity and adolescents' intake of sugar-sweetened beverages, healthy and unhealthy snack, and the moderating role of (parent-reported) health-promoting parenting practices ($n = 131$).

Outcomes	Model 1		Model 2		Model 3		Model 4	
	B (95% CI)	p-Value	B (95% CI)	p-Value	B (95% CI)	p-Value	B (95% CI)	p-Value
Outcome: Sugar-Sweetened Beverages	Adjusted $R^2 = 0.014$		Adjusted $R^2 = 0.006$		Adjusted $R^2 = 0.093$		Adjusted $R^2 = 0.071$	
BAS total [#]	0.164 (−0.009, 0.336)	0.06	0.166 (−0.009, 0.341)	0.06	0.182 (0.011, 0.353)	0.04	0.189 (0.013, 0.364)	0.04
Health-promoting parenting practices	0.022 (−0.136, 0.180)	0.8	0.021 (−0.138, 0.180)	0.8	0.051 (−0.106, 0.208)	0.5	0.048 (−0.114, 0.210)	0.6
BAS total * Health-promoting parenting practices			−0.017 (−0.201, 0.167)	0.9	−0.035 (−0.214, 0.145)	0.7	−0.043 (−0.23, 0.143)	0.6
Age child					0.156 (−0.102, 0.415)	0.2	0.143 (−0.124, 0.410)	0.3
Age parent					−0.017 (−0.056, 0.022)	0.4	−0.017 (−0.057, 0.023)	0.4
Gender [Ref: boy]					−0.298 (−0.592, −0.004)	0.05	−0.287 (−0.592, 0.018)	0.07
Gender parent [Ref: father]					−0.113 (−0.490, 0.263)	0.6	−0.116 (−0.499, 0.267)	0.5
SES [Ref: Lower SES]					−0.387 (−0.77, −0.004)	0.05	−0.371 (−0.782, 0.040)	0.08

Table A5. Cont.

Outcomes	Model 1		Model 2		Model 3		Model 4	
	B (95% CI)	p-Value	B (95% CI)	p-Value	B (95% CI)	p-Value	B (95% CI)	p-Value
Family type [Ref: not traditional]					−0.188 (−0.577, 0.201)	0.4	−0.156 (−0.565, 0.253)	0.5
School type General [Ref: Vocational]					0.468 (−0.312, 1.248)	0.2	0.450 (−0.363, 1.263)	0.3
School type Technical [Ref: Vocational]					0.614 (−0.146, 1.375)	0.1	0.581 (−0.239, 1.401)	0.2
Breakfast [Ref: Not daily]							−0.118 (−0.468, 0.232)	0.5
Lunch [Ref: Not daily]							0.107 (−0.377, 0.590)	0.7
Dinner [Ref: Not daily]							−0.067 (−0.821, 0.686)	0.9
	Adjusted R² = −0.009		Adjusted R² = −0.016		Adjusted R² = 0.014		Adjusted R² = 0.014	
Outcome: Healthy Snack Intake								
BAS total	0.070 (−0.157, 0.297)	0.5	0.078 (−0.152, 0.308)	0.5	0.062 (−0.170, 0.294)	0.6	0.056 (−0.179, 0.291)	0.6
Health-promoting parenting practices	0.075 (−0.133, 0.283)	0.5	0.072 (−0.137, 0.281)	0.5	0.099 (−0.115, 0.312)	0.4	0.112 (−0.105, 0.329)	0.3
BAS total * Health-promoting parenting practices			−0.063 (−0.305, 0.179)	0.6	−0.030 (−0.273, 0.213)	0.8	−0.033 (−0.282, 0.217)	0.8
Age child					−0.084 (−0.435, 0.266)	0.6	−0.098 (−0.456, 0.260)	0.6
Age parent					0.001 (−0.051, 0.054)	1.0	−0.004 (−0.057, 0.050)	0.9
Gender [Ref: boy]					−0.018 (−0.417, 0.380)	0.9	−0.079 (−0.487, 0.329)	0.7
Gender parent [Ref: father]					−0.082 (−0.592, 0.428)	0.8	−0.041 (−0.554, 0.472)	0.9
SES [Ref: Lower SES]					−0.585 (−1.104, −0.066)	0.03	−0.524 (−1.074, 0.027)	0.06
Family type [Ref: not traditional]					0.233 (−0.295, 0.760)	0.4	0.195 (−0.352, 0.743)	0.5
School type General [Ref: Vocational]					1.092 (0.035, 2.150)	0.04	1.260 (0.171, 2.349)	0.02
School type Technical [Ref: Vocational]					0.592 (−0.440, 1.623)	0.3	0.812 (−0.286, 1.910)	0.1
Breakfast [Ref: Not daily]							0.111 (−0.358, 0.579)	0.6
Lunch [Ref: Not daily]							−0.565 (−1.212, 0.083)	0.09
Dinner [Ref: Not daily]							0.108 (−0.902, 1.117)	0.8
	Adjusted R² = 0.022		Adjusted R² = 0.013		Adjusted R² = 0.009		Adjusted R² = 0.001	
Outcome: Unhealthy Snack Intake								
BAS total	0.265 (0.018, 0.513)	0.04	0.269 (0.018, 0.520)	0.04	0.243 (−0.015, 0.501)	0.07	0.228 (−0.034, 0.490)	0.09
Health-promoting parenting practices	0.016 (−0.210, 0.243)	0.9	0.015 (−0.213, 0.243)	0.9	0.044 (−0.193, 0.281)	0.7	0.024 (−0.218, 0.267)	0.8
BAS total * Health-promoting parenting practices			−0.028 (−0.291, 0.236)	0.8	0.009 (−0.262, 0.279)	1.0	0.026 (−0.253, 0.304)	0.9
Age child					−0.112 (−0.502, 0.277)	0.6	−0.144 (−0.543, 0.255)	0.5
Age parent					0.010 (−0.048, 0.069)	0.7	0.004 (−0.056, 0.063)	0.9
Gender [Ref: boy]					−0.308 (−0.751, 0.135)	0.2	−0.304 (−0.759, 0.152)	0.2
Gender parent [Ref: father]					0.138 (−0.428, 0.705)	0.6	0.151 (−0.421, 0.723)	0.6
SES [Ref: Lower SES]					−0.588 (−1.165, −0.011)	0.05	−0.619 (−1.233, −0.005)	0.05
Family type [Ref: not traditional]					0.218 (−0.368, 0.803)	0.5	0.271 (−0.340, 0.882)	0.4
School type General [Ref: Vocational]					0.446 (−0.728, 1.621)	0.5	0.658 (−0.557, 1.873)	0.3
School type Technical [Ref: Vocational]					0.281 (−0.865, 1.427)	0.6	0.590 (−0.635, 1.815)	0.3
Breakfast [Ref: Not daily]							−0.059 (−0.582, 0.464)	0.8
Lunch [Ref: Not daily]							−0.336 (−1.059, 0.387)	0.4
Dinner [Ref: Not daily]							0.676 (−0.450, 1.802)	0.2

* Results in the table are for complete cases ($n = 131$); Model 1 includes the main independent variables (BAS total, Health-promoting parenting practices); Model 2 includes the main independent variables (BAS total, Health-promoting parenting practices) and the interaction term; Model 3 includes adjustments for age, gender, family type (traditional versus other), and school type (general, technical, vocational); and for age of parent, gender of parent, and family SES; Model 4 includes model 3 adjustments plus additional adjustment for breakfast, lunch, and dinner patterns. # BAS total (Behavioral Activation System) is an indicator of Reward sensitivity.

Table A6. Associations between reward sensitivity and adolescents' intake of sugar-sweetened beverages, healthy and unhealthy snacks, and the moderating role of (parent-reported) health-reducing parenting practices.

Outcomes	Model 1		Model 2		Model 3		Model 4	
	B (95% CI)	p-Value	B (95% CI)	p-Value	B (95% CI)	p-Value	B (95% CI)	p-Value
Outcome: Sugar-Sweetened Beverages	Adjusted R^2 = 0.048		Adjusted R^2 = 0.068		Adjusted R^2 = 0.140		Adjusted R^2 = 0.120	
BAS total [#]	0.152 (−0.018, 0.322)	0.08	0.147 (−0.021, 0.316)	0.09	0.166 (0.001, 0.331)	0.05	0.172 (0.003, 0.340)	0.05
Health-reducing parenting practices	0.145 (0.002, 0.289)	0.05	0.169 (0.025, 0.313)	0.02	0.146 (0.000, 0.291)	0.05	0.150 (0.002, 0.298)	0.05
BAS total * Health-reducing parenting practices			0.145 (−0.009, 0.299)	0.07	0.148 (−0.006, 0.301)	0.06	0.149 (−0.011, 0.310)	0.07
Age child					0.222 (−0.035, 0.479)	0.09	0.216 (−0.052, 0.483)	0.1
Age parent					−0.014 (−0.052, 0.023)	0.5	−0.013 (−0.052, 0.026)	0.5
Gender [Ref: boy]					−0.277 (−0.563, 0.009)	0.06	−0.265 (−0.562, 0.033)	0.08
Gender parent [Ref: father]					−0.065 (−0.434, 0.304)	0.7	−0.069 (−0.445, 0.306)	0.7
SES [Ref: Lower SES]					−0.364 (−0.730, 0.002)	0.05	−0.352 (−0.749, 0.044)	0.08
Family type [Ref: not traditional]					−0.152 (−0.528, 0.223)	0.4	−0.127 (−0.523, 0.269)	0.5
School type General [Ref: Vocational]					0.477 (−0.294, 1.248)	0.2	0.430 (−0.375, 1.235)	0.3
School type Technical [Ref: Vocational]					0.571 (−0.175, 1.318)	0.1	0.496 (−0.313, 1.305)	0.2
Breakfast [Ref: Not daily]							−0.095 (−0.433, 0.243)	0.6
Lunch [Ref: Not daily]							0.153 (−0.320, 0.626)	0.5
Dinner [Ref: Not daily]							−0.139 (−0.868, 0.590)	0.7
Outcome: Healthy Snack Intake	Adjusted R^2 = −0.014		Adjusted R^2 = 0.023		Adjusted R^2 = 0.041		Adjusted R^2 = 0.041	
BAS total	0.076 (−0.152, 0.304)	0.5	0.068 (−0.156, 0.292)	0.5	0.056 (−0.170, 0.283)	0.6	0.055 (−0.174, 0.283)	0.6
Health-reducing parenting practices	−0.015 (−0.207, 0.177)	0.9	0.024 (−0.168, 0.215)	0.8	0.076 (−0.124, 0.275)	0.5	0.058 (−0.143, 0.259)	0.6
BAS total * Health-reducing parenting practices			0.238 (0.032, 0.443)	0.02	0.208 (−0.004, 0.419)	0.05	0.219 (0.002, 0.437)	0.05
Age child					−0.016 (−0.369, 0.338)	0.9	−0.025 (−0.388, 0.338)	0.9
Age parent					0.004 (−0.048, 0.056)	0.9	−0.001 (−0.053, 0.052)	1.0
Gender [Ref: boy]					−0.016 (−0.409, 0.377)	0.9	−0.087 (−0.491, 0.317)	0.7
Gender parent [Ref: father]					−0.057 (−0.564, 0.450)	0.8	−0.021 (−0.531, 0.488)	0.9
SES [Ref: Lower SES]					−0.513 (−1.016, −0.011)	0.05	−0.432 (−0.970, 0.106)	0.1
Family type [Ref: not traditional]					0.252 (−0.264, 0.767)	0.4	0.197 (−0.341, 0.735)	0.5
School type General [Ref: Vocational]					1.010 (−0.048, 2.069)	0.06	1.130 (0.037, 2.223)	0.04
School type Technical [Ref: Vocational]					0.495 (−0.530, 1.520)	0.3	0.663 (−0.434, 1.761)	0.2
Breakfast [Ref: Not daily]							0.140 (−0.319, 0.599)	0.5
Lunch [Ref: Not daily]							−0.546 (−1.188, 0.096)	0.1
Dinner [Ref: Not daily]							0.001 (−0.988, 0.991)	1.0
Outcome: Unhealthy Snack Intake	Adjusted R^2 = 0.055		Adjusted R^2 = 0.116		Adjusted R^2 = 0.113		Adjusted R^2 = 0.096	
BAS total	0.248 (0.004, 0.492)	0.05	0.238 (0.001, 0.474)	0.05	0.219 (−0.023, 0.460)	0.08	0.212 (−0.034, 0.458)	0.09
Health-reducing parenting practices	0.206 (0.001, 0.412)	0.05	0.259 (0.057, 0.461)	0.01	0.285 (0.072, 0.498)	0.009	0.275 (0.059, 0.491)	0.01
BAS total * Health-reducing parenting practices			0.324 (0.107, 0.540)	0.004	0.315 (0.090, 0.540)	0.007	0.297 (0.062, 0.531)	0.01

Table A6. Cont.

Outcomes	Model 1		Model 2		Model 3		Model 4	
	B (95% CI)	p-Value	B (95% CI)	p-Value	B (95% CI)	p-Value	B (95% CI)	p-Value
Age child					0.040 (−0.336, 0.417)	0.8	0.013 (−0.377, 0.404)	0.9
Age parent					0.015 (−0.041, 0.070)	0.6	0.010 (−0.047, 0.067)	0.7
Gender [Ref: boy]					−0.266 (−0.684, 0.153)	0.2	−0.272 (−0.706, 0.163)	0.2
Gender parent [Ref: father]					0.234 (−0.306, 0.775)	0.4	0.244 (−0.304, 0.792)	0.4
SES [Ref: Lower SES]					−0.552 (−1.088, −0.017)	0.4	−0.564 (−1.143, 0.015)	0.06
Family type [Ref: not traditional]					0.268 (−0.281, 0.818)	0.3	0.292 (−0.286, 0.871)	0.3
School type General [Ref: Vocational]					0.459 (−0.670, 1.588)	0.4	0.606 (−0.570, 1.783)	0.3
School type Technical [Ref: Vocational]					0.185 (−0.907, 1.277)	0.7	0.396 (−0.785, 1.577)	0.5
Breakfast [Ref: Not daily]							−0.030 (−0.524, 0.464)	0.9
Lunch [Ref: Not daily]							−0.259 (−0.950, 0.431)	0.5
Dinner [Ref: Not daily]							0.391 (−0.674, 1.456)	0.5

* Results in the table are for complete cases (n = 131); Model 1 includes the main independent variables (BAS total, Health-reducing parenting practices); Model 2 includes the main independent variables (BAS total, Health-promoting parenting practices) and the interaction term; Model 3 includes adjustments for age, gender, family type (traditional versus other), and school type (general, technical, vocational); and for age of parent, gender of parent, and family SES; Model 4 includes model 3 adjustments plus additional adjustment for breakfast, lunch, and dinner patterns. # BAS total (Behavioral Activation System) is an indicator of Reward sensitivity.

References

1. Martens, M.K.; van Assema, P.; Brug, J. Why do adolescents eat what they eat? Personal and social environmental predictors of fruit, snack and breakfast consumption among 12–14-year-old Dutch students. *Public Health Nutr.* **2005**, *8*, 1258–1265. [CrossRef] [PubMed]
2. Janssen, I.; Katzmarzyk, P.T.; Boyce, W.F.; Vereecken, C.; Mulvihill, C.; Roberts, C.; Currie, C.; Pickett, W.; Health Behaviour in School-Aged Children Obesity Working Group. Comparison of overweight and obesity prevalence in school-aged youth from 34 countries and their relationships with physical activity and dietary patterns. *Obes. Rev.* **2005**, *6*, 123–132. [CrossRef] [PubMed]
3. Rodriguez, G.; Moreno, L.A. Is dietary intake able to explain differences in body fatness in children and adolescents? *Nutr. Metab. Cardiovasc. Dis.* **2006**, *16*, 294–301. [CrossRef] [PubMed]
4. Phillips, S.M.; Bandini, L.G.; Naumova, E.N.; Cyr, H.; Colclough, S.; Dietz, W.H.; Must, A. Energy-dense snack food intake in adolescence: Longitudinal relationship to weight and fatness. *Obe. Res.* **2004**, *12*, 461–472. [CrossRef] [PubMed]
5. Ludwig, D.S.; Peterson, K.E.; Gortmaker, S.L. Relation between consumption of sugar-sweetened drinks and childhood obesity: A prospective, observational analysis. *Lancet* **2001**, *357*, 505–508. [CrossRef]
6. Swinburn, B.; Egger, G.; Raza, F. Dissecting obesogenic environments: The development and application of a framework for identifying and prioritizing environmental interventions for obesity. *Prev. Med.* **1999**, *29*, 563–570. [CrossRef]
7. Booth, K.M.; Pinkston, M.M.; Carlos Poston, W.S. Obesity and the built environment. *J. Am. Diet. Assoc.* **2005**, *105*, 110–117. [CrossRef]
8. De Cock, N.; Van Lippevelde, W.; Vervoort, L.; Vangeel, J.; Maes, L.; Eggermont, S.; Braet, C.; Lachat, C.; Huybregts, L.; Goossens, L.; et al. Sensitivity to reward is associated with snack and sugar-sweetened beverage consumption in adolescents. *Eur. J. Nutr.* **2016**, *55*, 1623–1632. [CrossRef]
9. Franken, I.H.A.; Muris, P. Individual differences in reward sensitivity are related to food craving and relative body weight in healthy women. *Appetite* **2005**, *45*, 198–201. [CrossRef]
10. Davis, C.; Fox, J. Sensitivity to reward and body mass index (BMI): Evidence for a non-linear relationship. *Appetite* **2008**, *50*, 43–49. [CrossRef]
11. Gray, J.A.; McNaughton, N. *The Neuropsychology of Anxiety: An Enquiry into the Functions of the Septo-Hippocampal System*, 2nd ed.; Oxford University Press: Oxford, UK, 2000.
12. Davis, C.; Patte, K.; Levitan, R.; Reid, C.; Tweed, S.; Curtis, C. From motivation to behaviour: A model of reward sensitivity, overeating, and food prefs in the risk profile for obesity. *Appetite* **2007**, *48*, 12–19. [CrossRef] [PubMed]
13. Verbeken, S.; Braet, C.; Lammertyn, J.; Goossens, L.; Moens, E. How is reward sensitivity related to bodyweight in children? *Appetite* **2012**, *58*, 478–483. [CrossRef] [PubMed]
14. Story, M.; Neumark-Sztainer, D.; French, S. Individual and environmental influences on adolescent eating behaviors. *J. Am. Diet. Assoc.* **2002**, *102*, S40–S51. [CrossRef]
15. Vaughn, A.E.; Ward, D.S.; Fisher, J.O.; Faith, M.S.; Hughes, S.O.; Kremers, S.P.J.; Musher-Eizenman, D.R.; O'Connor, T.M.; Patrick, H.; Power, T.G. Fundamental constructs in food parenting practices: a content map to guide future research. *Nutr. Rev.* **2016**, *74*, 98–117. [CrossRef]
16. Patrick, H.; Nicklas, T.A.; Hughes, S.O.; Morales, M. The benefits of authoritative feeding style: caregiver feeding styles and children's food consumption patterns. *Appetite* **2005**, *44*, 243–249. [CrossRef]
17. Birch, L.L.; Fisher, J.O.; Davison, K.K. Learning to overeat: maternal use of restrictive feeding practices promotes girls' eating in the absence of hunger. *Am. J. Clin. Nutr.* **2003**, *78*, 215–220. [CrossRef]
18. Yee, A.Z.H.; Lwin, M.O.; Ho, S.S. The influence of parental practices on child promotive and preventive food consumption behaviors: A systematic review and meta-analysis. *Int. J. Behav. Nutr. Phys. Act.* **2017**, *14*, 47. [CrossRef]
19. Van Durme, K.; Goossens, L.; Bosmans, G.; Braet, C. The Role of Attachment and Maladaptive Emotion Regulation Strategies in the Development of Bulimic Symptoms in Adolescents. *J. Abnorm. Child Psychol.* **2018**, *46*, 881–893. [CrossRef]
20. Kremers, S.P.; Brug, J.; de Vries, H.; Engels, R. Parenting style and adolescent fruit consumption. *Appetite* **2003**, *41*, 43–50. [CrossRef]

21. Pearson, N.; Atkin, A.J.; Biddle, S.J.H.; Gorely, T.; Edwardson, C. Parenting styles, family structure and adolescent dietary behaviour. *Public Health Nutr.* **2010**, *13*, 1245–1253. [CrossRef]
22. Loth, K.A.; MacLehose, R.F.; Fulkerson, J.A.; Crow, S.; Neumark-Sztainer, D. Food-Related Parenting Practices and Adolescent Weight Status: A Population-Based Study. *Pediatrics* **2013**, *131*, E1443–E1450. [CrossRef] [PubMed]
23. Fleary, S.A.; Ettienne, R. The relationship between food parenting practices, parental diet and their adolescents' diet. *Appetite* **2019**, *135*, 79–85. [CrossRef] [PubMed]
24. Berge, J.M.; Wall, M.; Larson, N.; Forsyth, A.; Bauer, K.W.; Neumark-Sztainer, D. Youth dietary intake and weight status: Healthful neighborhood food environments enhance the protective role of supportive family home environments. *Health Place* **2014**, *26*, 69–77. [CrossRef] [PubMed]
25. Bauer, K.W.; Neumark-Sztainer, D.; Fulkerson, J.A.; Hannan, P.J.; Story, M. Familial correlates of adolescent girls' physical activity, television use, dietary intake, weight, and body composition. *Int. J. Behav. Nutr. Phys. Act.* **2011**, *8*, 25. [CrossRef] [PubMed]
26. Thomas, A.; Chess, S. *Temperament and Development*; Brunner/Mazel: New York, NY, USA, 1977.
27. De Cock, N.; van Lippevelde, W.; Goossens, L.; De Clercq, B.; Vangeel, J.; Lachat, C.; Beullens, K.; Huybregts, L.; Vervoort, L.; Eggermont, S.; et al. Sensitivity to reward and adolescents' unhealthy snacking and drinking behavior: the role of hedonic eating styles and availability. *Int. J. Behav. Nutr. Phys. Act.* **2016**, *13*, 17. [CrossRef] [PubMed]
28. Huybrechts, I.; Vereecken, C.; De Bacquer, D.; Vandevijvere, S.; Van Oyen, H.; Maes, L.; Vanhauwaert, E.; Temme, L.; De Backer, G.; De Henauw, S. Reproducibility and validity of a diet quality index for children assessed using a FFQ. *Br. J. Nutr.* **2010**, *104*, 135–144. [CrossRef] [PubMed]
29. FSA. Nutrient Profiling Technical Guidance. 2020. Available online: https://www.gov.uk/government/publications/the-nutrient-profiling-model (accessed on 7 January 2020).
30. Muris, P.; Meesters, C.; De Kanter, E.; Timmerman, E. Behavioural inhibition and behavioural activation system scales for children: Relationships with Eysenck's personality traits and psychopathological symptoms. *Pers. Individ. Differ.* **2005**, *38*, 103–113. [CrossRef]
31. Vervoort, L.; Wolters, L.H.; Hogendoorn, S.M.; de Haan, E.; Boer, F.; Prins, P.J.M. Sensitivity of Gray's Behavioral Inhibition System in clinically anxious and non-anxious children and adolescents. *Pers. Individ. Differ.* **2010**, *48*, 629–633. [CrossRef]
32. Birch, L.L.; Fisher, J.O.; Grimm-Thomas, K.; Markey, C.N.; Sawyer, R.; Johnson, S.L. Confirmatory factor analysis of the Child Feeding Questionnaire: A measure of parental attitudes, beliefs and practices about child feeding and obesity proneness. *Appetite* **2001**, *36*, 201–210. [CrossRef]
33. Haszard, J.J.; Williams, S.M.; Dawson, A.M.; Skidmore, P.M.L.; Taylor, R.W. Factor analysis of the Comprehensive Feeding Practices Questionnaire in Cross Mark a large sample of children. *Appetite* **2013**, *62*, 110–118. [CrossRef]
34. Stok, F.M.; Hoffmann, S.; Volkert, D.; Boeing, H.; Ensenauer, R.; Stelmach-Mardas, M.; Kiesswetter, E.; Weber, A.; Rohm, H.; Lien, N.; et al. The DONE framework: Creation, evaluation, and updating of an interdisciplinary, dynamic framework 2.0 of determinants of nutrition and eating. *PLoS ONE* **2017**, *12*, e0171077. [CrossRef] [PubMed]
35. De Los Reyes, A.; Augenstein, T.M.; Wang, M.; Thomas, S.A.; Drabick, D.A.G.; Burgers, D.E.; Rabinowitz, J. The Validity of the Multi-Informant Approach to Assessing Child and Adolescent Mental Health. *Psychol. Bull.* **2015**, *141*, 858–900. [CrossRef] [PubMed]
36. Taylor, A.; Wilson, C.; Slater, A.; Mohr, P. Parent- and child-reported parenting. Associations with child weight-related outcomes. *Appetite* **2011**, *57*, 700–706. [CrossRef] [PubMed]
37. Moens, E.; Goossens, L.; Verbeken, S.; Vandeweghe, L.; Braet, C. Parental feeding behavior in relation to children's tasting behavior: An observational study. *Appetite* **2018**, *120*, 205–211. [CrossRef] [PubMed]
38. Gevers, D.W.M.; Kremers, S.P.J.; de Vries, N.K.; van Assema, P. Clarifying concepts of food parenting practices. A Delphi study with an application to snacking behavior. *Appetite* **2014**, *79*, 51–57. [CrossRef]
39. Wouters, E.J.; Larsen, J.K.; Kremers, S.P.; Dagnelie, P.C.; Geenen, R. Peer influence on snacking behavior in adolescence. *Appetite* **2010**, *55*, 11–17. [CrossRef]

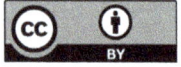

© 2020 by the authors. Licensee MDPI, Basel, Switzerland. This article is an open access article distributed under the terms and conditions of the Creative Commons Attribution (CC BY) license (http://creativecommons.org/licenses/by/4.0/).

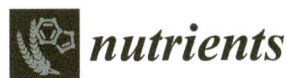

Article

Home Cooking and Child Obesity in Japan: Results from the A-CHILD Study

Yukako Tani, Takeo Fujiwara *, Satomi Doi and Aya Isumi

Department of Global Health Promotion, Tokyo Medical and Dental University (TMDU), 1-5-45, Yushima, Bunkyo-ku, Tokyo 113-8519, Japan; tani.hlth@tmd.ac.jp (Y.T.); doi.hlth@tmd.ac.jp (S.D.); isumi.hlth@tmd.ac.jp (A.I.)
* Correspondence: fujiwara.hlth@tmd.ac.jp; Tel.: +81-3-5803-5187; Fax: +81-3-5803-5190

Received: 1 October 2019; Accepted: 19 November 2019; Published: 21 November 2019

Abstract: This study aimed to investigate the association between the frequency of home cooking and obesity among children in Japan. We used cross-sectional data from the Adachi Child Health Impact of Living Difficulty study, a population-based sample targeting all fourth-grade students aged 9 to 10 in Adachi City, Tokyo, Japan. Frequency of home cooking was assessed by a questionnaire for 4258 caregivers and classified as high (almost every day), medium (4–5 days/week), or low (≤3 days/week). School health checkup data on height and weight were used to calculate body mass index z-scores. Overall, 2.4% and 10.8% of children were exposed to low and medium frequencies of home cooking, respectively. After adjusting for confounding factors, children with a low frequency of home cooking were 2.27 times (95% confidence interval: 1.16–4.45) more likely to be obese, compared with those with a high frequency of home cooking. After adjustment for children's obesity-related eating behaviors (frequency of vegetable and breakfast intake and snacking habits) as potential mediating factors, the relative risk ratio of obesity became statistically non-significant (1.90; 95% confidence interval: 0.95–3.82). A low frequency of home cooking is associated with obesity among children in Japan, and this link may be explained by unhealthy eating behaviors.

Keywords: home cooking; meal preparation; obesity; children; parenting

1. Introduction

The prevalence of childhood overweight and obesity has increased worldwide in recent decades, becoming a major public health epidemic [1]. In Organization for Economic Cooperation and Development (OECD) countries, the prevalence of childhood overweight and obesity is 25% [2]. Obese children are more likely to become obese adults [3] and are at a higher risk of a wide range of serious health complications [4]. To combat the obesity epidemic, it is important that prevention efforts are shaped by a solid evidence base regarding the risk factors for obesity in children.

Home cooking has been suggested as a key strategy to prevent obesity [5]. In developed countries, sociodemographic changes, such as an increasing numbers of working women and single-parent or small families, have led to less time being available for home cooking and an increased shift toward eating out or buying prepared meals [6–8]. In Japan, household expenditure for prepared food has increased in recent decades, and eating out is common among younger age groups [9]. Increased consumption of out-of-home foods, such as fast food and convenience food, is a major concern because these foods are higher in calories, fat, and sodium; lower in fiber and calcium [10–13]; and associated with poor diet quality and increased energy intake among children [12–15]. Several studies conducted in the United States have shown an association between fast food consumption and increased weight gain in adolescents [16,17]. However, these studies evaluated only the effect of eating out; they did not examine the effect of at-home consumption of prepared (precooked) meals, such as packed lunches, convenience foods, and ready-made meals. To account for the effects of both eating out and eating prepared meals at home, it is necessary to examine the frequency of home cooking.

Several studies of adults have suggested that home cooking improves diet quality and weight status [18–20]. However, there is limited evidence on the relationship between home cooking and children's weight status. Parents who report a low enjoyment of cooking, little meal planning, and fewer hours spent on food preparation are less likely to serve vegetable and fruits, whereas they are more likely to serve fast food for family dinners [21]. Furthermore, because children may model their parents' healthy eating habits, enjoy meal time more, and feel closer to their caregivers through having home-cooked meals, home cooking may be beneficial for healthy child development, including weight status, because it fosters a better relationship between the caregiver and the child [22–26]. Moreover, because dietary intake patterns established early in life tend to persist into adolescence and adulthood [27–29], it is also important to understand the associations between home-cooking habits and child weight status. Children who eat less home-cooked food may be vulnerable to the development of unhealthy dietary behaviors, which may, in turn, be linked to obesity. However, to the best of our knowledge, no studies have been conducted to examine the association between home cooking and child obesity in Japan.

The purpose of the present study was to examine the association between the frequency of home cooking and obesity among children in Japan.

2. Materials and Methods

2.1. Study Design and Subjects

The Adachi Child Health Impact of Living Difficulty (A-CHILD) project was established in 2015 to evaluate the determinants of health among children in Adachi City, Tokyo, Japan [30–32]. We used data from the 2018 wave of the A-CHILD study. The survey covered all 69 public elementary schools established in Adachi City, Tokyo, Japan. In 2018, self-reported questionnaires with anonymous unique identification numbers were distributed to 5311 children in the fourth grade (aged 9–10 years) in these elementary schools. The children were asked to pass on the questionnaires to their caregivers at home to complete. The children then returned the completed questionnaires to their schools. A total of 4605 caregivers completed the questionnaires (response rate: 86.7%), and 4290 provided informed consent and returned all the questionnaires. To examine child body mass index (BMI), we used school health checkup data on body height and weight, collected in April or May 2018, which was linked to the questionnaire responses using the anonymous unique identification number. Participants who did not indicate their body height, weight status, or month of birth ($n = 20$) were excluded from the analysis, as were participants who did not complete the questions related to home-cooking status ($n = 12$). After these exclusions, 4258 participants were included in the study. The final sample comprised information on 2151 boys and 2107 girls. Of the caregivers who completed the questionnaires, 91.5% were mothers and 7.7% were fathers. The A-CHILD protocol and the use of the data in this study were approved by the Ethics Committee at Tokyo Medical and Dental University (No. M2016-284).

2.2. Child Body Height and Weight Status

School teachers assessed child height and weight at elementary schools during a school health checkup, following a standardized protocol [33]. Height was measured to the nearest 0.1 cm using a portable stadiometer, and weight was measured to the nearest 0.1 kg on a digital scale, without shoes and in light clothing. BMI was calculated by dividing the child's weight (in kilograms) by the square of body height (in meters). BMI was expressed as a z-score representing the deviation in standard deviation units from the mean of a standard normal distribution of BMI specific to age and sex, according to the World Health Organization's Child Growth Standards. Children's BMIs were categorized as underweight/normal weight (<+1 SD), overweight (≥+1 SD and <+2 SD), or obese (≥+2 SD) using standard deviation cut-off points [34].

2.3. Home-Cooking Frequency

Following previous studies [35,36], home-cooking frequency over the past month was assessed using the following question: "How many times did you or someone else in your family cook meals at home? Include a simple meal, such as fried eggs, as a cooked meal". The five response categories were almost every day, 4–5 days/week, 2–3 days/week, a few days/month, and rarely. Considering the distribution of the answers to this question and based on categories previously used in other studies [35,36], we collapsed the responses into three groups of frequency of home cooking: (i) High (almost every day: 86.8%); (ii) medium (4–5 days/week: 10.8%); and (iii) low (≤3 days/week: 2.4%).

2.4. Covariates

Possible covariates, such as children's physical activity and eating behaviors, were also assessed using the caregiver-completed questionnaires. Children's physical activity was assessed using the frequency of physical activity for 30 min or more during the week (never/rarely, 1–2 times/week, 3–4 times/week, or ≥5 times/week). Children's eating behavior included frequency of vegetable intake (twice/day, once/day, or <3 times/week), frequency of breakfast intake (every day, often, or rarely/never), and snacking habits (no snacking, snacking at a set time (controlled), or snacking freely) [32]. Household characteristics included the caregiver's marital status (married or living with partner, single, divorced, or widowed), the child having siblings (yes or no), cohabitation with the child's grandparents (yes or no), and annual household income (<3.00, 3.00–5.99, 6.00–9.99, or ≥10.0 million yen). Caregiver characteristics included mother's age (<35, 35–44, or ≥45 years), mother's educational attainment (low (junior high school, dropped out of high school, or completed high school), middle (professional school, some college, or dropped out of college), or high (completed college or more), mother's employment and time of returning home from work (employed/returning home before 18:00, employed/returning home 18:00–20:00, employed/returning home after 20:00, employed/returning home at irregular times, or not employed), and mother's and father's BMIs calculated using self-reported height in centimeters and weight in kilograms. Standard categories of BMI [37] were used to characterize parents as obese (BMI ≥ 30.0 kg/m^2), overweight (BMI = 25.0–29.9 kg/m^2), normal weight (BMI = 18.5–24.9 kg/m^2), or underweight (BMI < 18.5 kg/m^2).

2.5. Statistical Analysis

First, the participants' characteristics were stratified by home-cooking status, and differences were tested using Pearson's chi-square test. Second, we calculated relative risk ratios (RRRs) and 95% confidence intervals (CIs) of overweight and obesity using multinomial logistic regression. Two models were constructed for both overweight and obesity. Model 1 adjusted for child's sex, physical activity, household characteristics (marital status, having siblings, living with grandparents, and household income), and caregiver characteristics (mother's age, education, employment, and BMI and father's BMI) as potential confounders. Model 2 additionally adjusted for the child's obesity-related eating behaviors (frequency of vegetable intake, frequency of breakfast consumption, and snacking habits) as potential mediating factors because children may learn to model their eating behaviors based on their caregivers through home cooking, which may affect children's weight status.

3. Results

The majority of the caregivers cooked at home for their children almost every day (86.8%), whereas 2.4% of the caregivers cooked at home less often than 3 days per week and 10.8% cooked at home 4 to 5 days per week. The breakdown of the distribution of cooking at home less often than 3 days per week was 1.8% for 2 to 3 days/week, 0.5% for a few days/month, and 0.1% for rarely. Overall, 14.7% of the children were overweight, and 5.9% were obese (Table 1). In terms of household status, 72.8% of the caregivers were married, 80.5% of the children had siblings, 10.2% lived with the child's grandparents, and 10.7% were poor households with annual incomes of less than three million yen. (Table 2) The most common maternal education level was professional school, some college, or dropped out of college. In 21% of the households, the mothers returned home from work after 18:00 or irregularly. When the mothers did not work or returned home from work before 18:00, the frequency of home cooking was high. The frequency of home cooking was low in households with a non-married parent and in those with low income. Children exposed to a low frequency of home cooking tended to have lower frequencies of vegetable and breakfast intake and snacked freely (Table 1).

Table 1. Characteristics of participating children (n = 4258).

	Total		Frequency of Home Cooking			x^2	p-Value
			High (n = 3695, 86.8%)	Medium (n = 461, 10.8%)	Low (n = 102, 2.4%)		
	n	%	%	%	%		
Child's status							
Sex							
Boy	2164	50.6	51.1	47.1	46.6	3.4	0.18
Girl	2114	49.4	48.9	52.9	53.4		
Body weight status (BMI for age z-score)							
Normal weight/ underweight (<1 SD)	3384	79.5	80.1	76.8	67.6	11.8	0.003
Overweight (≥1 SD and <2 SD)	624	14.7	14.3	15.8	20.6		
Obese (≥2 SD)	250	5.9	5.5	7.4	11.8		
Physical activity							
Never/rarely	501	11.7	10.8	16.3	25.2	38.8	<0.001
1–2 times/week	1600	37.4	37.5	38.1	32.0		
3–4 times/week	1189	27.8	28.6	22.2	23.3		
≥5 times/week	969	22.7	22.7	23.0	17.5		
Missing	19	0.4	0.4	0.4	1.9		
Eating behaviors							
Frequency of vegetable intake							
Twice/day	1748	40.9	43.6	22.8	24.3	259.6	<0.001
Once/day	2072	48.4	48.2	54.0	31.1		
<3 times/week	446	10.4	8.0	22.8	42.7		
Missing	12	0.3	0.2	0.4	1.9		
Frequency of breakfast intake							
Every day	3822	89.3	91.1	78.7	75.7	113.2	<0.001
Often	330	7.7	6.4	17.2	13.6		
Rarely/never	82	1.9	1.6	2.8	9.7		
Missing	44	1.0	1.0	1.3	1.0		
Snacking habits							
Not snacking	278	6.5	6.4	6.5	8.7	43.2	<0.001
Snacking at a set time (controlled)	1856	43.4	45.3	31.4	29.1		
Snacking freely	2104	49.2	47.4	61.1	61.2		
Missing	40	0.9	0.9	1.1	1.0		

BMI: body mass index; SD: standard deviation.

Table 2. Characteristics of participating households and caregivers (n = 4258).

	Total		Frequency of Home Cooking			χ^2	p-Value
			High (n = 3695, 86.8%)	Medium (n = 461, 10.8%)	Low (n = 102, 2.4%)		
	n	%	%	%	%		
Household status							
Marital status							
Married/common-law marriage	3098	72.8	74.6	61.8	53.9	84.7	<0.001
Single/divorced/widowed	352	8.3	7	15	24.5		
Other/missing	808	19	18.4	23.2	21.6		
Other children in the household							
No	836	19.5	18.1	27.7	35.0	39.9	<0.001
Yes	3442	80.5	81.9	72.3	65.0		
Living with the child's grandparents							
No	3840	89.8	89.4	92.7	90.3	4.7	0.10
Yes	438	10.2	10.6	7.3	9.7		
Household income (million yen)							
<3.00	457	10.7	9.7	15.7	22.3	35.7	<0.001
3.00–5.99	1275	29.8	29.7	30.1	33.0		
6.00–9.99	1411	33.0	34.0	27.3	20.4		
≥10.0	499	11.7	11.8	11.0	9.7		
Missing	636	14.9	14.7	15.9	14.6		
Caregiver's status							
Mother's age (years)							
<35	470	11.0	10.2	15.3	18.4	26.6	<0.001
35–44	2573	60.1	60.7	57.6	51.5		
≥45	1098	25.7	26.1	23.2	22.3		
Missing	137	3.2	3.0	3.9	7.8		
Mother's education							
Low	1098	25.7	25.0	29.0	34.0	33.2	<0.001
Middle	1381	32.3	33.2	26.9	24.3		
High	646	15.1	15.8	10.5	8.7		
Other/missing	1153	27.0	26.0	33.5	33.0		
Mother's employment and time of returning home from work							
Employed/returning home before 18:00	1949	45.8	47.1	37.3	35.3	74.0	<0.001
Employed/returning home 18:00–20:00	622	14.6	13.8	20.2	17.6		
Employed/returning home after 20:00	143	3.4	2.8	6.3	11.8		
Employed/returning home irregularly	136	3.2	3.1	4.3	2.9		
Not employed	928	21.8	22.4	18.0	15.7		
Missing	480	11.3	10.8	13.9	16.7		
Parents' BMI							
Mother's BMI							
Underweight (<18.5 kg/m^2)	487	11.4	11.5	11.2	7.8	13.4	0.10
Normal weight (18.5–24.9 kg/m^2)	2817	65.8	66.4	61.7	63.1		
Overweight (25.0–29.9 kg/m^2)	428	10.0	9.7	12.5	8.7		
Obese (≥30 kg/m^2)	89	2.1	2.0	2.2	2.9		
Missing	457	10.7	10.3	12.5	17.5		
Father's BMI							
Underweight (<18.5 kg/m^2)	63	1.5	1.3	2.4	3.9	35.3	<0.001
Normal weight (18.5–24.9 kg/m^2)	2286	53.4	54.7	45.8	41.7		
Overweight (25.0–29.9 kg/m^2)	909	21.2	21.2	21.9	21.4		
Obese (≥30 kg/m^2)	169	4.0	4.1	3.0	2.9		
Missing	851	19.9	18.7	26.9	30.1		

BMI: body mass index.

After adjusting for potential confounding factors, children who were exposed to a low frequency (≤3 days/week) of home cooking were 2.27 times (95% CI: 1.16–4.45) more likely to be obese, compared with children who were exposed to home cooking almost every day (Table 3, Model 1). After adjustment for children's obesity-related eating behaviors as potential mediators, this RRR was reduced and became statistically non-significant (RRR = 1.90; 95% CI: 0.95–3.82) (Table 3, Model 2).

Table 3. Adjusted relative risk ratios of overweight and obesity according to the frequency of home cooking among school children in Japan ($n = 4258$).

	Overweight		Obesity	
	RRR (95% CI)	p-Value	RRR (95% CI)	p-Value
Model 1				
Frequency of home cooking				
High (Almost every day)	ref		ref	
Medium (4–5 times/week)	1.07 (0.81–1.41)	0.60	1.33 (0.89–1.99)	0.20
Low (≤3 times/week)	1.46 (0.87–2.46)	0.16	**2.27 (1.16–4.45)**	**0.02**
Model 2				
Frequency of home cooking				
High (Almost every day)	ref		ref	
Medium (4–5 times/week)	1.09 (0.82–1.44)	0.52	1.31 (0.87–1.98)	0.24
Low (≤3 times/week)	1.46 (0.86–2.48)	0.17	1.90 (0.95–3.82)	0.08

RRR: relative risk ratio; CI: confidence interval; ref: reference. Boldface indicates statistical significance ($p < 0.05$). Model 1 adjusted for child's sex, physical activity, household status (parents' marital status, siblings, living with grandparents, and household income), and caregiver's status (mother's age, education, employment, and BMI and father's BMI). Model 2 adjusted for child's eating behaviors (frequency of vegetable and breakfast intake and snacking habits), as well as all variables in Model 1.

4. Discussion

To our knowledge, this is the first study to examine the association between the frequency of home cooking and obesity among children aged 9 to 10 years. We found that a low frequency (<3 days per week) of home cooking doubled the risk of obesity for children, even after controlling for child's sex, physical activity, household characteristics (parents' marital status, siblings, living with grandparents, and household income), and parents' individual characteristics (maternal age, education, and employment, and BMI for both parents). This association was attenuated after controlling for potential mediating factors (i.e., child's obesity-related eating behaviors), suggesting that children's eating behaviors partially mediated the association between home cooking and children's obesity.

Three possible factors may explain the link between less frequent home cooking and child obesity: (i) Caregivers' food choices; (ii) healthy eating practices; and (iii) children eating similar foods to those eaten by their caregivers. These potential mechanisms could play a role in determining whether the association between home cooking and obesity in children is direct (i.e., home cooking is directly associated with child obesity) or indirect (i.e., home cooking influences children's eating behavior, which, in turn, is associated with child obesity). We found that the association between home cooking and the child's obesity became non-significant after adjusting for the child's frequency of vegetable and breakfast intake and snacking habits in Model 2. This finding may be explained by the caregiver's food choice: Caregivers who usually cook at home may be more likely to select healthier foods, compared with caregivers who provide out-of-home food. Consistent with this idea, a previous study found that home cooking was associated with higher vegetable consumption among children [38]. Two other studies demonstrated that, among adults, a higher frequency of home-cooked meals was associated with indicators of a healthier diet, including fruit and vegetable intake, Mediterranean diet score, and Dietary Approaches to Stop Hypertension (DASH) score [20,39]. Compared with food prepared at home, food prepared outside of the home is higher in calories as well as total and saturated fats and has less fiber, calcium, and iron [10]. Alexy et al. argued that convenience foods have a high fat content and contain many flavorings and food additives [12]. Previous research has suggested that the presence of children in the household might be protective for family body weight: Sobal et al. reported an inverse association between the frequency of family meals and body weight for adults with children at home, but no such association was found among adults without children [40]. These results may indicate that cooking at home with children is beneficial for creating a healthy food environment.

A second explanation is that the frequency of home cooking may be a proxy for caregivers' healthy eating practices. For example, caregivers who cook at home infrequently might be less likely to prepare breakfast for their children, which is associated with an increased risk of children becoming obese [41,42]. This is supported by our finding that children who have a low frequency of home-cooked meals are more likely to skip breakfast and to eat snacks freely (Table 1). We also found that the significant association between home cooking and obesity disappeared after adjusting for children's eating behaviors, including skipping breakfast and snacking habits (Table 3, Model 2). In previous systematic reviews examining the association between parental practices and children's consumption of unhealthy foods (including snacks and sugar-sweetened beverages), restrictive parental guidance/rulemaking and control of the availability of unhealthy foods were the practices that were most positively associated with children's consumption of unhealthy foods [43,44]. Children who snack frequently have been shown to consume higher total energy and energy from sugars [45]. Therefore, a low frequency of home cooking may be a proxy for less effective parental practice in terms of children eating healthy foods, which could explain the association with obesity in children.

A third potential explanation for this association is that home cooking may lead to a healthy diet because children eat foods similar to those consumed by their parents. When children eat home-cooked meals, they tend to eat the same foods as their parents. In contrast, when children eat outside the home or consume prepared meals, they select what they want and thus eat different foods from those eaten by their parents. Previous studies have reported that children who eat similar foods to those eaten by their parents are more likely to have healthy diets [38,46], suggesting that children may miss out on specific nutrients or food types, such as vegetables, if they are served a separate "child meal". Home cooking may also create a supportive and positive food environment for children. Creating a positive atmosphere at mealtime supports children's opportunities to try new foods and to develop their own food preferences [22].

Several limitations of this study should be mentioned. First, we assessed the frequency of cooking using a simple questionnaire based on previous studies, but the validity and reliability of the questionnaire were not examined here or in these existing studies. However, we confirmed the plausibility of the results by testing the association of the frequency of home cooking with the child's vegetable intake and breakfast skipping. Second, we defined home cooking as a basic and simple practice, such as frying an egg, and we did not assess the quality of the meals being prepared. Therefore, caregivers who cook low-quality meals (e.g., meals with little variety or unhealthy meals) may be included in the high frequency of home cooking category. This may have led to an underestimate of the association between home cooking and children's obesity. However, in large-scale surveys, it is difficult to evaluate the quality of meals because a great deal of time would be required for this assessment. Additionally, our study focused on parents engaging in the behavior of preparing meals for their children rather than on the quality of the meals they prepared. Third, we did not account for caregivers' food knowledge, which is particularly important for preventing obesity in children; this topic warrants further research. Fourth, because our sample of school children was from only one city, the generalizability of the results may be low. Furthermore, the caregivers in the present study were well educated, and most of the respondents were mothers. Low parental socioeconomic status was linked to children's obesity, and we also found that low maternal educational attainment was significantly associated with children's obesity (data not shown); this may have led to an underestimate of the association between home cooking and children's obesity. Finally, because this was a cross-sectional study, we were unable to assess causality. Longitudinal studies or randomized controlled trials are needed in the future to clarify the effectiveness of home cooking in preventing obesity in children. Despite these limitations, we were able to demonstrate a significant association between a low frequency of home cooking and children's obesity, controlling for potential confounding factors, and our findings may be useful for identifying potential targets for interventions aimed at improving children's body weight management.

5. Conclusions

Our study has provided novel findings regarding the association between home cooking and children's body weight status. Home cooking presents an opportunity for parents to offer a model of healthy eating to their children and to pass on food traditions from their own culture. When children participate in meal preparation, they tend to eat healthy diets [47]. Future studies are needed to clarify the causal relationship and mechanisms through which home cooking influences children. Although the present study focused on body weight, future studies should also examine other physical, psychological, and social outcomes that may be associated with home cooking for children.

Author Contributions: Conceptualization, Y.T. and T.F.; Data Curation, Y.T. and T.F.; Methodology, Y.T.; Formal Analysis, Y.T.; Investigation, Y.T., T.F., S.D., and A.I.; Writing—Original Draft Preparation, Y.T.; Writing—Review and Editing, T.F.; Supervision, T.F., S.D., and A.I.; Project Administration, Y.T.; Funding Acquisition, Y.T. and T.F.

Funding: This research was funded by Grants-in-Aid for Scientific Research from the Japan Society for the Promotion of Science (JSPS KAKENHI Grant Numbers 16H03276 and 19K14029).

Acknowledgments: We are particularly grateful to the staff members and the central office of Adachi City Hall for conducting the survey. We would also like to thank everyone who participated in the surveys. We would especially like to thank M.Y.K., S.A., and Y.B. from Adachi City Hall, who contributed significantly to the completion of this study.

Conflicts of Interest: The authors declare no conflict of interest.

References

1. Ng, M.; Fleming, T.; Robinson, M.; Thomson, B.; Graetz, N.; Margono, C.; Mullany, E.C.; Biryukov, S.; Abbafati, C.; Abera, S.F.; et al. Global, regional, and national prevalence of overweight and obesity in children and adults during 1980–2013: A systematic analysis for the Global Burden of Disease Study 2013. *Lancet* **2014**, *384*, 766–781. [CrossRef]
2. Organisation for Economic Co-operation and Development. *Overweight and Obesity among Children, in Health at a Glance 2017: OECD Indicators*; OECD Publishing: Paris, France, 2017.
3. Simmonds, M.; Llewellyn, A.; Owen, C.G.; Woolacott, N. Predicting adult obesity from childhood obesity: A systematic review and meta-analysis. *Obes. Rev.* **2016**, *17*, 95–107. [CrossRef] [PubMed]
4. Llewellyn, A.; Simmonds, M.; Owen, C.G.; Woolacott, N. Childhood obesity as a predictor of morbidity in adulthood: A systematic review and meta-analysis. *Obes. Rev.* **2016**, *17*, 56–67. [CrossRef] [PubMed]
5. Lichtenstein, A.H.; Ludwig, D.S. Bring back home economics education. *JAMA* **2010**, *303*, 1857–1858. [CrossRef] [PubMed]
6. Smith, L.P.; Ng, S.W.; Popkin, B.M. Trends in US home food preparation and consumption: Analysis of national nutrition surveys and time use studies from 1965–1966 to 2007–2008. *Nutr. J.* **2013**, *12*, 45. [CrossRef] [PubMed]
7. Moser, A. Food preparation patterns in German family households. An econometric approach with time budget data. *Appetite* **2010**, *55*, 99–107. [CrossRef] [PubMed]
8. Nielsen, S.J.; Siega-Riz, A.M.; Popkin, B.M. Trends in food locations and sources among adolescents and young adults. *Prev. Med.* **2002**, *35*, 107–113. [CrossRef]
9. Statistics Bureau, Ministry of Internal Affairs and Communications. Family Income and Expenditure Survey FY2015. 2016. Available online: http://www.stat.go.jp/data/kakei/longtime/ (accessed on 13 August 2019).
10. Guthrie, J.F.; Lin, B.H.; Frazao, E. Role of food prepared away from home in the American diet, 1977–1978 versus 1994–1996: Changes and consequences. *J. Nutr. Educ. Behav.* **2002**, *34*, 140–150. [CrossRef]
11. Scourboutakos, M.J.; Semnani-Azad, Z.; L'Abbe, M.R. Restaurant meals: Almost a full day's worth of calories, fats, and sodium. *JAMA Intern. Med.* **2013**, *173*, 1373–1374. [CrossRef]
12. Alexy, U.; Sichert-Hellert, W.; Rode, T.; Kersting, M. Convenience food in the diet of children and adolescents: Consumption and composition. *Br. J. Nutr.* **2008**, *99*, 345–351. [CrossRef]
13. Lachat, C.; Nago, E.; Verstraeten, R.; Roberfroid, D.; Van Camp, J.; Kolsteren, P. Eating out of home and its association with dietary intake: A systematic review of the evidence. *Obes. Rev. Off. J. Int. Assoc. Study Obes.* **2012**, *13*, 329–346. [CrossRef] [PubMed]

14. Poti, J.M.; Popkin, B.M. Trends in energy intake among US children by eating location and food source, 1977–2006. *J. Am. Diet. Assoc.* **2011**, *111*, 1156–1164. [CrossRef] [PubMed]
15. Powell, L.M.; Nguyen, B.T. Fast-food and full-service restaurant consumption among children and adolescents: Effect on energy, beverage, and nutrient intake. *JAMA Pediatr.* **2013**, *167*, 14–20. [CrossRef] [PubMed]
16. Niemeier, H.M.; Raynor, H.A.; Lloyd-Richardson, E.E.; Rogers, M.L.; Wing, R.R. Fast food consumption and breakfast skipping: Predictors of weight gain from adolescence to adulthood in a nationally representative sample. *J. Adolesc. Health Off. Publ. Soc. Adolesc. Med.* **2006**, *39*, 842–849. [CrossRef]
17. Thompson, O.M.; Ballew, C.; Resnicow, K.; Must, A.; Bandini, L.G.; Cyr, H.; Dietz, W.H. Food purchased away from home as a predictor of change in BMI z-score among girls. *Int. J. Obes. Relat. Metab. Disord. J. Int. Assoc. Study Obes.* **2004**, *28*, 282–289. [CrossRef]
18. Kant, A.K.; Whitley, M.I.; Graubard, B.I. Away from home meals: Associations with biomarkers of chronic disease and dietary intake in American adults, NHANES 2005–2010. *Int. J. Obes.* **2015**, *39*, 820–827. [CrossRef]
19. Zick, C.D.; Stevens, R.B.; Bryant, W.K. Time use choices and healthy body weight: A multivariate analysis of data from the American Time Use Survey. *Int. J. Behav. Nutr. Phys. Act.* **2011**, *8*, 84. [CrossRef]
20. Mills, S.; Brown, H.; Wrieden, W.; White, M.; Adams, J. Frequency of eating home cooked meals and potential benefits for diet and health: Cross-sectional analysis of a population-based cohort study. *Int. J. Behav. Nutr. Phys. Act.* **2017**, *14*, 109. [CrossRef]
21. Neumark-Sztainer, D.; MacLehose, R.; Loth, K.; Fulkerson, J.A.; Eisenberg, M.E.; Berge, J. What's for dinner? Types of food served at family dinner differ across parent and family characteristics. *Pub. Health Nutr.* **2014**, *17*, 145–155. [CrossRef]
22. Birch, L.L.; Ventura, A.K. Preventing childhood obesity: What works? *Int. J. Obes.* **2009**, *33*, S74–S81. [CrossRef]
23. Benton, D. Role of parents in the determination of the food preferences of children and the development of obesity. *Int. J. Obes. Relat. Metab. Disord. J. Int. Assoc. Study Obes.* **2004**, *28*, 858–869. [CrossRef] [PubMed]
24. Campbell, K.J.; Crawford, D.A.; Ball, K. Family food environment and dietary behaviors likely to promote fatness in 5-6 year-old children. *Int. J. Obes.* **2006**, *30*, 1272–1280. [CrossRef] [PubMed]
25. Pearson, N.; Biddle, S.J.; Gorely, T. Family correlates of fruit and vegetable consumption in children and adolescents: A systematic review. *Pub. Health Nutr.* **2009**, *12*, 267–283. [CrossRef] [PubMed]
26. Berge, J.M.; Rowley, S.; Trofholz, A.; Hanson, C.; Rueter, M.; MacLehose, R.F.; Neumark-Sztainer, D. Childhood obesity and interpersonal dynamics during family meals. *Pediatrics* **2014**, *134*, 923–932. [CrossRef] [PubMed]
27. Mikkila, V.; Rasanen, L.; Raitakari, O.T.; Pietinen, P.; Viikari, J. Consistent dietary patterns identified from childhood to adulthood: The cardiovascular risk in Young Finns Study. *Br. J. Nutr.* **2005**, *93*, 923–931. [CrossRef] [PubMed]
28. Movassagh, E.Z.; Baxter-Jones, A.D.G.; Kontulainen, S.; Whiting, S.J.; Vatanparast, H. Tracking Dietary Patterns over 20 Years from Childhood through Adolescence into Young Adulthood: The Saskatchewan Pediatric Bone Mineral Accrual Study. *Nutrients* **2017**, *9*, 990. [CrossRef] [PubMed]
29. Lien, N.; Lytle, L.A.; Klepp, K.I. Stability in consumption of fruit, vegetables, and sugary foods in a cohort from age 14 to age 21. *Prev. Med.* **2001**, *33*, 217–226. [CrossRef]
30. Doi, S.; Fujiwara, T.; Ochi, M.; Isumi, A.; Kato, T. Association of sleep habits with behavior problems and resilience of 6- to 7-year-old children: Results from the A-CHILD study. *Sleep Med.* **2018**, *45*, 62–68. [CrossRef]
31. Tani, Y.; Fujiwara, T.; Ochi, M.; Isumi, A.; Kato, T. Does Eating Vegetables at Start of Meal Prevent Childhood Overweight in Japan? A-CHILD Study. *Front. Pediatr.* **2018**, *6*, 134. [CrossRef]
32. Morita, A.; Ochi, M.; Isumi, A.; Fujiwara, T. Association between grandparent coresidence and weight change among first-grade Japanese children. *Pediatr. Obes.* **2019**, *14*, e12524. [CrossRef]
33. Education and Science in Ministry of Sports and Youth Bureau of School Health Education. *Children's Health Diagnostic Manual*, Revised ed.; Japanese Society of School Health: Tokyo, Japan, 2006. (In Japanese)
34. de Onis, M.; Onyango, A.W.; Borghi, E.; Siyam, A.; Nishida, C.; Siekmann, J. Development of a WHO growth reference for school-aged children and adolescents. *Bull. World Health Organ.* **2007**, *85*, 660–667. [CrossRef] [PubMed]
35. Wolfson, J.A.; Bleich, S.N. Is cooking at home associated with better diet quality or weight-loss intention? *Pub. Health Nutr.* **2015**, *18*, 1397–1406. [CrossRef] [PubMed]

36. Virudachalam, S.; Long, J.A.; Harhay, M.O.; Polsky, D.E.; Feudtner, C. Prevalence and patterns of cooking dinner at home in the USA: National Health and Nutrition Examination Survey (NHANES) 2007–2008. *Pub. Health Nutr.* **2014**, *17*, 1022–1030. [CrossRef] [PubMed]
37. World Health Organization. *Obesity: Preventing and Managing the Global Epidemic*; WHO: Geneva, Switzerland, 2000.
38. Sweetman, C.; McGowan, L.; Croker, H.; Cooke, L. Characteristics of family mealtimes affecting children's vegetable consumption and liking. *J. Am. Diet. Assoc.* **2011**, *111*, 269–273. [CrossRef]
39. Crawford, D.; Ball, K.; Mishra, G.; Salmon, J.; Timperio, A. Which food-related behaviours are associated with healthier intakes of fruits and vegetables among women? *Pub. Health Nutr.* **2007**, *10*, 256–265. [CrossRef]
40. Sobal, J.; Hanson, K. Family meals and body weight in US adults. *Public Health Nutr.* **2011**, *14*, 1555–1562. [CrossRef]
41. Szajewska, H.; Ruszczynski, M. Systematic review demonstrating that breakfast consumption influences body weight outcomes in children and adolescents in Europe. *Crit. Rev. Food Sci. Nutr.* **2010**, *50*, 113–119. [CrossRef]
42. Pereira, M.A.; Erickson, E.; McKee, P.; Schrankler, K.; Raatz, S.K.; Lytle, L.A.; Pellegrini, A.D. Breakfast frequency and quality may affect glycemia and appetite in adults and children. *J. Nutr.* **2011**, *141*, 163–168. [CrossRef]
43. Blaine, R.E.; Kachurak, A.; Davison, K.K.; Klabunde, R.; Fisher, J.O. Food parenting and child snacking: A systematic review. *Int. J. Behav. Nutr. Phys. Act.* **2017**, *14*, 146. [CrossRef]
44. Yee, A.Z.; Lwin, M.O.; Ho, S.S. The influence of parental practices on child promotive and preventive food consumption behaviors: A systematic review and meta-analysis. *Int. J. Behav. Nutr. Phys. Act.* **2017**, *14*, 47. [CrossRef]
45. Larson, N.; Story, M. A review of snacking patterns among children and adolescents: What are the implications of snacking for weight status? *Child. Obes.* **2013**, *9*, 104–115. [CrossRef] [PubMed]
46. Skafida, V. The family meal panacea: Exploring how different aspects of family meal occurrence, meal habits and meal enjoyment relate to young children's diets. *Sociol. Health Illn.* **2013**, *35*, 906–923. [CrossRef] [PubMed]
47. Chu, Y.L.; Storey, K.E.; Veugelers, P.J. Involvement in meal preparation at home is associated with better diet quality among Canadian children. *J. Nutr. Educ. Behav.* **2014**, *46*, 304–308. [CrossRef] [PubMed]

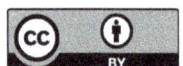

© 2019 by the authors. Licensee MDPI, Basel, Switzerland. This article is an open access article distributed under the terms and conditions of the Creative Commons Attribution (CC BY) license (http://creativecommons.org/licenses/by/4.0/).

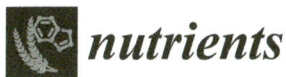

Article
Modern Transference of Domestic Cooking Skills

Fiona Lavelle [1], Tony Benson [1], Lynsey Hollywood [2], Dawn Surgenor [2], Amanda McCloat [3], Elaine Mooney [3], Martin Caraher [4] and Moira Dean [1,*]

[1] Institute for Global Food Security, School of Biological Sciences, Queen's University Belfast, Belfast BT9 5DL, UK; flavelle01@qub.ac.uk (F.L.); t.benson@qub.ac.uk (T.B.)
[2] Department of Hospitality and Tourism Management, Ulster Business School, Ulster University, Ulster BT52 1SA, UK; l.hollywood@ulster.ac.uk (L.H.); d.surgenor@ulster.ac.uk (D.S.)
[3] Department of Home Economics, St. Angela's College, F91 C634 Sligo, Ireland; amccloat@stangelas.nuigalway.ie (A.M.); emooney@stangelas.nuigalway.ie (E.M.)
[4] Centre for Food Policy, Department of Sociology, School of Arts and Social Sciences, City University London, London EC1R 0JD, UK; M.caraher@city.ac.uk
* Correspondence: moira.dean@qub.ac.uk; Tel.: +44-(0)28-9097-6561

Received: 13 March 2019; Accepted: 15 April 2019; Published: 18 April 2019

Abstract: As the primary source of learning cooking skills; it is vital to understand what mothers think about the transference of cooking skills to their children. The current analysis aimed to highlight mothers' perceptions of children's involvement and cooking practices within the home setting. Sixteen focus group discussions were conducted on the island of Ireland (Republic of Ireland and Northern Ireland [UK]) with 141 mothers aged 20–39 years old. All focus groups were transcribed verbatim and an inductive thematic analysis using NVivo software was undertaken. Seven themes emerged from the dataset; (1) "How we learned to cook"; (2) "Who's the boss"; (3) "Children in the way"; (4) "Keep kids out"; (5) "Involvement means eating"; (6) "Intentions versus reality"; and (7) "Kids' 'interest' in cooking". These themes illustrate a lack of cooking skill transference in relation to everyday meal preparation in modern times. The culture of children in the kitchen has vastly changed; and opportunities for children to learn basic skills are currently limited. Further research is required to confirm the findings that emerged from this analysis.

Keywords: cooking; learning; mothers; children; adolescents; obesity; qualitative; environmental influences

1. Introduction

The possession and application of cooking skills can have numerous health benefits including a greater diet quality, weight control, and even longevity of life [1–4]. In light of this, there has been a resurgence in cooking skills education and a push for the re-skilling of the general population to reinvigorate meal preparation in the home environment [5–7]. Cooking skills interventions are also being increasingly implemented as childhood obesity prevention strategies or as essential components in multidisciplinary prevention approaches [8–10] as recommended by the World Health Organization [11]. These interventions are utilized as a means of enabling children and adolescents to prepare healthy meals as alternatives to the use of ready meals and the consumption of food outside the home [2,4,11,12]. The need for children and adolescents to learn these cooking skills has been highlighted as an important life skill [11]. Research suggests that adolescents who are involved in home meal preparation present with a higher diet quality than their non-food preparing counterparts [13]. In addition, learning cooking skills at younger ages has also been linked to skill maintenance through to adulthood, cooking confidence and a better diet quality [14].

Despite understanding the importance of cooking skills development at a young age, the optimal source for learning these skills has been debated. While a substantial emphasis has been placed on teachers through the education system [14–17], other sources are also important. The mother has been consistently identified as the primary source for learning cooking skills [14,18]. In addition, mothers have been identified as key influencers of children's weight status [19–21] and learning from the mother is associated with greater cooking confidence and less consumption of unhealthy foods, emphasizing the valuable role of the mother as a primary source of learning [14]. However, due to the increasing demand of current modern lifestyles and external pressures, some research suggests that mothers may no longer possess the necessary skills or time to prepare a healthy diet [22] and, therefore, may no longer be able to pass on cooking skills to their children. Anecdotally, it has been suggested that there is a lack of skill transference occurring from mothers to children, however, this phenomenon has not been explored qualitatively in order to understand why this may be happening. Thus, the role of the mother as a current source of learning must be examined.

Given their key role as influencers on children's weight status and the primary source for learning skills that enable the preparation of a healthy diet, it is vital to understand what mothers think about the importance of cooking skills development in their children and how this can be best modeled in the home setting to promote confidence and learning and the passing on of these skills to their children. A greater understanding of mothers' attitudes, behaviors and feelings could help to inform strategies to promote and encourage the learning of cooking skills. Therefore, this analysis aimed to highlight mothers' perceptions of children's involvement and cooking practices within the home setting.

2. Materials and Methods

2.1. Focus Group Recruitment

The participants were recruited to partake in a cooking from "scratch" experiment [23], with an immediate follow up focus group, in a room adjacent to the kitchens, to discuss their perceptions of the cooking experiment and experiences of cooking in general. They were recruited by Social Market Research (a market research company based in the United Kingdom and Republic of Ireland (ROI)). Overall, 160 mothers (20–39 years old), both employed and unemployed, who were responsible for the main meal preparation at least 3 times per week, and who had at least one child (under the age of 16 years) currently living in their household, with a range of children's ages, were recruited, with the final sample consisting of 141 (due to non-attendance). Participants could also not have any strict dietary requirements (such as lactose intolerant or vegetarian, for the purposes of partaking in the cooking experiment). Sixteen focus groups were conducted, with eight held in Sligo, ROI and eight held in Coleraine, Northern Ireland (NI). Each group had six to ten participants. Participants were recruited from a 30-mile radius of both sites and included both urban and rural participants. Results are treated as one island of Ireland sample. Sociodemographic and food-related characteristics were collected before the beginning of the cooking experiment and focus groups.

2.2. Focus Group Procedures

The focus groups were conducted in line with the principles outlined in Kreuger and Casey [24]. The discussions were facilitated by an experienced moderator (DS) and an assistant moderator (FL). The focus groups followed a guided open-ended questioning route relating to experiences of the cooking experiment and cooking habits and behaviors in general, an outline of the topic guide can be seen in Table 1. Probing questions relating to children's involvement in cooking were used for all mentions of children. The focus group topic guide was developed from a literature review [25] and earlier individual interviews conducted on the island of Ireland relating to cooking behaviors and habits [26]. Additionally, the guide was piloted with two focus groups, one group who had not conducted the cooking experiment (for general flow of the question route and the wording of the questions) and one group after piloting of the cooking experiment. The moderator emphasized the importance of all participants contributing to the discussion, and that all opinions and points were equally valid. The assistant moderator was present to take notes and facilitate the direction and flow of the discussion. All participants were assured of their confidentiality and all discussions were audio recorded. Each focus group discussion lasted between 50 and 65 min. Upon completion of the focus group, each participant was thanked and given an honorarium (£50/€50) and a cookbook to compensate for their time (including the cooking experiment) and travel.

Table 1. Outline of the focus group topic guide.

Topic	Description/Question
Introduction	• Facilitator introduction • Boundaries of the focus group and contracting including recording consent
Confidence Levels	• What was your perceived confidence ability in cooking lasagne from scratch prior to the task? • Has this confidence changed? How?
Barriers/facilitators to cooking from scratch	• How challenging did you find the task? What were the most/least challenging aspects? • What would encourage/discourage you to cook using fresh ingredients at home? • What additional barriers do you consider prevent you from cooking in the home environment?
Identification of skills used	• What skills can you identify in cooking lasagne? • Do you consider these skills achievable in your home? • Which skills did you consider most challenging? • Would you practise these to enable you to cook this or a similar dish at home?
Use of Technology	• Do you have home access to the internet? • Do you use the internet to assist with learning practical skills? • Can you think of an example? • Would you consider using technology to assist with home cooking? • What part do you consider technology can play in promoting cooking from scratch in your own homes?
Transferability of skills/learning to the home setting	• Considering the skills you identified earlier—can you think of other meals where you might incorporate skills developed today, or different ingredients, for example, you may like to change or incorporate ingredients to make the dish healthier or more preferable for the family's taste? • What would you do differently next time?
Summary and ending	• Do you have anything else you would like to add or feel we have missed? • Thank you and close

2.3. Institutional Review Board

The study was conducted in line with the guidelines laid down in the declaration of Helsinki. All participants provided written and verbal consent and were aware that they could withdraw from the research study at any point. The study was approved by the Research Ethics Committee within The School of Biological Sciences at Queen's University Belfast.

2.4. Analysis of Focus Group Transcripts

Focus group discussions were professionally, independently transcribed verbatim and checked for accuracy by the moderator and then imported into Nvivo 11 (QSR International Pty Ltd, Doncaster,

Victoria, Australia) for analysis. An inductive thematic analysis in line with Braun and Clarke [27,28] was undertaken. The dataset used in this analysis involved all instances where participants discussed children in the kitchen environment including discussion of when they were children.

All transcripts were read and re-read by two of the authors in order to achieve data immersion. Subsequently, all data relating to "children" were coded for this analysis. The next phases involved grouping codes together to form potential themes, inspecting these themes for overlap and where necessary refining the themes. This refinement ensured that there were "clear and identifiable distinctions" between the themes and that there was no overlap [27].

An inter-rater process was used throughout the entirety of the analysis. Initially, two researchers (FL, a sport and health scientist, and TB, a health psychologist) independently coded 3 randomly selected transcripts (18% of the transcripts). The coders had an initial agreement of 90% on the coding of the transcripts. The codes were discussed to verify their applicability to the data, and agreement was reached on all codes upon discussion. Following this, FL coded the remaining transcripts and TB coded a further 5 transcripts, leading to 97% coding agreement across these 8 transcripts. Then, FL grouped codes to form potential themes. The themes were inspected for overlap and consensus was reached on all themes through discussion (TB and MD, a consumer food choice psychologist). Illustrative quotes were then extracted from the data to demonstrate typical views within each theme. Data saturation was reached within this topic area as no new codes appeared after the first ten transcripts. Sociodemographic data was summarized using SPSS v22 (IBM Corporation, Armonk, NY, USA, 2013).

3. Results

3.1. Participant Characteristics

The characteristics of the 141 participants can be seen in Table 2. Mean age was 30.45 years (SD 5.70).

Table 2. Demographic and Sociodemographic Characteristics of Focus Group Participants ($N = 141$).

Characteristic	N = 141	
	N	%
Country of Residence		
Northern Ireland (NI)	77	54.6
Republic of Ireland (ROI)	64	45.4
Highest Level of Education		
None/Primary School	4	2.8
Junior cert/GCSE *	17	12.1
Leaving cert/A level **	18	12.8
Additional training	67	47.5
Undergraduate University Degree	24	17.0
Postgraduate University Degree	9	6.4
Number of Children in household under 16		
1	69	48.9
2	43	30.5
3	21	14.9
4+	6	4.2

Table 2. *Cont.*

Characteristic	N = 141	
	N	%
Perceptions of their weight status		
Very underweight	1	0.7
Slightly underweight	5	3.5
About the right weight	51	36.2
Slightly overweight	57	40.4
Very overweight	26	18.4
Follow a special diet		
No	99	70.2
Yes—self determined	39	27.7
Yes—prescribed by medical professional	3	2.1
Work or has worked in the "food or hospitality industry" preparing food		
Yes	50	35.5
No	91	64.5

* Junior Cert (ROI)/GCSE (NI)—Age 15/16 years, exams taken midway through secondary school. ** Leaving Cert (ROI)/A level—Age 17/18 years, final exams taken in secondary school.

Mothers with a wide range of food related behaviors and levels of cooking and food skills confidence were recruited, as shown in Table 3.

Table 3. Food Related Characteristics of Participants (*N* = 141).

Food Related Variables	Number	%
	141	100
Typical ingredients used in meal preparation		
Mostly pre-prepared ingredients and assemble	5	3.5
Mostly pre-prepared ingredients, some fresh, basic or raw ingredients	68	48.2
Mostly fresh, basic or raw ingredients, some pre-prepared ingredients	59	41.8
Only fresh, basic or raw ingredients	9	6.4
Consumption of meals prepared outside the home (e.g. restaurant takeaway food, Chinese, fish and chips, etc.)		
Everyday	6	4.3
4–6 times per week	6	4.3
2–3 times per week	7	5.0
Once per week	62	44.0
Less than once per week	54	38.3
Never	6	4.3
*Breakfast (*N* = 138)		
Never	8	5.8
Weekdays	16	11.6
Weekends	18	13.0
Both	96	69.6

Table 3. Cont.

Food Related Variables	Number		%	
	141		100	
Lunch (N = 137)				
Never	4		2.9	
Weekdays	25		18.2	
Weekends	9		6.6	
Both	99		72.3	
Dinner (N = 136)				
†Never	1		0.7	
Weekdays	13		9.6	
Weekends	3		2.2	
Both	119		87.5	
	Minimum	Maximum	Mean	SD
‡Cooking Skills Confidence (N = 139)	30	97	65.74	14.66
Food Skills Confidence (N = 140)	14	124	84.15	20.41
Cooking Identity (N = 138)	7	30	16.67	3.82
Food Neophilia (N = 140)	3	14	6.33	2.28

* Participants were asked "Do you prepare/cook Breakfast/Lunch/Dinner during weekdays, weekends or both? (including preparing cold dishes like salads, or reheating ready-made foods)" † This participant was responsible for the meal preparation of their household, however, this consisted of collecting the takeaway. ‡ Cooking and food skills confidence were measured using a paper pen version of the validated measure in Lavelle et al. [29].

3.2. Overview of Themes

Through thematic analysis of the focus group transcripts, seven themes were constructed: (1) "How we learned to cook"; (2) "Who's the boss?"; (3) "Children in the way"; (4) "Keep kids out"; (5) "Involvement means eating"; (6) "Intentions versus reality"; and (7) "Kids' interest".

The culture of children being present in the kitchen appeared to revolve around the mother–child dynamic, with an underlying shift in this dynamic, from mothers being in control in previous generations to currently the child dictating meal choice. This shift appeared in two themes, "How we learned to cook" and "Who's the boss?", as described below.

(1) **How we learned to cook.** Here, participants discussed how they were present in the kitchen from a young age and how they learnt to cook from their mothers.

"When I was younger mum always had us in the kitchen and teaching us how to cook and that." ROI FG2

The majority of participants claimed that they had to help with the dinner. There was no choice and it was what was expected of them and part of their family dynamics.

"When we were younger my mum was out working an awful lot and I was minding the younger ones ... I just remember cooking at a really young age..."

"Oh yeah I'd have done that stand on the chair [because] you couldn't reach." ROI FG6

Some of the mothers noted that in some instances they had to assume the role as meal preparer in its entirety for their families. This is a sharp contrast to current practices where only two mothers of the 141 involved in the focus groups mentioned their older children helping with every day meal preparation. Thus, the culture of children helping in the kitchen and "doing jobs" in the kitchen is a rarity.

(2) **Who's the boss?** This theme highlights how the power of food choice has shifted to the child. This shift has put extra pressure and stress on the mother and has changed the 'cooking a meal' experience as well as what preparing a meal actually entails. Mothers claim that children dictate

what type of food is prepared by being fussy eaters or liking different textures or by how food is eaten (for example with their hands).

"We all have different dinners in our house. So, because my wee (small/young) boy is like three so he's like 'I don't like that, I don't like that' and my wee girl she would rather sit with like salads, like she just loves all that so it's really difficult in my house ... .My wee girl hates mince so like, you know your spag bol (spaghetti Bolognese) that you would love really quick or like cottage pie or anything like that she's 'no' so I know she's not going to eat it ... There's always one with something different in my house." NI FG5

In every focus group, it was mentioned that the participants cook to cater to their children's wants and needs, *"What the wee ones [the children] want to eat"* (NI, FG 8). Sometimes they are unaware of this level of control, and believe that they are making "compromises", although still preparing what the child wants.

"[There] might be something that you want to cook but you know they're not going to eat it so you just have [to] compromise and go with what you know is going to be eaten as well." ROI FG6

If mothers do not want to eat what their children are eating, they make multiple dinners to avoid arguments, tantrums or revolt. To cope with the demand of having to make multiple dishes, some participants resorted to the use of convenience products instead of deciding what is to be eaten.

From these added stresses and pressures in the kitchen, two negative themes arose, "Children in the way" and "Keep kids out" with over three quarters of the focus groups having discussed children being in the way of their cooking and not wanting the children in the kitchen when they are cooking.

(3) **Children in the way.** This strongly presented theme revolves around the impact of having children present in the kitchen on the mother's current cooking practices. It highlights how children, *"little tigers"*, are in the way when mothers are trying to prepare a meal, hanging on to the mothers or shouting and pulling at them.

"I have 2 kids running about pulling me grabbing me mummy, mummy, mummy ... then babies looking fed and it's just madness." NI FG2

Some of the mothers mentioned that they would like a *"babysitter"* to occupy the children so that the participants were able to cook a meal. When children have disabilities requiring extra time or can have problems with food, this results in less time for the mother to cook. When faced with these situations, mothers tend to cope by cooking quickly, and by taking shortcuts, such as using convenience products, or by cooking food when the children are out of the way in school or in another room playing.

"Like I have 5 kids fluttering around and you just don't have time to be standing with a flipping wooden spoon ... " ROI FG1

(4) Keep kids out. This theme revolves around what stops mothers having their kids in the kitchen and involving them in the cooking process. The participants stated that they are too busy to deal with the mess children create in the kitchen as at times children can leave the kitchen looking like a *"bomb site"*.

"See because they'll just create such a mess." NI FG8

Along with the potential mess of letting the children in the kitchen, participants also noted concerns over the safety of having children in the kitchen.

"Do you not be worried about them using a baker [oven] and things at that age?"

"Well I don't let my 4 year old use the cooker."

"Oh no obviously."

"The 13 year old she says yeah they have to use the cooker in school and stuff so."

"Oh I see now aye it just sounds really young still doesn't it though." NI FG4

While not as prevalent, there were also positive themes relating to the transference of skills from the mother to the child—"Involvement means eating" and "Intentions versus reality". The themes were mentioned multiple times within a smaller number of focus group discussions. While some transference of skills to the child occurring may happen as a result of these themes, the skill level being transferred may not occur frequently, not happen in all situations, and the type of skills transferred may not be optimal for everyday living.

(5) Involvement means eating. The "involvement means eating and trying foods" theme highlights the participants' perceptions about their children eating different types of food or food they have previously refused when they are involved in the preparation of the food.

"My wee girl doesn't like vegetables or anything I think 2 or 3 weeks ago I got her to help me make lasagne, she loves pasta. I got her to help me make it and oh my god there was a clear plate so she loved it, she doesn't like peas or carrots or courgettes (zucchinis) or onions or anything like that everything in and then she ate it all, no questions asked." NI FG5

Some of the participants felt that children experiencing the food ingredients in the kitchen rather than it being presented to them as a complete dish to eat removes the fear of the unknown.

"Whereas if she was actually helping to make (dinner) ... She'll eat anything if she kind of knows what it is but whenever they don't seem to know what it is they are just a bit wary of it." NI FG3

(6) **Intentions versus reality.** This theme addresses the concept of cooking with children. Mothers in general expressed a desire for their children to be able to cook to help them in their future.

"Yeah and you want them to be able to know how to cook, so that when they hit 18 they wouldn't just live on little packets of you know pasta or takeaway, that they have some idea, they can come in they can make a Spaghetti Bolognese or they can do the basics." ROI FG1

However, when mothers discuss instances of when they cook with their children they mention baking, which is seen as a fun activity or random dishes that children pick to cook rather than everyday dishes that form their diet.

"My little one loves to bake and stir and she'll make pizza for her friends, you know, she loves doing stuff like that and all sorts of nonsense." NI FG8

Participants also referred to the occasional instances where they had the children make the meal with them, to try and encourage them to eat the food, as discussed in the previous theme. In addition, the participants mentioned eating food they do not like that children have prepared to encourage the children to cook.

In the final theme, participants discussed their child's interest or stated that they were not interested in cooking. It was unclear whether children showed an interest in cooking due to greater cooking exposure or whether children were naturally interested. This theme is detailed below.

(7) **Kids' "interest" in cooking.** This theme was present in eight of the 16 focus groups, however, not all instances were positive, as some reported that their children had no interest in cooking.

"(Cooking) bores my 10 year old, (they're) not interested." NI FG4

Some mothers commented on their children's interest in cooking and that they wanted to cook and learn to cook at home or in home economics.

"Well he's doing home economics and all in school and he loves to cook yeah." ROI FG5

Some participants proposed that the child's interest in cooking arises as a way of gaining a sense of independence instead of just having their *'dinner set down in front of them'* and that they gained a sense of pride and achievement.

4. Discussion

This analysis investigated the phenomenon of transgenerational cooking skills transference in modern times. The findings indicate that the culture of children being in the kitchen has vastly changed, and opportunities for children to learn basic and fundamental food related skills are not present in the current climate. Recently, home economics teachers in Australia highlighted how children "don't have a clue" about food skills when they enter schools due to parents' time constraints and perhaps due to parents' limited skills [30]. They stressed the importance of adolescents learning cooking and food skills to enable them to make informed food choices [30].

In line with recent research showing that the mother is the primary source of learning [14,18], the transference of cooking skills from the mothers' mothers was found. This relates to past behaviors and learning and is therefore logical that these participants report the same source that has been discussed previously in the literature. Mothers reported how they were involved in the cooking process in the kitchen and were sometimes responsible for cooking when they were children. This is in contrast to current practices, with a minority of mothers mentioning their children helping with the everyday meal preparation. The mothers' felt a lack of control when the children were in the kitchen and the children distract the mothers from cooking. This caused extra stress and negativity to the whole cooking experience. In addition, mothers did not want their children in the kitchen because of safety concerns, not considering that they themselves had previously been in the kitchen at a similar young age. Additionally, although there was a mention of children using different appliances at certain ages in school, some participants still showed a hesitancy about this and there appeared to be uncertainty over the appropriate age for including children in cooking. Furthermore, the participants did not want to have to clean up the mess created by having children in the kitchen. This idea of having to clean up after the children may be a misunderstanding because, as part of learning basic food skills, children need to learn about cleaning up after cooking and about learning to cook in a neat and safe manner [31]. However, this may also reflect a societal change, where more women are in employment and may have limited time to undertake household responsibilities [32] and, therefore, removing children from the kitchen may be seen as a means to reduce their workload. However, the removal of the children from the kitchen may result in a lack of skill transference.

Furthermore, children are currently dominating meal choice, which in turn influences the type of cooking that occurs and increases the pressure on mothers through the cooking of multiple meals. This is in direct contrast to Lai-Yeung [33] who found that Hong Kong mothers dictate food choice decisions. However, this theme is in line with other western studies [26,34,35] where there has been an emergence of the "junior consumer" deciding on the food to be purchased and prepared, suggesting the existence of cross-cultural differences in this area.

The "rareness" of skill transference occurring from parent to child was alluded to by Lai-Yeung [33] and minimal transference may have been occurring from a minority of participants to their children. Cooking experiences mentioned tended to be fun activities, not daily occurrences and not daily meal preparation. Although any level or element of cooking is positive, the infrequency and type of cooking contribute to the lack of transference of skills.

These changes in cooking practices may have detrimental effects on the learning of cooking skills, where children do not perform the everyday tasks in meal preparation (including food skills such as cleaning up safely after creating a mess in the kitchen), or are being removed from the kitchen and in turn are missing crucial opportunities to learn basic, fundamental skills. This may be contributing to the disappearance of important life skills.

Involving children in cooking has been used previously as a successful strategy to overcome picky eating [36], increase consumption of healthier foods [37] and to increase willingness to taste unfamiliar foods [38]. This strategy has the potential to combat the lack of transference of skills. In addition, it may help to reduce the impact of the child dictating the meal choice, as the child would be more open to and aware of different foods, potentially increasing their food neophilia (i.e., their openness/willingness to trying new and novel foods). Greater willingness to try new foods could be promoted as a key benefit in learning cooking skills.

Not everyone is interested in cooking; however, as it is a valued life skill, it would be appropriate to encourage it across all genders. Parents have been previously found to be supportive of this skill transference [33]. Mothers in this research felt that cooking could be a way for their children to assert their independence and achieve a sense of pride. The ability for cooking skills to be empowering in adult settings has been proposed in previous research [22] and from our results it is suggested that the sense of achievement and empowering element of having cooking skills is not only found in adults but across all ages. Teaching children skills in other domains such as in research has been shown to empower children to become engaged researchers and that the greater is the participation, the more experienced and competent the child becomes, and the greater is the sense of empowerment as the child becomes more effective in the execution of skills [39]. How cooking skills can provide a sense of independence and pride could be a key focus for the promotion of cooking skills in combination with health benefits.

4.1. Limitations

A limitation to this research is that the sample consisted only of mothers. However, mothers have been reported as the primary source of learning cooking skills [14] and an investigation into the current situation was therefore warranted. As some of the participants were in employment, further research is needed into the role of the primary daytime carer of the child, for example grandparents, in the transference of cooking skills. Additionally, there may be some cross-cultural differences in the findings. While there may be limited generalizability (as is inherent in qualitative research), the large number of focus groups with a broad range of mothers with varying food-related behaviors and practices allowed for an extensive range of descriptive ideas that may contribute towards reducing these differences. Further quantitative research in this area could help with the generalizability of the results.

4.2. Implications for Research and Practice

From the above findings, the authors propose two key recommendations: (1) upskilling of mothers' food skills in relation to organizing meals and preparation time, to allow for children to be involved and to reduce stress; and 2) creating an awareness of the importance of kids being in the kitchen and helping with everyday meal preparation. These recommendations may have implications for future interventions and future research. Recommendations 1 and 2 could be implemented through increased numbers of family inclusive interventions, to help parents to acclimatize to children cooking alongside them. This may show parents that children can be involved and assist with everyday meal preparation and highlight different age appropriate cooking skills and tasks. Our findings support the idea of having interventions that focus on the mother–child dyad. Inclusive family interventions may promote the use of these cooking skills to prepare healthy and nutritious meals.

The inclusion of practical cooking skills in any nutrition component of an obesity prevention program is key, to provide individuals with the necessary skills to prepare healthy food [22]. Future longitudinal research could investigate the use of cooking skills over the life course and its impact on weight status. Additionally, the influence of parenting styles on the learning of cooking skills is a key novel area that requires further investigation, as some of the findings in this analysis show children dictating food choices instead of parents which could suggest a shift from the more authoritarian/authoritative parenting approaches in the past to a more permissive/uninvolved style [40]. This could be problematic as a recent review of parenting styles and future weight status [41] suggests that an authoritative parenting style may have a protective role against future overweight and obesity [41]. Although mothers currently have the responsibility of passing on cooking skills, with shifting family dynamics and the increase in the "stay at home husband", future research could investigate if fathers are currently involved in meal preparation and whether this impacts on children's involvement in meal preparation.

Previous research has stressed the importance of cooking skills education through the educational system [14–17], however, initially the role played by the educational system was to expand upon the skills learned in the home environment [17]. Presently, the lack of skills that children present with at school has been highlighted [31] and a push for compulsory practical education can be seen in numerous countries [14,15,31]. It is suggested that a combination of the above methods is essential to promote the use of cooking skills and to empower individuals to prepare healthy nutritious meals to improve their diet quality as a strategy for obesity and other diet-related disease prevention and management.

5. Conclusions

The findings suggest that the culture of children cooking in the kitchen has vastly changed, and opportunities for children to learn basic and fundamental skills are currently lacking which may have detrimental effects on their diet quality. The qualitative nature of the study provides insights into why mothers may not involve their children in cooking including children creating a mess and distracting the mothers from their own cooking and may help with the design of future interventions targeting these behaviors. In addition, a greater awareness of age-related skills and tasks for children in the kitchen should be promoted.

Author Contributions: Conceptualization, F.L. and M.D.; data curation, F.L.; methodology, F.L., L.H., D.S., A.M., E.M., M.D. and M.C.; project administration, M.D.; formal analysis, F.L., T.B. and M.D.; investigation, F.L. and D.S.; resources, M.D., A.M., E.M. and L.H.; supervision, M.D.; writing—original draft, F.L.; writing—review and editing, F.L., T.B., M.D., A.M., E.M., L.H., D.S. and M.C.; and funding acquisition, M.D., A.M., E.M., L.H., and M.C.

Funding: This material was based upon work supported by safefood, The Food Safety Promotion Board, under Grant No. 11/2013 for the period May 2014–October 2015.

Conflicts of Interest: The authors declare no conflict of interest. The funders had no role in the design of the study; in the collection, analyses, or interpretation of data; in the writing of the manuscript, or in the decision to publish the results.

References

1. McGowan, L.; Pot, G.K.; Stephen, A.M.; Lavelle, F.; Spence, M.; Raats, M.; Hollywood, L.; McDowell, D.; McCloat, A.; Mooney, E.; et al. The influence of socio-demographic, psychological and knowledge-related variables alongside perceived cooking and food skills abilities in the prediction of diet quality in adults: A nationally representative cross-sectional study. *Int. J. Behav. Nutr. Phys. Act.* **2016**, *13*, 111. [CrossRef] [PubMed]
2. Wolfson, J.A.; Bleich, S.N. Is cooking at home associated with better diet quality or weight-loss intention? *Public Health Nutr.* **2015**, *18*, 1397–1406. [CrossRef] [PubMed]
3. Chen, R.C.Y.; Lee, M.S.; Chang, Y.H.; Wahlqvist, M.L. Cooking frequency may enhance survival in Taiwanese elderly. *Public Health Nutr.* **2012**, *15*, 1142–1149. [CrossRef] [PubMed]
4. Van der Horst, K.; Brunner, T.A.; Siegrist, M. Ready-meal consumption: Associations with weight status and cooking skills. *Public Health Nutr.* **2011**, *14*, 239–245. [CrossRef]
5. U.S. Department of Health and Human Services; National Institutes of Health; National Cancer Institute. Down Home Healthy Cooking. 2016. Available online: http://www.cancer.gov/about-cancer/causes-prevention/risk/diet/down-home-healthy-cooking.pdf (accessed on 10 September 2016).

6. Reicks, M.; Trofholz, A.C.; Stang, J.S.; Laska, M.N. Impact of cooking and home food preparation interventions among adults: Outcomes and implications for future programs. *J. Nutr. Educ. Behav.* **2014**, *46*, 259–276. [CrossRef] [PubMed]
7. Jones, M.; Dailami, N.; Weitkamp, E.; Salmon, D.; Kimberlee, R.; Morley, A.; Orme, J. Food sustainability education as a route to healthier eating: Evaluation of a multi-component school programme in English primary schools. *Health Educ. Res.* **2012**, *27*, 448–458. [CrossRef]
8. Davis, J.N.; Ventura, E.E.; Cook, L.T.; Gyllenhammer, L.E.; Gatto, N.M. LA Sprouts: A gardening, nutrition, and cooking intervention for Latino youth improves diet and reduces obesity. *J. Am. Diet. Assoc.* **2011**, *111*, 1224–1230. [CrossRef]
9. Morgan, P.J.; Collins, C.E.; Plotnikoff, R.C.; Callister, R.; Burrows, T.; Fletcher, R.; Okely, A.D.; Young, M.D.; Miller, A.; Lloyd, A.B.; et al. The 'Healthy Dads, Healthy Kids' community randomized controlled trial: A community-based healthy lifestyle program for fathers and their children. *Prev. Med.* **2014**, *61*, 90–99. [CrossRef]
10. Isoldi, K.K.; Calderon, O.; Dolar, V. Cooking up energy: Response to a youth-focused afterschool cooking and nutrition education program. *Top. Clin. Nutr.* **2014**, *29*, 123–131. [CrossRef]
11. World Health Organisation. Report of the Commission on Ending Childhood Obesity. 2016. Available online: http://apps.who.int/iris/bitstream/10665/204176/1/9789241510066_eng.pdf?ua=1&ua=1 (accessed on 24 May 2017).
12. Nelson, S.A.; Corbin, M.A.; Nickols-Richardson, S.M. A call for culinary skills education in childhood obesity-prevention interventions: Current status and peer influences. *J. Acad. Nutr. Diet.* **2013**, *113*, 1031–1036. [CrossRef]
13. Larson, N.I.; Perry, C.L.; Story, M.; Neumark-Sztainer, D. Food preparation by young adults is associated with better diet quality. *J. Am. Diet. Assoc.* **2006**, *106*, 2001–2007. [CrossRef] [PubMed]
14. Lavelle, F.; Spence, M.; Hollywood, L.; McGowan, L.; Surgenor, D.; McCloat, A.; Mooney, E.; Caraher, M.; Raats, M.; Dean, M. Learning cooking skills at different ages: A cross-sectional study. *Int. J. Behav. Nutr. Phys. Act.* **2016**, *13*, 119. [CrossRef] [PubMed]
15. Wolfson, J.A.; Frattaroli, S.; Bleich, S.N.; Smith, K.C.; Teret, S.P. Perspectives on learning to cook and public support for cooking education policies in the United States: A mixed methods study. *Appetite* **2017**, *108*, 226–237. [CrossRef] [PubMed]
16. Hartmann, C.; Dohle, S.; Siegrist, M. Importance of cooking skills for balanced food choices. *Appetite* **2013**, *65*, 125–131. [CrossRef] [PubMed]
17. Caraher, M.; Lang, T. Can't cook, won't cook: A review of cooking skills and their relevance to health promotion. *Int. J. Health Promot. Educ.* **1999**, *37*, 89–100. [CrossRef]
18. Caraher, M.; Dixon, P.; Lang, T.; Carr-Hill, R. The state of cooking in England: The relationship of cooking skills to food choice. *Br. Food J.* **1999**, *101*, 590–609. [CrossRef]
19. Golan, M.; Crow, S. Parents are key players in the prevention and treatment of weight-related problems. *Nutr. Rev.* **2004**, *62*, 39–50. [CrossRef]
20. Faith, M.S.; Scanlon, K.S.; Birch, L.L.; Francis, L.A.; Sherry, B. Parent-child feeding strategies and their relationships to child eating and weight status. *Obes. Res.* **2004**, *12*, 1711–1722. [CrossRef]
21. Spruijt-Metz, D.; Lindquist, C.H.; Birch, L.L.; Fisher, J.O.; Goran, M.I. Relation between mothers' child-feeding practices and children's adiposity. *Am. J. Clin. Nutr.* **2002**, *75*, 581–586. [CrossRef]
22. Lang, T.; Caraher, M. Is there a culinary skills transition? Data and debate from the UK about changes in cooking culture. *J. HEIA* **2001**, *8*, 2–14.
23. Lavelle, F.; Hollywood, L.; Caraher, M.; McGowan, L.; Spence, M.; Surgenor, D.; McCloat, A.; Mooney, E.; Raats, M.; Dean, M. Increasing intention to cook from basic ingredients: A randomised controlled study. *Appetite* **2017**, *116*, 502–510. [CrossRef]
24. Krueger, R.A.; Casey, M.A. *Focus Groups: A Practical Guide for Applied Research*; Sage Publications: Thousand Oaks, CA, USA, 2014.
25. McGowan, L.; Caraher, M.; Raats, M.; Lavelle, F.; Hollywood, L.; McDowell, D.; Spence, M.; McCloat, A.; Mooney, E.; Dean, M. Domestic cooking and food skills: A review. *Crit. Rev. Food Sci. Nutr.* **2017**, *57*, 2412–2431. [CrossRef] [PubMed]

26. Lavelle, F.; McGowan, L.; Spence, M.; Caraher, M.; Raats, M.M.; Hollywood, L.; McDowell, D.; McCloat, A.; Mooney, E.; Dean, M. Barriers and facilitators to cooking from 'scratch' using basic or raw ingredients: A qualitative interview study. *Appetite* **2016**, *107*, 383–391. [CrossRef]
27. Braun, V.; Clarke, V. Using thematic analysis in psychology. *Qual. Res. Psychol.* **2006**, *3*, 77–101. [CrossRef]
28. Braun, V.; Clarke, V. What can "thematic analysis" offer health and wellbeing researchers? *Int. J. Qual. Stud. Health Well-Being* **2014**, *9*. [CrossRef] [PubMed]
29. Lavelle, F.; McGowan, L.; Hollywood, L.; Surgenor, D.; McCloat, A.; Mooney, E.; Caraher, M.; Raats, M.; Dean, M. The development and validation of measures to assess cooking skills and food skills. *Int. J. Behav. Nutr. Phys. Act.* **2017**, *14*, 118. [CrossRef]
30. Ronto, R.; Ball, L.; Pendergast, D.; Harris, N. Environmental factors of food literacy in Australian high schools: Views of home economics teachers. *Int. J. Consum. Stud.* **2017**, *41*, 19–27. [CrossRef]
31. Lai-Yeung, T.W. Hong Kong parents' perceptions of the transference of food preparation skills. *Int. J. Consum. Stud.* **2015**, *39*, 117–124. [CrossRef]
32. Soliah, L.A.; Walter, J.M.; Jones, S.A. Benefits and barriers to healthful eating: What are the consequences of decreased food preparation ability? *Am. J. Lifestyle Med.* **2012**, *6*, 152–158. [CrossRef]
33. Dixon, J.; Banwell, C. Heading the table: Parenting and the junior consumer. *Br. Food J.* **2004**, *106*, 182–193. [CrossRef]
34. Trepka, M.J.; Murunga, V.; Cherry, S.; Huffman, F.G.; Dixon, Z. Food safety beliefs and barriers to safe food handling among WIC program clients, Miami, Florida. *J. Nutr. Educ. Behav.* **2006**, *38*, 371–377. [CrossRef] [PubMed]
35. Jabs, J.; Devine, C.M. Time scarcity and food choices: An overview. *Appetite* **2006**, *47*, 196–204. [CrossRef] [PubMed]
36. van der Horst, K. Overcoming picky eating. Eating enjoyment as a central aspect of children's eating behaviors. *Appetite* **2012**, *58*, 567–574. [CrossRef] [PubMed]
37. Russell, C.G.; Worsley, A.; Campbell, K.J. Strategies used by parents to influence their children's food preferences. *Appetite* **2015**, *90*, 123–130. [CrossRef] [PubMed]
38. Allirot, X.; da Quinta, N.; Chokupermal, K.; Urdaneta, E. Involving children in cooking activities: A potential strategy for directing food choices toward novel foods containing vegetables. *Appetite* **2016**, *103*, 275–285. [CrossRef]
39. Kellett, M.; Forrest, R.; Dent, N.; Ward, S. 'Just teach us the skills please, we'll do the rest': Empowering ten-year-olds as active researchers. *Child. Soc.* **2004**, *18*, 329–343. [CrossRef]
40. Baumrind, D. Parenting styles and adolescent development. In *The Encyclopedia of Adolescence*; Brooks-Gunn, J., Lerner, R., Petersen, A.C., Eds.; Garland Publishing: New York, NY, USA, 1991; pp. 746–758.
41. Sokol, R.L.; Qin, B.; Poti, J.M. Parenting styles and body mass index: A systematic review of prospective studies among children. *Obes. Rev.* **2017**, *18*, 281–292. [CrossRef]

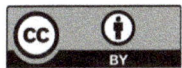

© 2019 by the authors. Licensee MDPI, Basel, Switzerland. This article is an open access article distributed under the terms and conditions of the Creative Commons Attribution (CC BY) license (http://creativecommons.org/licenses/by/4.0/).

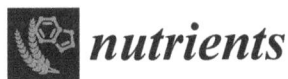

Article

A Cross-Sectional Study on the Relationship between the Family Nutrition Climate and Children's Nutrition Behavior

Sacha Verjans-Janssen [1,*], Dave Van Kann [1,2], Stef Kremers [1], Steven Vos [2,3], Maria Jansen [4,5] and Sanne Gerards [1]

1. Department of Health Promotion, NUTRIM School of Nutrition and Translational Research in Metabolism, Maastricht University, 6229 HA Maastricht, The Netherlands; d.vankann@fontys.nl (D.V.K.); s.kremers@maastrichtuniversity.nl (S.K.); sanne.gerards@maastrichtuniversity.nl (S.G.)
2. School of Sport Studies, Fontys University of Applied Sciences, 5644 HZ Eindhoven, The Netherlands; steven.vos@fontys.nl
3. Department of Industrial Design, Eindhoven University of Technology, 5612 AZ Eindhoven, The Netherlands
4. Academic Collaborative Center for Public Health, Public Health Service South-Limburg, 6400 AA Heerlen, The Netherlands; maria.jansen@ggdzl.nl
5. Department of Health Services Research, Maastricht University, CAPHRI Care and Public Health Research Institute, 6229 GT Maastricht, The Netherlands
* Correspondence: s.verjans@maastrichtuniversity.nl; Tel.: +31-433-884-278

Received: 5 August 2019; Accepted: 25 September 2019; Published: 2 October 2019

Abstract: Background: Parents influence their children's nutrition behavior. The relationship between parental influences and children's nutrition behavior is often studied with a focus on the dyadic interaction between the parent and the child. However, parents and children are part of a broader system: the family. We investigated the relationship between the family nutrition climate (FNC), a family-level concept, and children's nutrition behavior. Methods: Parents of primary school-aged children (N = 229) filled in the validated family nutrition climate (FNC) scale. This scale measures the families' view on the consumption of healthy nutrition, consisting of four different concepts: value, communication, cohesion, and consensus. Parents also reported their children's nutrition behavior (i.e., fruit, vegetable, water, candy, savory snack, and soda consumption). Multivariate linear regression analyses, correcting for potential confounders, were used to assess the relationship between the FNC scale (FNC-Total; model 1) and the different FNC subscales (model 2) and the child's nutrition behavior. Results: FNC-Total was positively related to fruit and vegetable intake and negatively related to soda consumption. FNC-value was a significant predictor of vegetable (positive) and candy intake (negative), and FNC-communication was a significant predictor of soda consumption (negative). FNC-communication, FNC-cohesion, and FNC-consensus were significant predictors (positive, positive, and negative, respectively) of water consumption. Conclusions: The FNC is related to children's nutrition behavior and especially to the consumption of healthy nutrition. These results imply the importance of taking the family-level influence into account when studying the influence of parents on children's nutrition behavior. Trial registration: Dutch Trial Register NTR6716 (registration date 27 June 2017, retrospectively registered), METC163027, NL58554.068.16, Fonds NutsOhra project number 101.253.

Keywords: family; parents; health; nutrition; children

1. Introduction

Worldwide, children's body mass index (BMI) and the prevalence of overweight and obesity among children increased in the last 40 years [1]. Although the trend concerning the age-standardized

BMI of children in the northwestern part of Europe is flattening, numbers remain high. In 2018, almost 12% of Dutch children between the ages of four and 11 years were overweight or obese [2]. Overweight and obesity in childhood are associated with physical and psychological morbidity in the short and long term [3]. A cause of overweight and obesity is high-energy intake, in the form of energy-dense, nutrient-poor foods and soft drinks [4]. Many children consume too much sugar, e.g., sugar-containing beverages and energy-dense snacks [5], and consume insufficient amounts of healthy foods, such as fruits and vegetables [4]. Healthy eating behaviors in childhood decrease the risk of health-related diseases at a later age, and are related to having healthy eating habits as an adult [6,7].

During childhood, parents decide what children eat, gradually shaping the child's nutritional behavior. Parents do this by exhibiting specific, goal-directed behaviors, i.e., food parenting practices [8,9]. Certain food parenting practices, such as controlling the availability of healthy or unhealthy foods, and parental modeling of eating behaviors, are most consistently related to children's nutrition behavior [10,11]. On the other hand, other food parenting practices, such as pressuring to eat, monitoring, and rewarding food consumption, are not consistently related to children's nutrition behavior [10,11]. This is probably due to the influence of general parenting on these parent–child interactions [8,11–13]. General parenting refers to the emotional climate in which the parenting practices are expressed [8]. Children show a healthier nutrition behavior as a result of certain parenting practices (e.g., encouragement) when the parents provide a positive parenting climate [13]. A positive parenting climate is characterized by nurturance, structure, and behavioral control [14].

Many studies on the relationship between food parenting practices, general parenting, and children's nutrition behavior assume a unidirectional communication in which the child is the mere recipient [15]. However, in reality, parents and children are part of a family in which family members influence each other's behaviors, indicating a reciprocal influence [16]. Focusing only on individual parenting practices and general parenting, and not considering this family-level influence can lead to important information being missed when studying the parents' influence on children's nutrition behavior [15,17].

Very little research was conducted on the family-level influence on children's nutrition behavior. It is hypothesized that the family's emphasis on healthy nutrition and their interactions concerning nutrition behavior (e.g., parents discussing whether it is important to eat healthy as a family, consuming meals together as a family) influence whether and how much healthy nutrition is consumed by the child. These familial interactions and views are part of a family's health climate. To capture this family climate concerning healthy nutrition, Niermann and colleagues [18] developed the family nutrition climate (FNC) scale (as part of the family health climate scale). The FNC is considered "the [family's] shared perceptions and cognitions" concerning healthy nutrition behavior on a daily basis [18] (p. 31).

The FNC is a relatively new construct and, to our knowledge, only two studies were conducted using this validated instrument to measure the relationship between the family and individual nutrition behavior [19,20]. Both studies found a relationship between the FNC and individual nutrition behavior: families with healthy behavioral patterns (consuming high levels of healthy nutrition and showing high levels of physical activity) rated their FNC higher compared to families with unhealthier behavioral patterns [20]. In the second study, it was found that a higher score on the FNC was related to a higher consumption of children's healthy foods (i.e., fruit, vegetables, and salad) [19]. In both studies, the children were adolescents with a mean age of 14 years. It is unknown whether these results are similar for a population of younger children. Therefore, this study aimed to investigate the relationship between the FNC and the nutrition behavior of Dutch children aged 7–10 years old.

2. Methods

2.1. Study Design and Procedure

For the current study, baseline data of a quasi-experimental study were used. The protocol of this quasi-experimental intervention study was described in Verjans-Janssen et al. [21]. Ethical approval for the study was provided by the Medical Ethics Committee of the Maastricht University Medical Centre and Maastricht University (METC163027, national number: NL58554.068.16). After being informed about the study, all participants consented to participate before the start of the study. The parents of the participants signed an informed consent form. The questionnaires are available in Dutch from the corresponding author upon request.

Primary school children in grades 4–6 (Dutch educational system: between the ages of seven and 10 years) were eligible for inclusion. Eleven primary schools participated in the study. The schools were located in low socio-economic neighborhoods in two cities in the southern region of the Netherlands.

The children were provided with oral and written information by a researcher. Their parents received written information about the study and were given the opportunity to ask questions during scheduled information hours or via phone or e-mail. The children were included in the study if both parents provided written consent. Of the eligible children, 60.4% consented to participate in the study.

2.2. Measurements

Data were collected in March and April 2017. Data collection tools included a child questionnaire, a parent questionnaire (both paper-based), and anthropometric measurements. The child questionnaire was filled in on paper in the classroom during school hours. The child's anthropometric measurements were taken by trained researchers at school. Parents filled in the parent questionnaire at home and returned the questionnaire via the child to school. The questionnaires are available in Dutch from the corresponding author upon request.

2.2.1. Children's Nutrition Behavior

The child's nutrition behavior was measured with the parent questionnaire. For this, items of a validated food frequency questionnaire for Dutch children was used [22]. Children's fruit, vegetable, water, candy (i.e., sweets, licorice, candy bars), savory snack (e.g., cheese, crisps), and soda intake were measured. For water intake, the consumption of tea without sugar was also included. For soda, only sugar-containing drinks were included (diet soda sweetened with artificial sweeteners was excluded from the analysis). The frequency (from zero to seven days a week) and the amount per day of these foods and drinks were measured. The amount was measured in natural units: pieces for fruit, serving spoons for vegetables, portions for candy (i.e., a handful of sweets or one normal-sized candy bar), portions for savory snacks (i.e., a handful of cheese or a bowl of crisps), and glasses for water and soda. The frequency and the amount were multiplied and divided by seven to calculate an average daily consumption.

2.2.2. Family Health Climate

The FNC scale is a validated questionnaire [18], which was translated into Dutch [17]. It can be completed by one family member or by multiple family members, after which an aggregated FNC score can be calculated [18,19]. In this study, one parent filled out the FNC. The higher the score is on the FNC scale, the more importance is placed on eating healthy as a family [18]. The FNC scale consists of four subscales: FNC-value, FNC-communication, FNC-cohesion, and FNC-consensus. FNC-value (four items) encompasses the family's interest in healthy nutrition in daily life and whether healthy nutrition is a norm within the family (e.g., "In our family, a healthy diet plays an important role in our lives") ($\alpha = 0.87$). FNC-communication (five items) comprises the family's talks about healthy nutrition and support regarding eating healthy foods (e.g., "In our family, we are interested in articles (e.g., magazines) on healthful nutrition") ($\alpha = 0.81$). FNC-cohesion (five items) encompasses whether consuming meals together as a family is common and whether eating together is considered important (e.g., "In our family, we appreciate spending time together during meals") ($\alpha = 0.67$). FNC-consensus (three items) refers to the agreement within a family concerning nutrition (e.g., "In our family, we rarely argue about food- or diet-related matters") ($\alpha = 0.80$). All items were assessed on a four-point Likert scale ("strongly disagree" to "strongly agree"). The average of the four FNC-subscale scores was taken to obtain the FNC overall score (FNC-Total; 17 items) ($\alpha = 0.86$). Missing data for the FNC scale were imputed when there was 10% or less of missing items. A missing value was replaced by the mean of the available FNC subscale items for that particular participant. If a subscale had only one valid item, data were not imputed, and the participant was excluded from analysis. Imputation on the FNC scale was applied for nine participants.

2.2.3. Children's Weight Status

The children were weighed and measured during the schools' physical education lessons. They wore light sports clothes during the anthropometric measurements, but shoes were taken off. Weight was measured to the nearest 0.1 kg with a digital weighing scale (Seca 803), and height was measured to the nearest 0.1 cm with a portable stadiometer (Seca 213). For the children with missing data due to absence on the day of measurement, data were imputed from the parent questionnaire (i.e., self-reported data); this was the case for five children. Children's BMI z-scores were calculated using a Dutch reference population and adjusting for the child's age and gender [23].

2.2.4. Socio-Demographic Characteristics

Socio-demographic characteristics of the child were measured with the child questionnaire. Children reported their date of birth, their gender, and the number of brothers and sisters. This was used to calculate the number of children within a family. Children reported the birth country of both parents, which was used to define the children's ethnicity. Ethnicity was based on the definition of Western and non-Western by Statistics Netherlands [24]; the child's ethnicity was non-Western when at least one parent was born in a non-Western country.

In the parent questionnaire, the parents reported on their educational level, parent relationship (married/having a partner or single), and weight and height. Educational level was recoded into three categories based on the International Standard Classification of Education 2011 [25]: no or primary educational level (no education or primary school), secondary educational level (pre-vocational school, secondary education, or lower vocational education), and tertiary educational level (higher vocational education or university degree). Parent's body mass index (BMI) was calculated and used to define the weight status of the parent (i.e., BMI <20: underweight, BMI 20–25: normal weight, BMI 25–30: overweight, and BMI >30: obese).

2.3. Participants

In total, 523 children participated in the study. Only data of parent–child dyads were used. Of the 523 children, 329 parents (62.9%) provided data on their child(ren)'s nutrition behavior and the family nutrition climate. To ensure that independent samples were included, the data of one sibling of a sibling pair were excluded; the sibling with the lowest birth month was excluded. In the case of twins, the child who was first in the dataset (sorted by subject identifier) was excluded. In total, 18 siblings were excluded. Only cases with complete data were included in the analyses.

2.4. Statistical Analysis

Data were analyzed with SPSS version 24.0 (IBM Corp., Armonk, NY, USA). Descriptive statistics were used to describe the characteristics of the study population and the mean values and standard deviations of FNC-Total, the FNC subscales, and the nutrition behavior outcomes. Differences in the FNC between different types of families, based on the child's ethnicity (Western versus non-Western) and the parent's education level (low versus high), were analyzed. As the FNC data were not normally distributed, differences between these groups were analyzed with a Mann–Whitney U-Test.

Data of the nutrition behaviors were square-root-transformed due to violation of the normality assumption of the residuals in the regression analyses. Pearson correlation analyses were conducted to obtain the correlations between the FNC-Total/FNC subscales and nutrition behavior outcomes. Multivariate linear regression analyses were used to examine the relationship between the FNC and the individual nutrition behavior outcomes, while correcting for potential confounders: age, gender, ethnicity, and BMI z-score of the child, and parent's educational level, BMI, and age. These covariates were entered simultaneously into the linear regression models.

Two types of linear regression models were built. Firstly, regression models were built for all foods and drinks, separately, with FNC-Total as an independent variable (model 1). Secondly, the regression models were restructured by replacing FNC-Total with the FNC subscales (i.e., FNC-value, FNC-communication, FNC-cohesions, FNC-consensus), which were added simultaneously as independent variables to the models (model 2). A two-sided p-value of less than 0.05 was considered statistically significant.

3. Results

3.1. Characteristics of the Study Population

In total, 229 (69.6%) parent–child dyads were included in the analyses. The mean age of the children was 8.3 years (SD = 1.0). More girls (62.0%) than boys participated in the study. Mainly mothers filled in the questionnaire (83.8%). The mean age of the parents was 38.6 years (SD = 5.4). Of the parents, 35.4% had a secondary educational level, and 38.9% had a tertiary educational level (higher vocational degree or higher). Of the remaining parents, 22.7% finished primary education, and 3.1% ($N = 7$) reported having no education. Of all children, slightly more than one-quarter (27.1%) had a non-Western ethnicity, with one or both parents born in a non-Western country. Overall, 17.9% of the children and 42.8% of the parents were overweight and obese. Regarding the family situation, the majority of the parents had a partner (81.7%) and two or more children (83.4%) (Table 1).

Table 1. Characteristics of the target population ($N = 229$).

	Number	%	Mean	SD
Parent characteristics				
Parent				
Mother	192	83.8		
Father	37	16.2		
Age			38.6	5.4
Educational level				
No or primary education	59	25.8		
Secondary education	81	35.4		
Tertiary education	89	38.9		
Weight status				
Underweight or normal weight	131	57.2		
Overweight or obese	98	42.8		
Child characteristics				
Age			8.3	1.0
Gender				
Male	87	38.0		
Female	142	62.0		
Ethnicity				
Western	167	72.9		
Non-Western	62	27.1		
Weight status				
Underweight or normal weight	188	82.1		
Overweight or obese	41	17.9		

Table 1. Cont.

	Number	%	Mean	SD
Family situation				
Relationship				
Living together with a partner	187	81.7		
Single	42	18.3		
Number of children				
1 child	38	16.6		
2 or more children	191	83.4		

3.2. Means of the Child's Nutrition Behavior and the Family Nutrition Climate

Children consumed on average 1.4 pieces of fruit (SD = 0.6), 1.8 portions (±90 g) of vegetables (SD = 0.9), and 2.3 glasses of water daily. On average, they consumed a little less than one portion of candy (mean (M) = 0.9, SD = 0.7), a little less than half a portion of savory snacks (M = 0.4, SD = 0.4), and 1.4 glasses of soda (SD = 1.3) daily (Table 2).

The average scores on the FNC subscales were high (>3), except for FNC-communication (M = 2.9, SD = 0.6), see Table 2. Parents scored highest on FNC-cohesion (M = 3.7, SD = 0.4).

FNC-Total did not differ significantly for families of different ethnicity (U = 4735.0, p = 0.32), but it did differ significantly between less well-educated and highly educated parents (U = 4121.5, p = 0.04). Highly educated parents scored higher on the FNC (M = 3.3, SD = 0.4) compared to less well-educated parents (M = 3.2, SD = 0.4).

3.3. Relationship between the Family Nutrition Climate and the Child's Nutrition Behavior

FNC-Total correlated positively with healthy food consumption, i.e., fruit and vegetable intake, and negatively with unhealthy food and drink consumption, i.e., candy intake and soda consumption (Table 2). FNC-value correlated with the same food and drink consumption as FNC-Total, and in the same direction, i.e., positively with fruit and vegetable intake and negatively with candy intake and soda consumption. FNC-communication correlated positively with all healthy foods (fruit intake, vegetable intake, and water consumption) and negatively with soda consumption. There were no significant correlations between FNC-cohesion and nutrition behavior or between FNC-consensus and nutrition behavior.

Adjusting for child and parent characteristics, FNC-Total was a significant predictor of fruit intake (standardized β = 0.15), vegetable intake (β = 0.23), and soda consumption (β = −0.20) (Table 3). FNC-value was positively related to vegetable intake (β = 0.34) and negatively to candy consumption (β = −0.19). FNC-communication was positively related to water consumption (β = 0.19) and negatively to soda consumption (β = −0.24). Regarding water consumption, FNC-cohesion and FNC-consensus were also predictors, but in opposite directions (β = 0.15 and β = −0.20, respectively).

Table 2. Correlation coefficients between family nutrition climate and the child's individual nutrition behavior.

		M (SD)	1	2	3	4	5	6	7	8	9	10
	Family Nutrition Climate											
1	Total	3.3 (0.4)	-									
2	Value	3.4 (0.6)	**0.83**	-								
3	Communication	2.9 (0.6)	**0.81**	**0.59**	-							
4	Cohesion	3.7 (0.4)	**0.56**	**0.33**	**0.21**	-						
5	Consensus	3.1 (0.7)	**0.68**	**0.46**	**0.30**	**0.33**	-					
	Individual nutrition behavior [a]											
6	Fruit (pieces/day)	1.4 (0.6)	**0.18**	**0.16**	**0.21**	0.08	0.01	-				
7	Vegetables (portions/day) [b]	1.8 (0.9)	**0.26**	**0.32**	**0.19**	0.10	0.12	0.12	-			
8	Water (glasses/day)	2.3 (1.7)	0.10	0.07	**0.17**	0.11	-0.10	**0.17**	**0.23**	-		
9	Candy (portions/day) [c]	0.9 (0.7)	**-0.15**	**-0.19**	-0.09	-0.12	-0.05	0.06	-0.11	0.02	-	
10	Snacks (portions/day) [d]	0.4 (0.4)	-0.05	-0.08	0.01	-0.04	-0.06	**0.17**	-0.06	-0.07	**0.30**	-
11	Soda (glasses/day)	1.4 (1.3)	**-0.23**	**-0.21**	**-0.29**	-0.04	-0.07	-0.07	**-0.14**	**-0.39**	**0.11**	0.12

Note: M: mean, SD: standard deviation; bold numbers are statistically significant ($p < 0.05$). [a] The data for the nutrition behaviors were transformed (square root). [b] One serving spoon is approximately 50 g. [c] One portion is a handful of sweets or a normal-sized candy bar, for example. [d] One portion is a handful of cheese or a bowl of crisps, for example.

Table 3. Associations between the family nutrition climate (FNC) and the child's individual nutrition behavior (linear regression models).

		Model 1			Model 2		
	FNC	Unst. B	(SE)	St. β	Unst. B	(SE)	St. β
Individual nutrition behavior [a]							
Fruit (pieces/day)	FNC-Total	**0.11**	(0.05)	**0.15**			
	Value				0.07	(0.10)	0.06
	Communication				0.15	(0.08)	0.15
	Cohesion				0.15	(0.13)	0.08
	Consensus				-0.10	(0.07)	-0.10
	R^2			0.12			0.15

Table 3. Cont.

	FNC	Model 1			Model 2		
		Unst. B	(SE)	St. β	Unst. B	(SE)	St. β
Vegetables (serving spoons/day) [b]	FNC-Total	**0.19**	**(0.05)**	**0.23**			
	Value				**0.20**	**(0.05)**	**0.34**
	Communication				−0.02	(0.04)	−0.04
	Cohesion				−0.01	(0.07)	−0.01
	Consensus				0.00	(0.04)	0.00
	R^2			0.12			0.16
Water (glasses/day)	FNC-Total	0.13	(0.10)	0.09			
	Value				−0.03	(0.10)	−0.03
	Communication				**0.18**	**(0.08)**	**0.19**
	Cohesion				**0.26**	**(0.12)**	**0.15**
	Consensus				**−0.17**	**(0.07)**	**−0.20**
	R^2			0.06			0.11
Candy (portions/day) [c]	FNC-Total	−0.10	(0.06)	−0.12			
	Value				**−0.11**	**(0.06)**	**−0.19**
	Communication				0.03	(0.04)	0.05
	Cohesion				−0.09	(0.07)	−0.09
	Consensus				0.03	(0.04)	0.06
	R^2			0.07			0.09
Snacks (portions/day) [d]	FNC-Total	−0.04	(0.13)	−0.02			
	Value				−0.07	(0.12)	−0.06
	Communication				0.13	(0.10)	0.11
	Cohesion				−0.04	(0.16)	−0.02
	Consensus				−0.09	(0.09)	−0.08
	R^2			0.05			0.06
Soda (glasses/day)	FNC-Total	**−0.31**	**(0.10)**	**−0.20**			
	Value				−0.06	(0.10)	−0.06
	Communication				**−0.23**	**(0.08)**	**−0.24**
	Cohesion				0.04	(0.13)	0.02
	Consensus				0.02	(0.07)	0.02
	R^2			0.13			0.15

Note: Model 1: FNC-Total as independent variable. Model 2: FNC-value, FNC-communication, FNC-cohesions, and FNC-consensus as independent variables. All models were adjusted for child's age, gender, body mass index (BMI) z-score, and ethnicity, and parent's educational level, BMI, and age. Bold numbers are significant, $p < 0.05$. Unst. = unstandardized, St. = standardized. [a] The data for the nutrition behaviors were transformed (square root). [b] One serving spoon is approximately 50 g. [c] One portion is a handful of sweets or a normal-sized candy bar, for example. [d] One portion is a handful of cheese or a bowl of crisps, for example.

4. Discussion

The current study investigated the relationship between the FNC and the nutrition behavior of primary school-aged children. We found that FNC-Total was a positive predictor of the consumption of healthy nutrition (i.e., fruit and vegetable intake) and a negative predictor of the consumption of one unhealthy nutrition (i.e., soda consumption). The results were in line with our expectation that the FNC is mainly a predictor of children's healthy nutrition consumption. Our results show that a family-level influence is present on children's nutrition behavior. Other research already showed that family members influence each other's nutrition behaviors. For example, families have similar dietary intakes [26,27], especially regarding the consumption of healthy nutrition [26]. Our study specifically shows the influence of shared values, routines, and interaction patterns concerning healthy nutrition within a family (defined as the family nutrition climate) on the child's nutrition behavior.

In this study, the parents rated FNC-cohesion the highest, indicating that consuming meals together as a family was common and considered important. Family meals are related to a healthier nutrition behavior of children [28]. However, in our study, we only found a significant association between FNC-cohesion and water consumption. It can be that, although family meals were common, these moments did not consist of interpersonal contact. Research showed that distractions during family meals, such as having the television on, is negatively related to group enjoyment during the meals (even when the family is not paying attention to the television) [29]. The quality of the time spent together during family meals, e.g., talking about each other's day and discussing the importance of healthy nutrition during family meals, is likely a more important part of the family nutrition climate and of more influence on children's nutrition behavior than merely sitting together at the dinner table. In our study, we indeed found a stronger association between the communication within the family concerning healthy nutrition and FNC-Total than between FNC-cohesion and FNC-Total.

FNC-Total was associated the strongest with children's vegetable consumption. In the Netherlands, children consume vegetables mainly during dinner in the form of cooked vegetables [30,31]. Dinner is most of the times consumed at home with the family and more regularly compared to breakfast and lunch [32,33], which explains the strong association between FNC-Total and children's vegetable consumption. Research showed that parents highly value the consumption of vegetables by their child because of the health benefits [34]. Our results showed that FNC-value was the only significant predictor of the child's vegetable intake.

While vegetables are mainly consumed during meals, fruit, candy, and snacks are mainly consumed in between meals [5,31]. However, this does not imply that the family influence is not present regarding the consumption of fruit. On the contrary, FNC-total was also related to the child's fruit consumption, but to a lesser extent than vegetable consumption. This can be explained by the fact that Dutch primary school-aged children consume at least 70% of their fruit intake at home, and about 20% at school [31]. Since the schools in this study participated in the "European Union (EU) school fruit" program, in which children were provided with fruit at least three days a week during morning recess [35], there was also an influence of the school environment on the children's fruit consumption.

The third association between FNC-Total and children's nutrition behavior involved children's soda consumption. The FNC refers to the importance of a healthy diet within the family. Although soda is not a healthy food, the FNC was associated with soda consumption; however, this was in the preferred direction (i.e., lower soda intake). This desirable family influence on soda intake was present because Dutch primary school children consume soda mainly at home. Furthermore, 11.3% of the daily soda consumption takes place during dinner [5], which is mainly consumed at home and with the family, as mentioned earlier. Our results showed that the family influence on soda consumption was present in the communication within the family concerning healthy nutrition (FNC-communication). Based on these results and the positive relationship between FNC-communication and water consumption, we hypothesize that the family supports each other in refraining from soda and talks about water as being a healthy drink.

This positive relationship between FNC-communication and children's water consumption and between FNC-cohesion and children's water consumption countered the negative relationship between FNC-consensus and children's water consumption. These contrasting results explain the non-significant relationship between FNC-Total and children's water consumption. Although a higher score on FNC-consensus was assumed to positively relate to a healthier nutrition behavior, the negative association between FNC-consensus and water consumption might be explained by the framing of the items, i.e., "In our family, we rarely argue about food- or diet-related matters". The unexpected relationship could either imply that there is no arguing about drinking water or that water consumption is insufficiently considered to be part of "food- or diet-related matters".

There was no association between FNC-Total and candy and savory snacks. It may be that the family influence on the consumption of these foods is less present compared to the other foods. One-third of the time, Dutch primary school-aged children consume candy and snacks at a friend's place or when outside [5] and, thus, away from the family environment. Another explanation may be that snacks and candies are not healthy foods and are, thus, not taken into consideration when thinking about consuming healthy nutrition within the family.

Our results are in line with the study on the FNC and adolescents' nutrition behavior [19]. Niermann and colleagues [19] found a positive association between the aggregated FNC and adolescents' healthy dietary behavior, consisting of the intake of salads, vegetables, and fruits. The effect size of their association was medium. The associations found in the current study were less strong, while the influence of the family on the nutrition behavior of younger children was expected to be stronger. A likely explanation for the stronger associations found in the study by Niermann et al. [19] is that they included more highly educated parents (41.9% of the mothers and 58.4% of the fathers). In our study, highly educated parents had a significantly higher FNC-Total score compared to less well-educated parents. Additional interaction analysis was conducted to see whether educational level had an influence on the relation between the FNC and the children's nutrition behavior, but no significant interaction between FNC-Total and the parent's educational level was found (data not shown). However, our sample was rather small, and further research is required to investigate whether different types of families (e.g., based on ethnicity, educational level, socioeconomic status) differ in the FNC and how this difference is related to the children's nutrition behavior.

The family can be considered a social dynamic system consisting of different subsystems (e.g., individuals, spouse subsystem, parent–child subsystem) that interact with each other. To understand a family's properties and their influence, the different parts of a family cannot simply be combined because they are interdependent (e.g., family functioning depends on an interplay of communication patterns and role fulfillment) [15,36]. Given the complexity of the family influences on the children's energy balance-related behaviors, it is quite challenging to study this family system [15]. The FNC is a part of this complex family system and, by the use of the FNC-scale, we aimed to capture some of the influence of this complex family system on children's nutrition behavior.

The rather weak associations found between the FNC and the children's nutrition behaviors in this study can be explained by the fact that the FNC operates on a more distal level within the family system [15]. However, these weak associations do not imply that this family-level influence is less relevant. On the contrary, the FNC is an important part of the family system, which is associated with the children's nutrition behavior, as shown in our study, via mediated paths (e.g., through intrinsic motivation), as shown in the study of Niermann et al. [19], and as a higher-level moderator (i.e., stronger relationships were found between food parenting practices and children's BMI z-score when the family nutrition climate was healthier), as shown in the study of Gerards et al. [17].

4.1. Strengths and Limitations

To our knowledge, this is the first study to investigate the relationship between the FNC and the nutrition behavior of primary school-aged children. The strengths of this study were the diversity of the sample regarding the children's ethnicity and the educational level of the parents.

A limitation of the study was the underrepresentation of paternal views on the FNC. Paternal views on FNC may differ from maternal views [37]. The underrepresentation of fathers in studies is a common limitation of observational studies on parenting and children's obesity-related behaviors, especially nutrition behavior [38]. This possibly limits the generalizability of the results.

Another limitation possibly affecting generalizability of the results might be the slight overrepresentation of girls in the sample. However, in the study on the association between the FNC and adolescents' consumption of healthy foods, the correlations did not differ significantly between boys and girls [19].

Other limitations were the cross-sectional design and the use of a self-reporting instrument to measure the children's nutrition behavior. Longitudinal studies should be conducted between the FNC and the children's energy balance-related behaviors to study the stability of the FNC over time and how the FNC influences the children's energy balance-related behaviors over time. We also recommend objective measurements of the children's nutrition behavior, such as the use of wearables [39], because self-reporting instruments for nutrition behavior are prone to social desirability.

Finally, it is debatable whether our choice of nutrition behaviors is the best representation of children's healthy and unhealthy nutrition behaviors, since other behaviors such as breakfast consumption or other foods and drinks such as milk are also part of the children's daily nutrition behavior.

4.2. Implications and Recommendations

Our results add to the existing knowledge of the family influence on children's nutrition behavior. The results underline the importance of addressing the whole family system instead of focusing merely on the parent–child subsystem [15,40]. Addressing the family environment should be done by involving all family members [19]. The healthy family environment can be assessed by the individual evaluations of the FNC. Ideally, the FNC is measured by assessing the views of all family members (the parents, the child, and siblings) [18].

To inform intervention developers, we recommend further research into the interaction between the more proximal parent-level influences (e.g., parenting practices) and the more distal family-level factors (e.g., the FNC) and their interacting influence on the children's nutrition behavior. To be able to study these interacting influences, we advocate studying general parental influences, i.e., general parenting, and more specific parenting, i.e., nutrition parenting practices, as well as the broader family context, i.e., the family nutrition climate.

To measure general parenting, we recommend the use of the validated comprehensive general parenting questionnaire for caregivers of 5–13-year-old children of Sleddens et al. [41]. This questionnaire was developed after a thorough search of the literature and assesses five parenting constructs: nurturance, structure, behavioral control, overprotection, and coercive control [41]. Unfortunately, there is little consensus on how to best measure food parenting practices [42]. There are at least 71 instruments measuring food parenting practices [43]. In most cases, these instruments measure a small part of the spectrum of food parenting practices [43]. Fortunately, a comprehensive food parenting practices item bank is currently being developed, which will allow a more consistent and comprehensive measurement of food parenting practices in the future [42]. For the measurement of the family-level influence, we recommend the use of the FNC.

5. Conclusions

The climate within a family concerning healthy nutrition (e.g., valuing healthy nutrition within a family, and communicating about eating healthy as a family) is a predictor of the children's nutrition behavior, especially the consumption of healthy foods. These results indicate the importance of considering family-level influences when aiming to improve children's nutrition behavior.

Author Contributions: S.V.-J. drafted and revised the manuscript. S.V.-J., D.V.K., and S.G. designed the study, and S.V.-J. carried out the study. S.V.-J. analyzed the data. S.G. helped draft the manuscript. S.K., D.V.K., and S.V.

initiated the project and obtained funding. D.V.K., S.K., S.V., and M.J. read the manuscript and provided feedback. All authors read and approved the final manuscript.

Funding: The present study was funded by Fonds NutsOhra (project number 101.253). Fonds NutsOhra had no role in the writing of this manuscript.

Acknowledgments: We are grateful to the parents and children participating in this study.

Conflicts of Interest: The authors declare no conflict of interest.

Abbreviations

NTR	Netherlands Trial Register
METC	Medical Ethical Research Committee
BMI	Body mass index
FNC	Family nutrition climate
M	Mean
SD	Standard deviation
Unst. B	Unstandardized beta
SE	Standard error
St. β	Standardized beta

References

1. NCD Risk Factor Collaboration. Worldwide trends in body-mass index, underweight, overweight, and obesity from 1975 to 2016: A pooled analysis of 2416 population-based measurement studies in 128.9 million children, adolescents, and adults. *Lancet* **2017**, *390*, 2627–2642. [CrossRef]
2. Statistics Netherlands. Kinderen Met Overgewicht en Obesitas Naar Leeftijd 2018. [Children with Overweight and Obesity by Age 2018]. 2019. Available online: https://www.volksgezondheidenzorg.info/onderwerp/overgewicht/cijfers-context/huidige-situatie#node-overgewicht-kinderen (accessed on 25 June 2019).
3. Reilly, J.J.; Kelly, J. Long-term impact of overweight and obesity in childhood and adolescence on morbidity and premature mortality in adulthood: Systematic review. *Int. J. Obes.* **2011**, *35*, 891–898. [CrossRef] [PubMed]
4. World Health Organization (WHO). *Diet, Nutrition, and the Prevention of Chronic Diseases. Joint WHO/FAO Expert Consultation*; WHO Technical Report Series No. 916; WHO: Geneva, Switzerland, 2003.
5. Gevers, D.W.M.; Kremers, S.P.J.; de Vries, N.K.; van Assema, P. Intake of energy-dense snack foods and drinks among Dutch children aged 7–12 years: How many, how much, when, where and which? *Public Health Nutr.* **2016**, *19*, 83–92. [CrossRef] [PubMed]
6. Kelder, S.H.; Perry, C.L.; Klepp, K.-I.; Lytle, L.L. Longitudinal tracking of adolescent smoking, physical activity, and food choice behaviors. *Am. J. Public Health* **1994**, *84*, 1121–1126. [CrossRef] [PubMed]
7. Craigie, A.M.; Lake, A.A.; Kelly, S.A.; Adamson, A.J.; Mathers, J.C. Tracking of obesity-related behaviours from childhood to adulthood: A systematic review. *Maturitas* **2011**, *70*, 266–284. [CrossRef]
8. Darling, N.; Steinberg, L. Parenting style as context: An integrative model. *Psychol. Bull.* **1993**, *113*, 487–496. [CrossRef]
9. Scaglioni, S.; Salvioni, M.; Galimberti, C. Influence of parental attitudes in the development of children eating behavior. *Br. J. Nutr.* **2008**, *99* (Suppl. 1), S22–S25. [CrossRef]
10. Blaine, R.E.; Kachurak, A.; Davison, K.K.; Klabunde, R.; Fisher, J.O. Food parenting and child snacking: A systematic review. *Int. J. Behav. Nutr. Phys. Act.* **2017**, *14*, 146. [CrossRef]
11. Yee, A.Z.H.; Lwin, M.O.; Ho, S.S. The influence of parental practices on child promotive and preventive food consumption behaviors: A systematic review and meta-analysis. *Int. J. Behav. Nutr. Phys. Act.* **2017**, *14*, 47. [CrossRef]
12. Rodenburg, G.; Oenema, A.; Kremers, S.P.J.; van de Mheen, D. Parental and child fruit consumption in the context of general parenting, parental education and ethnic background. *Appetite* **2012**, *58*, 364–372. [CrossRef]
13. Sleddens, E.F.C.; Kremers, S.P.J.; Stafleu, A.; Dagnelie, P.C.; de Vries, N.K.; Thijs, C. Food parenting practices and child dietary behavior. Prospective relations and the moderating role of general parenting. *Appetite* **2014**, *79*, 42–50. [CrossRef] [PubMed]

14. Skinner, E.; Johnson, S.; Snyder, T. Six dimensions of parenting: A motivational model. *Parent. Sci. Pract.* **2005**, *5*, 175–235. [CrossRef]
15. Niermann, C.Y.N.; Gerards, S.M.P.L.; Kremers, S.P.J. Conceptualizing family influences on children's energy balance-related behaviors: Levels of Interacting Family Environmental Subsystems (The LIFES Framework). *Int. J. Environ. Res. Public Health* **2018**, *15*, 2714. [CrossRef] [PubMed]
16. Roach, E.; Viechnicki, G.B.; Retzloff, L.B.; Davis-Kean, P.; Lumeng, J.C.; Miller, A.L. Family food talk, child eating behavior, and maternal feeding practices. *Appetite* **2017**, *117*, 40–50. [CrossRef]
17. Gerards, S.M.P.L.; Niermann, C.; Gevers, D.W.M.; Eussen, N.; Kremers, S.P.J. Context matters! The relationship between mother-reported family nutrition climate, general parenting, food parenting practices and children's BMI. *BMC Public Health* **2016**, *16*, 1018. [CrossRef] [PubMed]
18. Niermann, C.Y.N.; Krapf, F.; Renner, B.; Reiner, M.; Woll, A. Family health climate scale (FHC-scale): Development and validation. *Int. J. Behav. Nutr. Phys. Act.* **2014**, *11*, 30. [CrossRef]
19. Niermann, C.Y.N.; Kremers, S.P.J.; Renner, B.; Woll, A. Family Health Climate and adolescents' physical activity and healthy eating: A cross-sectional study with mother-father-adolescent triads. *PLoS ONE* **2015**, *10*, e0143599. [CrossRef] [PubMed]
20. Niermann, C.Y.N.; Spengler, S.; Gubbels, J.S. Physical activity, screen time, and dietary intake in families: A cluster-analysis with mother-father-child triads. *Front. Public Health* **2018**, *6*, 276. [CrossRef]
21. Verjans-Janssen, S.R.B.; Van Kann, D.H.H.; Gerards, S.M.P.L.; Vos, S.B.; Jansen, M.W.J.; Kremers, S.P.J. Study protocol of the quasi-experimental evaluation of "KEIGAAF": A context-based physical activity and nutrition intervention for primary school children. *BMC Public Health* **2018**, *18*, 842. [CrossRef]
22. Dutman, A.E.; Stafleu, A.; Kruizinga, A.; Brants, H.A.M.; Westerterp, K.R.; Kistemaker, C.; Meuling, W.J.A.; Goldbohm, R.A. Validation of an FFQ and options for data processing using the doubly labelled water method in children. *Public Health Nutr.* **2010**, *14*, 410–417. [CrossRef]
23. Schönbeck, Y.; Talma, H.; van Dommelen, P.; Bakker, B.; Buitendijk, S.E.; Hirasing, R.A.; van Buuren, S. Increase in prevalence of overweight in Dutch children and adolescents: A comparison of nationwide growth studies in 1980, 1997 and 2009. *PLoS ONE* **2011**, *6*, e27608. [CrossRef] [PubMed]
24. Statistics Netherlands. Niet-Westers Allochtoon [Non-Western Immigrant]. 2019. Available online: https://www.cbs.nl/nl-nl/dossier/_links%20oude%20site/niet-westers-allochtoon/ (accessed on 11 January 2019).
25. UNESCO Institute for Statistics. *International Standard Classification of Education*; ISCED 2011; UNESCO: Paris, France; UIS: Montreal, QC, Canada, 2012.
26. Bogl, L.H.; Mehlig, K.; Intemann, T.; Masip, G.; Keski-Rahkonen, A.; Russo, P.; Michels, N.; Reisch, L.; Pala, V.; Johnson, L.; et al. on behalf of the I.Family Consortium. A within-sibling pair analysis of lifestyle behaviours and BMI z-score in the multi-centre I.Family Study. *Nutr. Metab. Cardiovasc. Dis.* **2019**, *29*, 580–589. [CrossRef] [PubMed]
27. Hebestreit, A.; Intemann, T.; Siani, A.; De Henauw, S.; Eiben, G.; Kourides, Y.A.; Kovacs, E.; Moreno, L.A.; Veidebaum, T.; Krogh, V.; et al. Dietary patterns of European children and their parents in association with family food environment: Results from the I.Family Study. *Nutrients* **2017**, *9*, 126. [CrossRef] [PubMed]
28. Fulkerson, J.A.; Larson, N.; Horning, M.; Neumark-Sztainer, D. A review of associations between family or shared meal frequency and dietary and weight status outcomes across the lifespan. *J. Nutr. Educ. Behav.* **2017**, *46*, 2–19. [CrossRef] [PubMed]
29. Trofholz, A.C.; Tate, A.D.; Miner, M.H.; Berge, J.M. Associations between TV viewing at family meals and the emotional atmosphere of the meal, meal healthfulness, child dietary intake, and child weight status. *Appetite* **2017**, *108*, 361–366. [CrossRef]
30. Ray, C.; Roos, E.; Brug, J.; Behrendt, I.; Ehrenblad, B.; Yngve, A.; te Velde, S.J. Role of free school lunch in the associations between family-environmental factors and children's fruit and vegetable intake in four European countries. *Public Health Nutr.* **2012**, *16*, 1109–1117. [CrossRef] [PubMed]
31. Van Rossum, C.T.M.; Buurma-Rethans, E.J.M.; Vennemann, F.B.C.; Beukers, M.; Brants, H.A.M.; de Boer, E.J.; Ocké, M.C. *The Diet of the Dutch. Results of the First Two Years of the Dutch National Food Consumption Survey 2012–2016*; National Institute for Public Health and the Environment: Bilthoven, The Netherlands, 2016.
32. Wijtzes, A.I.; Jansen, W.; Jaddoe, V.W.V.; Franco, O.H.; Hofman, A.; van Lenthe, F.J.; Raat, H. Social inequalities in young children's meal skipping behaviors: The Generation R Study. *PLoS ONE* **2015**, *10*, e0134487. [CrossRef]

33. Totland, T.H.; Knudsen, M.D.; Paulsen, M.M.; Bjelland, M.; van 't Veer, P.; Brug, J.; Klepp, K.I.; Andersen, L.F. Correlates of irregular family meal patterns among 11-year-old children from the Pro Children study. *Food Nutr. Res.* **2017**, *61*, 1339554. [CrossRef]
34. Hingle, M.; Beltran, A.; O'Connor, T.; Thompson, D.; Baranowski, J.; Baranowski, T. A model of goal directed vegetable parenting practices. *Appetite* **2012**, *58*, 444–449. [CrossRef]
35. Barnekow Rasmussen, V. The European Network of Health Promoting Schools- from Iceland to Kyrgyzstan. *Promot. Educ.* **2005**, *12*, 167–172.
36. Cox, M.J.; Paley, B. Understanding families as systems. *Curr. Dir. Psychol. Sci.* **2003**, *12*, 193–196. [CrossRef]
37. Berge, J.M.; MacLehose, R.F.; Meyer, C.; Didericksen, K.; Loth, K.A.; Neumark-Sztainer, D. He said, she said: Examining parental concordance on home environment factors and adolescent health behaviors and weight status. *J. Acad. Nutr. Diet* **2016**, *116*, 46–60. [CrossRef] [PubMed]
38. Davison, K.K.; Gicvic, S.; Aftosmes-Tobio, A.; Ganter, C.; Simon, C.L.; Newlan, S.; Manganello, J.A. Fathers' representation in observational studies on parenting and childhood obesity: A systematic review and content analysis. *Am. J. Public Health* **2016**, *106*, e14–e21. [CrossRef] [PubMed]
39. Gemming, L.; Rush, E.; Maddison, R.; Doherthy, A.; Gant, N.; Utter, J.; Ni Mhurchu, C. Wearable cameras can reduce dietary under-reporting: Doubly labelled water validation of a camera-assisted 24h recall. *Br. J. Nutr.* **2015**, *113*, 284–291. [CrossRef] [PubMed]
40. Sung-Chan, P.; Sung, Y.W.; Zhao, X.; Brownson, R.C. Family-based models for childhood-obesity intervention: A systematic review of randomized controlled trials. *Obes. Rev.* **2013**, *14*, 265–287. [CrossRef] [PubMed]
41. Sleddens, E.F.; O'Connor, T.M.; Watson, K.B.; Hughes, S.O.; Power, T.G.; Thijs, C.; De Vries, N.K.; Kremers, S.P.J. Development of the Comprehensive General Parenting Questionnaire for caregivers of 5–13 year olds. *Int. J. Behav. Nutr. Phys. Act.* **2014**, *11*, 15. [CrossRef] [PubMed]
42. O'Connor, T.M.; Mässe, L.C.; Tu, A.W.; Watts, A.W.; Hughes, S.O.; Beauchamp, M.R.; Baranowski, T.; Pham, T.; Berge, J.R.; Fiese, B.; et al. Food parenting practices for 5 to 12 year old children: A concept map analysis of parenting and nutrition experts input. *Int. J. Behav. Nutr. Phys. Act.* **2017**, *14*, 122. [CrossRef]
43. Vaughn, A.E.; Tabak, R.G.; Bryant, M.J.; Ward, D.S. Measuring parent food practices: A systematic review of existing measures and examination of instruments. *Int. J. Behav. Nutr. Phys. Act.* **2013**, *10*, 61. [CrossRef] [PubMed]

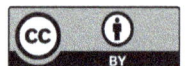

© 2019 by the authors. Licensee MDPI, Basel, Switzerland. This article is an open access article distributed under the terms and conditions of the Creative Commons Attribution (CC BY) license (http://creativecommons.org/licenses/by/4.0/).

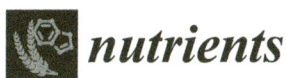

Article

The Contribution of Preschool Meals to the Diet of Finnish Preschoolers

Liisa Korkalo [1,*], Kaija Nissinen [1,2], Essi Skaffari [1], Henna Vepsäläinen [1], Reetta Lehto [1,3], Riikka Kaukonen [1,3], Leena Koivusilta [4], Nina Sajaniemi [5,6], Eva Roos [1,3,7] and Maijaliisa Erkkola [1]

1. Department of Food and Nutrition, University of Helsinki, P.O. Box 66, 00014 Helsinki, Finland
2. Seinäjoki University of Applied Sciences, Kampusranta 11, 60101 Seinäjoki, Finland
3. Folkhälsan Research Center, Topeliuksenkatu 20, 00250 Helsinki, Finland
4. Department of Social Research, Faculty of Social Sciences, Assistentinkatu 7, University of Turku, 20014 Turku, Finland
5. Faculty of Educational Sciences, P.O. Box 8, University of Helsinki, 00014 Helsinki, Finland
6. School of Applied Educational Sciences and Teacher Education, Philosophical Faculty, University of Eastern Finland, P.O. Box 111, 80101 Joensuu, Finland
7. Department of Public Health, Clinicum, University of Helsinki, P.O. Box 20, 00014 Helsinki, Finland
* Correspondence: liisa.korkalo@helsinki.fi

Received: 23 May 2019; Accepted: 26 June 2019; Published: 5 July 2019

Abstract: Preschool meals may influence the formation of children's dietary habits and health. We assessed the contribution of preschool meals to the diet of Finnish children. We used food record data from the cross-sectional DAGIS survey and selected recording days which included all three meals (breakfast, lunch, afternoon snack) at preschool. We analyzed the diet of three- to four-year-olds (n = 324) and five- to six-year-olds (n = 233). Preschool meals accounted for 54% of the weekday's energy intake in both age groups, and provided ≥60% of total fiber, polyunsaturated fatty acids, and vitamins D and E. More than 60% of fish dishes but only one third of total daily fresh fruit were consumed at preschool. The mean (SD) percentages of energy from protein and fat at preschool were 17% (3%) and 30% (7%) in the younger and 17% (3%) and 31% (6%) in the older age group, respectively. The mean proportions of energy from added sugar at preschool were below 5% in both age groups. On average, salt intake exceeded recommendations and 60% of salt came from preschool food. Tackling high salt intake should be a future goal of guidance for early childhood education and care food services.

Keywords: preschool-aged children; kindergarten; day care center; catering; food consumption; dietary intake

1. Introduction

Food behaviors are learnt during childhood and track into adulthood [1,2]. Dietary habits influence health over the long term [3,4] and for this reason, ensuring health-promoting food habits both at home and in early childhood education and care (ECEC) is of vital importance. Studies reporting the food consumption and/or nutrient intake of the same children both at home and in ECEC are limited [5–9] and only a few have been conducted in Europe [6,8]. A study in Finland [10] found that the diet of three-year-old children attending ECEC outside the home was closer to the Finnish nutrition recommendations than the diet of home-cared children. Studies conducted in the USA have reported that lunches at ECEC are, regarding some micronutrients, more nutrient-dense than lunches at home or away [11] or dinners at home [9]. In contrast, Gubbels et al. [8] reported that more vegetables were consumed at home than in day care in the Netherlands. The same study found that sweet snacks were mostly eaten in day care. In the study by Gubbels et al. [8], all food in the participating day care centers was provided by the center (Jessica Gubbels, personal communication 9 May 2019). The results regarding the contribution of ECEC to food consumption and nutrient intake are contradictory. The discrepancies may be due to differences in food culture and food service systems, regulations, recommendations, and laws, which need to be taken into account when comparing studies.

The aim of this study was to assess the contribution of preschool meals to the diet of children who attend full-time care in municipal preschools in Finland. We specifically aimed to calculate what is the percentage contribution of each meal to the total daily intake of energy and nutrients on weekdays when the child eats three meals at preschool and to describe the amounts of foods consumed and the sources of nutrients at preschool and at outside preschool. In this paper, we use the term preschool to mean municipally arranged center-based ECEC, which in Finland is voluntary until the age of six, and compulsory for one year before school starts at the age of seven.

2. Materials and Methods

2.1. Early Childhood Education and Care and Food Services in Finland

In Finland, parents can choose municipal (public) or private ECEC. In addition to preschools, children can attend to group family day care, or family day care, which is typically in the caregiver's home. Of one- to six-year old Finnish children in ECEC, 76% are in preschools [12]. The ECEC fee is moderate but depends on family's size and income level. Children from all socio-economic backgrounds are entitled to high-quality ECEC throughout the country. Early education is based on the Act on Early Childhood Education and Care [13] and the National Core Curriculum for Early Childhood Education and Care [14].

According to Finnish law, municipal preschools must provide healthy food which fulfils the child's nutritional requirements [13]. If a child is in full-time care, three meals (breakfast, lunch, and afternoon snack) must be offered. A target has been set that these three meals should cover two thirds of a child's daily energy intake [15]. Food for preschool is provided by either the municipality's own food service or an external food service provider. Food recommendations with meal-specific nutritional criteria are available to guide ECEC food services. The recent updates to children's food recommendations [16] and the first national food recommendations for ECEC [15] were not yet in effect at the time of the data collection for this study, but older nutrition recommendations for families with children were valid [17].

Lunch generally consists of typical Finnish foods: a warm main course with salad or a main course soup; bread and spreadable fat; and a drink (milk, sour milk, or non-dairy milk substitute suitable for special diets). Breakfast typically consists of porridge with milk and/or berry soup, fruit puree, or jam; and/or bread, spreadable fat and a cold cut; and possibly a piece of fruit or vegetable. A typical afternoon snack is a combination of two or more of the following: bread, yogurt, Finnish cultured milk ('*viili*'), quark ('*rahka*', also a cultured milk product), smoothie, berry soup, flavored porridge, pancakes, a piece of fruit or vegetable, a cold cut, and milk or juice. All meals are included in the client fee and no separate fees can be charged. This catering is part of the national effort to establish good nutrition, health, and welfare for children. According to the guidelines [15], mealtimes are part of early childhood education. They must be appropriately organized and supervised. The health-related and social role of meals, the objectives of nutritional education and learning manners and food culture, as well as the recreational aspect of eating occasions should be taken into account when arranging mealtimes. Meals are used as a pedagogical tool. The entire educational community should have commonly determined objectives and implementation policies for food education [15].

2.2. Study Participants

We used data from the Increased Health and Wellbeing in Preschools (DAGIS) research project. As a part of the larger DAGIS study, a cross-sectional survey of preschool children was conducted in 2015–2016. Details of the sampling process are described in open access format elsewhere [18]. In short, the cross-sectional survey was conducted in eight municipalities. Five of these were in Southern Finland and three were in Western Finland. Altogether 86 municipal (public) preschools consented to participate (Figure 1). From these preschools, all children in the target age of three to six years ($n = 3592$) and their families were invited to participate through an invitation letter. Children in preschools with a low participation rate ($\leq 30\%$ in each of the preschool groups for three- to six-year-olds) were excluded. The final sample consisted of 864 children (24% of those invited) from 66 preschools. These preschools operated from Monday to Friday. We excluded preschools operating 24 h a day from the sample.

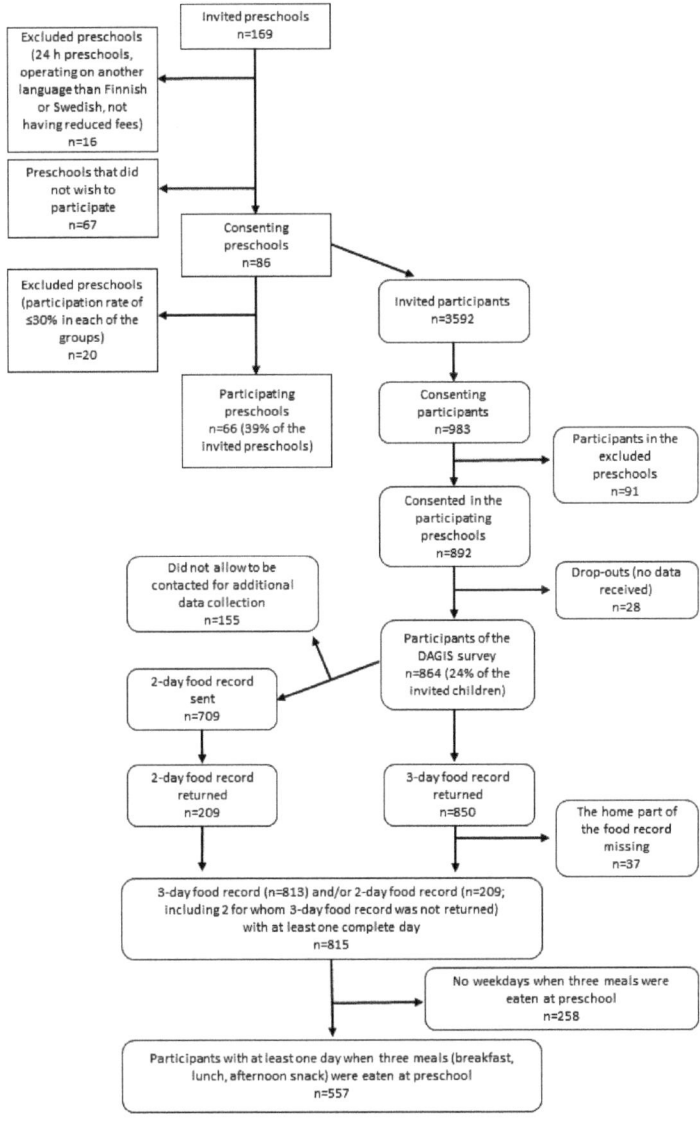

Figure 1. Participation of preschools and children in the DAGIS survey and the selection of participants for this paper.

A parent or legal guardian of each participating child provided written informed consent. We asked each family if we could contact them again for additional data collection. All procedures involving human subjects were approved by the University of Helsinki Ethical Review Board in the Humanities and Social and Behavioral Sciences on 24 February 2015 (Statement 6/2015).

2.3. Anthropometric and Background Data

Trained researchers measured weight and height at the preschool. The children removed their shoes and heavy clothing. The clothes that the child was wearing during the weight measurement were recorded and later deducted accordingly, creating a corrected weight variable. Body weight was measured to the nearest 0.01 kg using CAS portable bench scales (CAS PB-100/200). Height was measured to the nearest 0.1 cm using stadiometers (SECA 217). We used the extended international body mass index cut-offs for thinness and overweight [19]. Other background data such as the parents' level of education and the child's special diets were gathered via questionnaires.

2.4. Food Record Data

We sent each participating family a three-day food record including instructions. Exact dates (two weekdays and one weekend day) for filling in the food record were assigned for each family. As the aim was that all the days of the week would be well-represented in the data, these three days were not always consecutive. In some cases, when the parents felt that the dates were unsuitable for keeping a food record (for example due to illness in the family or a holiday trip), they contacted the study group and renegotiated the dates. The three-day food records were kept between September 2015 and April 2016.

To capture seasonal variation in the diet, after about six months, the families who had agreed to be contacted for additional data collection were sent an invitation to fill in a second food record ($n = 709$). This time it was a two-day food record and the families were assigned a week during which they should choose two days for recording (with preferably at least one day being a weekday). When necessary, parents also took the record and instructions to preschool. The two-day food records were kept between June 2016 and September 2016. The time between the two food records ranged from 4 to 11 months.

The instruction page of the food records advised parents to record all foods and beverages that their child consumed during the recording days, except for what they consumed at preschool. An example page was also included. We provided the families with a validated [20] Children's Food Picture Book [21], specifically designed for use in this project to assist in portion size estimation. The parents were instructed to estimate the portion sizes eaten using the picture book, weighing, household measures such as teaspoons or tablespoons, or package labels. The instruction was to list all the ingredients of composite dishes. For packed food products, the exact brand and product name was required. They were also asked to record the place and time of consumption.

The preschool personnel were given a separate pre-coded food record for recording food consumption at the preschool on the dates matching the home food record. The researchers/research assistants instructed the early educators orally, and the food record included written instructions. Breakfast, lunch, afternoon snack, and possible additional snacks each had predefined sections. Different food groups, such as main courses, side dishes (potatoes, pasta, rice), and salad at lunch each had predetermined rows. The early educators were given the Children's Food Picture Book [21] to help them record the portion sizes eaten. They could also estimate the amounts in household measures.

The research assistants checked the returned food records and, if necessary, made follow-up phone calls to complete missing details of foods consumed. Special attention was paid to vegetable, fruit, and sugary product consumption in the food record checking process. As an example, if the parent had forgotten to record the type of yogurt product, we asked if it had been natural yogurt or sugar-sweetened yogurt; or if the portion size was missing, we asked for more details.

The food data were recorded using AivoDiet dietary software. This software included the Fineli Food Composition Database Release 16 (2013) of the National Institute for Health and Welfare. New food items were also added to the database when necessary. We checked that the vitamin D values of foods fortified with vitamin D (fluid milk products, spreadable fats, and non-dairy milk substitutes) corresponded with the products on the market at the time of study. The database includes recipes for typical Finnish mixed dishes. For each individual meal, the research assistant used a suitable recipe from the database, modified an existing recipe, or created a new recipe according to the parents' reports. The salt content of home dishes was also based on the recipes in the database and unless the parents stated otherwise in the record, main dishes, porridges, rice, pasta, and potatoes were assumed to have been cooked using salt. We asked the preschool food services if they were willing to give their recipes to the study group to enable more precise calculation of the children's dietary intake at preschool. Out of the eight municipalities, five gave their recipes, one gave a part of their recipes and two municipalities declined the request. In cases in which the recipe was not available, we made estimations based on the recipes used in the other municipalities.

During the data entry, the research assistants coded each meal with a tag that specified the name of the meal and the place at which it was eaten. These nametags were: breakfast, lunch, dinner, snack, evening snack, and other. The research assistants decided on these based on the recorded time of day, the content of the meal, and general knowledge of Finnish food habits. The place tags were home, preschool, restaurant, and other.

After the data were entered, we checked for outlying values of food consumption in grams and outlying energy and nutrient intakes. After extracting the data from the software, each food code (food item or mixed dish) appearing in the data set was assigned to a food group and nutrient retention factors [22] were applied using a single factor per nutrient per food group. The food composition database did not include values for added sugar. As previously described [23], we estimated added sugar intake by first assigning each food item to a food group and then giving each food group that contained significant amounts of sugar a formula that represented the foods in that group. To estimate the relative amounts of naturally occurring and added sugar in a certain food, we used the information from package labels, the national food composition database and commonly used recipes.

The home and/or preschool food records of 850 (98% of the DAGIS survey sample) and 206 (29% of those invited) children were returned in the first and second round of food record data collection, respectively. However, the home part of the 3-day food record was missing for 37 children. Individual days of data were also excluded due to unrealistically long pauses between consecutive meals (>8 h). After data checking and entry, 815 children (94% of the DAGIS survey sample) had at least one day of food record data available for analysis.

2.5. Data Processing and Analysis

To assess the dietary contribution of preschool meals among children attending full-time care, we defined a 'full preschool day' and selected a sub-sample of the participants as follows. We selected each singular food recording day when a child had eaten all three preschool meals (breakfast, lunch, and afternoon snack). We defined this as >0 grams of consumption of any food or beverage during all these three meals. Using this criterion, we, in effect, discarded data for all weekend days and those weekdays when: (1) the child was home-cared (it is common in Finland for a child to only attend preschool four days per week) (2) the child came to preschool after preschool breakfast serving time (3) the child was away from preschool for the whole day or part of the day for other reasons, such as being ill or on vacation. The three meals were provided daily in all the participating preschools. Sometimes, when an additional snack was served during excursions or special events, we collapsed these with the regular afternoon snack in the data analysis. This approach yielded a sample of 557 children (64% of the DAGIS survey sample). Each of these children contributed to the data with one to four full preschool days; the total number of days in the data for this paper was 966. These children were from 489 families (423 families had one child in the sample, 64 had two, and 2 had three children in the sample). For analysis, we divided the data into two age groups. We used age at recruitment for this categorization (even though the children grew older between the first and second food recording period).

We rearranged all the meals in the data to fall under one of the seven possible meal categories (1) breakfast outside preschool, (2) breakfast at preschool, (3) lunch at preschool, (4) afternoon snack at preschool, (5) dinner outside preschool, (6) evening snack outside preschool, and (7) other snack outside preschool. We did not consider a glass of water or a chewing gum alone to be a meal and collapsed these with another meal. We first calculated the percentage of individual days in the data that included each meal. After that, we calculated an average day for each child and used these to calculate the mean intakes and population proportions [24] of energy and nutrients during each meal, during the preschool day in total, and during the whole day. We also calculated the mean amounts of foods consumed and the food group sources of energy and nutrients. This was also done after calculating an average day for each child. Finally, since not all the days included all the seven meals, we calculated the mean intake of energy and nutrients for each meal during the days when the meal was consumed after selecting these days and calculating an average day for each child. We used R version 3.5.2 for all analyses.

3. Results

The analyses included 557 children from 66 preschools, 264 (47%) of whom were girls. The majority (98%) of these children were in the target age group of three to six years. However, nine children were two years old and one was seven years old; for analysis, we included them in the closest age group. Of all the participants, 81% were categorized as being of normal weight. The participating children attended preschool on four and a half days per week on average (Table 1).

Table 1. Characteristics of sample (total n = 557).

Characteristics	3- to 4-Year-Olds (n = 324)		5- to 6-Year-Olds (n = 233)	
	Data Available, n	% or Mean (SD)	Data Available, n	% or Mean (SD)
Child				
Gender	324		233	
Girls		47.2		47.6
Boys		52.8		52.4
Age, years	324	4.1 (0.6)	233	5.6 (0.5)
Weight status [19]	301		224	
Underweight		8.0		5.8
Normal weight		83.1		78.6
Overweight or obese		9.0		15.7
Days in preschool/week	312	4.5 (0.8)	219	4.5 (0.8)
Hours in preschool/day	305	8.2 (0.8)	211	8.1 (0.8)
Special diets	322		226	
Food allergy or intolerance		8.4		7.5
Low lactose/lactose free		7.6		5.7
Gluten-free		0.9		1.3
Vegetarian or pescovegetarian		0.3		0.4
Family				
Highest educational level in family	315		221	
High school level or lower		19.1		18.0
Bachelor's degree or equivalent		43.5		42.1
Master's degree or higher		37.3		39.9
Number of < 18-year-old children living in the household, including participating child	315		221	
1		11.7		11.8
2		58.7		55.7
3 or more		29.5		32.6
Preschool				
Number of children in day care group	278	20 (6.8)	200	21 (7.0)

3.1. Food Consumption

We found that the majority (≥60%) of skimmed milk, potatoes and potato dishes, fish dishes, poultry dishes, sausage dishes, margarine and fat spread (In this paper, we use the European Union's definitions [25] for the following spreadable fats: butter, margarine, fat spread, and blended spread. In short, fat spreads and margarines are similar to each other, but the total fat content differs. Blended spreads are obtained from a mixture of vegetable and animal fats and the milk-fat content is between 10% and 80%.), porridge, fruit and berry soups, dairy-based desserts, rye crispbread, and multi-grain bread were consumed at preschool (Tables 2 and 3). The majority (≥60%) of fresh fruit, berries, sweet and savory bakery products, biscuits and muesli bars, blended spread, yogurt and Finnish cultured milk, and cheese were consumed at home (and elsewhere outside preschool). Furthermore, over 75% of the total amount of the 'sweets and sugar' group and sugar-sweetened juice and all soda were consumed outside preschool. Fresh vegetables and vegetable salads were consumed in roughly equal amounts at preschool and outside preschool.

Table 2. Mean food consumption on preschool days (Monday to Friday) of 3- to 4-year-old Finnish children who eat three meals at preschool (n = 324).

	Outside Preschool		Preschool		Total
	g/Day	%	g/Day	%	g/Day
Vegetables, vegetable dishes	50	50	50	50	100
fresh vegetables and vegetable salads	35	53	32	47	67
vegetarian dishes	9	37	15	63	24
side dish vegetables	5	60	3	40	8
Potatoes, potato dishes	20	32	42	68	62
Fruit, berries, fruit and berry products	93	52	85	48	179
fresh fruit	66	71	27	29	93
berries	4	91	0.4	9	5
fruit and berry soups	6	15	33	85	39
100% juice	9	56	7	44	16
Cereals, bakery products	93	34	180	66	273
rye bread	6	37	11	63	17
rye crispbread	1	12	11	88	12
multi-grain bread	9	31	21	69	30
white bread	3	52	3	48	6
porridge	33	22	115	78	147
rice, pasta, etc.	20	67	10	33	30
buns, sweet bakery products	4	90	0.5	10	5
biscuits and muesli bars	3	84	1	16	4
savory bakery products, hamburgers, pizza	7	76	2	24	10
pancakes, crêpes	3	34	5	66	8
Fats, oils, gravy	7	24	21	76	28
margarine and fat spread	2	12	16	88	18
blended spread	2	100	0	0	2
butter	0.2	100	0	0	0.2
Fish, fish dishes	11	30	25	70	35
Eggs, egg dishes	2	51	2	49	5
Meat, meat dishes	74	46	87	54	161
cold cuts	3	51	2	49	5
red meat dishes	51	51	48	49	99
poultry dishes	15	39	24	61	39
sausage dishes	5	29	12	71	17
Milk, dairy products	236	40	352	60	589
skimmed milk	79	23	265	77	344
milk with 1-1.5% fat content	84	63	50	37	134
whole milk	5	100	0	0	5
sour milk	3	37	5	63	8
milk with cocoa	10	77	3	23	14
yogurt and Finnish cultured milk	37	78	10	22	47
cheese	7	64	4	36	11
dairy-based desserts	7	35	14	65	21
ice-cream	3	84	1	16	4
Sugar, sweets	4	81	1	19	5
Drinks	100	68	47	32	147
water	55	66	29	34	83
sugar-sweetened juice	23	82	5	18	28
sugar-sweetened soda	4	100	0	0	4
non-dairy milk substitutes	10	47	12	53	22
Miscellaneous	7	74	2	26	9

Main food groups (bold) and selected sub-groups are presented.

At preschool, skimmed milk was the most commonly used milk. None of the preschools offered whole milk. Of the 66 preschools, 64 (97%) offered milk with and 2 (3%) without vitamin D fortification during the food recording days. The mean daily bread consumption was 65 g and 71 g among the three- to four-year-olds and five- to six-year-olds, respectively, and about two thirds of the bread consumption was at preschool (Tables 2 and 3). Preschools offered margarine or fat spread with bread and their consumption was relatively high (mean 16 and 18 g/day, among the three- to four-year-olds and five- to six-year-olds, respectively), which is in line with their bread consumption pattern. The most common spreadable fat offered at preschool was margarine with a fat content of 60 g/100 g (data not shown).

Table 3. Mean food consumption on preschool days (Monday to Friday) of 5- to 6-year-old Finnish children who eat three meals at preschool (n = 233).

	Outside Preschool		Preschool		Total
	g/Day	%	g/Day	%	g/Day
Vegetables, vegetable dishes	53	46	62	54	115
fresh vegetables and vegetable salads	38	49	39	51	77
vegetarian dishes	11	37	19	63	29
side dish vegetables	4	49	4	51	8
Potatoes, potato dishes	22	30	51	70	73
Fruit, berries, fruit and berry products	113	57	86	43	199
fresh fruit	64	68	30	32	93
berries	8	94	1	6	9
fruit and berry soups	12	31	28	69	40
100% juice	17	67	9	33	26
Cereals, bakery products	102	32	212	68	314
rye bread	7	43	10	57	17
rye crispbread	1	8	12	92	13
multi-grain bread	11	34	22	66	33
white bread	4	42	5	58	9
porridge	33	19	139	81	172
rice, pasta, etc.	22	66	11	33	34
buns, sweet bakery products	3	83	1	17	4
biscuits and muesli bars	3	70	1	30	4
savory bakery products, hamburgers, pizza	10	72	4	28	14
pancakes, crêpes	2	27	6	73	8
Fats, oils, gravy	7	22	24	78	31
margarine and fat spread	2	11	18	89	20
blended spread	2	99	0	1	2
butter	0.2	100	0	0	0.2
Fish, fish dishes	16	37	27	63	42
Eggs, egg dishes	3	57	2	42	5
Meat, meat dishes	82	44	103	56	185
cold cuts	3	47	3	53	6
red meat dishes	58	50	57	50	115
poultry dishes	15	32	31	68	46
sausage dishes	6	35	11	65	16
Milk, dairy products	258	40	391	60	649
skimmed milk	100	26	284	74	384
milk with 1-1.5% fat content	67	52	63	48	130
whole milk	6	100	0	0	6
sour milk	8	55	6	45	14
milk with cocoa	11	62	7	38	18
yogurt and Finnish cultured milk	44	83	9	17	53
cheese	8	65	4	35	12
dairy-based desserts	10	39	16	61	26
ice-cream	4	77	1	23	5
Sugar, sweets	8	83	2	17	10
Drinks	95	64	53	36	148
water	44	54	37	46	82
sugar-sweetened juice	29	77	9	23	38
sugar-sweetened soda	9	100	0	0	9
non-dairy milk substitutes	7	56	5	44	12
Miscellaneous	7	75	2	25	10

Main food groups (bold) and selected sub-groups are presented.

3.2. Energy and Macronutrients

The mean energy intake for Monday to Friday was 5.6 MJ among the three- to four-year-olds (Table 4) and 6.4 MJ among the five- to six-year-olds (Table 5). All preschool meals together accounted for 54% of the total energy intake in both age groups. Lunch and dinner were the two main meals regarding energy intake. Breakfast at preschool, afternoon snack at preschool, and evening snack at home were all of similar importance regarding energy intake. Most children did not have a home breakfast before going to preschool, and thus, on average, home breakfast was only 2–3% of the energy intake (Tables 4 and 5). Among those who did have a home breakfast, it contributed on average 0.50–0.57 MJ of energy (Supplementary Tables S1 and S2).

Table 4. Mean (SD) intake and population proportion [24] of energy and nutrients on weekdays among 3 to 4-year-old children who eat three meals at preschool (*n* = 324). Each child had data for 1 to 4 days; the total number of days was 561.

	Breakfast, Outside Preschool	Breakfast, Preschool	Lunch, Preschool	Afternoon Snack, Preschool	Dinner, Outside Preschool	Evening Snack, Outside Preschool	Other Snack, Outside Preschool	Preschool Food, Total	Total, per Day
% of days that included the meal	24	100	100	100	95	91	50		
Energy, MJ	0.13 (0.27)	0.77 (0.29)	1.37 (0.51)	0.90 (0.36)	1.15 (0.51)	0.89 (0.49)	0.37 (0.50)	3.04 (0.83)	5.59 (1.10)
Protein, g	1 (2)	7 (3)	15 (7)	8 (3)	15 (7)	8 (5)	2 (4)	31 (10)	56 (13)
Carbohydrates, g	4 (9)	24 (10)	35 (13)	29 (13)	26 (13)	28 (15)	13 (17)	88 (25)	159 (34)
Sucrose, g	1 (3)	2 (3)	2 (2)	7 (6)	3 (4)	7 (6)	5 (8)	11 (8)	27 (14)
Added sugar, g	1 (3)	1 (3)	1 (2)	6 (6)	2 (4)	6 (6)	5 (8)	8 (7)	21 (13)
Fiber, g	0.4 (0.9)	2.8 (1.5)	3.7 (1.5)	2.6 (1.5)	2.1 (1.4)	2.7 (2.0)	0.9 (1.5)	9.1 (3.1)	15.3 (4.6)
Fat, g	1 (2)	6 (4)	13 (6)	7 (4)	12 (6)	7 (6)	3 (5)	25 (9)	47 (13)
SAFA, g	0.4 (1.1)	1.8 (1.2)	4.1 (2.3)	2.5 (1.7)	4.3 (2.9)	2.9 (2.5)	1.3 (2.3)	8.4 (3.5)	17.3 (5.3)
MUFA, g	0.3 (0.8)	2 (1.5)	4.8 (2.6)	2.3 (1.4)	4.1 (2.5)	2.1 (2.1)	0.9 (1.8)	9.1 (3.7)	16.5 (5.1)
PUFA, g	0.1 (0.4)	1.2 (0.9)	2.5 (1.4)	1.3 (0.9)	1.6 (1.2)	0.9 (1.1)	0.4 (0.7)	4.9 (2.1)	8.0 (2.9)
Vitamin A, µg RAE	12 (52)	71 (56)	144 (126)	96 (104)	191 (517)	73 (104)	26 (79)	311 (185)	613 (568)
Vitamin D, µg	0.2 (0.6)	2.4 (1.2)	2.8 (1.5)	2.2 (1.1)	1.6 (1.5)	1.4 (1.2)	0.3 (0.7)	7.4 (2.8)	10.9 (3.7)
Vitamin E, mg	0.1 (0.4)	1.0 (0.6)	1.8 (1.0)	1.1 (0.7)	1.3 (0.8)	0.9 (0.9)	0.3 (0.6)	3.9 (1.5)	6.5 (2.1)
Thiamine, mg	0.02 (0.04)	0.10 (0.05)	0.27 (0.14)	0.11 (0.05)	0.20 (0.12)	0.12 (0.08)	0.03 (0.06)	0.47 (0.17)	0.84 (0.22)
Riboflavin, mg	0.04 (0.10)	0.29 (0.13)	0.39 (0.15)	0.30 (0.14)	0.37 (0.22)	0.28 (0.19)	0.07 (0.13)	0.98 (0.33)	1.74 (0.51)
Niacin eq., mg	0.4 (0.9)	2.5 (1.1)	5.5 (2.8)	2.4 (1.0)	5.6 (2.9)	2.5 (1.6)	0.7 (1.2)	10.4 (3.6)	19.5 (4.8)
Vitamin B6, mg	0.0 (0.1)	0.1 (0.1)	0.3 (0.2)	0.2 (0.1)	0.3 (0.1)	0.2 (0.2)	0.1 (0.1)	0.6 (0.2)	1.2 (0.3)
Folate, µg	4 (9)	21 (11)	42 (19)	24 (11)	34 (37)	23 (17)	7 (12)	87 (29)	154 (55)
Vitamin B12, µg	0.1 (0.2)	0.6 (0.3)	1.1 (0.7)	0.6 (0.3)	1.5 (2.5)	0.6 (0.9)	0.1 (0.3)	2.3 (1.0)	4.5 (2.9)
Vitamin C, mg	2 (6)	8 (9)	14 (9)	12 (18)	14 (15)	11 (14)	5 (11)	33 (23)	65 (35)
Salt, g	0.1 (0.2)	1.0 (0.5)	1.6 (0.7)	0.6 (0.3)	1.3 (0.7)	0.6 (0.4)	0.2 (0.3)	3.2 (1.1)	5.3 (1.4)
Potassium, mg	62 (130)	338 (126)	813 (332)	371 (152)	583 (303)	373 (211)	117 (177)	1521 (462)	2656 (610)
Phosphorous, g	26 (62)	198 (79)	291 (103)	194 (84)	250 (124)	181 (114)	46 (79)	684 (197)	1187 (281)
Calcium, mg	26 (67)	178 (80)	206 (90)	190 (94)	186 (116)	179 (129)	44 (87)	573 (197)	1007 (306)
Magnesium, mg	6 (14)	42 (17)	65 (22)	39 (17)	47 (23)	38 (23)	12 (18)	147 (41)	250 (54)
Iron, mg	0.2 (0.5)	1.2 (0.6)	1.9 (0.8)	0.9 (0.5)	1.7 (1.1)	1.1 (0.8)	0.3 (0.5)	4.1 (1.4)	7.3 (2.0)
Zinc, mg	0.2 (0.5)	1.2 (0.6)	2.1 (0.9)	1.2 (0.6)	2.0 (1.0)	1.2 (0.8)	0.3 (0.5)	4.5 (1.5)	8.1 (2.0)
Iodine, µg	3 (10)	40 (19)	47 (27)	27 (14)	46 (25)	26 (18)	6 (12)	114 (43)	195 (57)
Energy, %	2	14	24	16	21	16	7	54	100
Protein, %	2	13	27	14	27	13	4	54	100
Carbohydrates, %	3	15	22	18	16	18	8	55	100
Sucrose, %	4	8	8	25	10	26	19	41	100
Added sugar, %	4	7	4	28	9	27	22	39	100
Fiber, %	3	19	25	17	14	18	6	60	100
Fat, %	2	12	27	14	24	15	6	53	100
SAFA, %	2	11	24	14	25	17	8	49	100
MUFA, %	2	12	29	14	25	13	6	55	100
PUFA, %	2	15	30	16	20	12	5	61	100
Vitamin A, %	2	12	23	16	31	12	4	51	100
Vitamin D, %	2	22	25	20	15	13	3	68	100
Vitamin E, %	2	15	28	17	20	13	5	60	100
Thiamine, %	2	12	32	13	24	14	4	56	100
Riboflavin, %	2	17	22	17	21	16	4	56	100
Niacin eq., %	2	13	28	12	29	13	3	53	100
Vitamin B6, %	3	12	28	13	23	16	5	52	100
Folate, %	2	14	27	15	22	15	4	56	100
Vitamin B12, %	2	13	25	13	33	13	3	50	100
Vitamin C, %	3	12	21	18	21	18	7	50	100
Salt, %	1	20	29	11	24	11	3	60	100
Potassium, %	2	13	31	14	22	14	4	57	100
Phosphorous, %	2	17	25	16	21	15	4	58	100
Calcium, %	3	18	20	19	18	18	4	57	100
Magnesium, %	2	17	26	16	19	15	5	59	100
Iron, %	2	16	27	13	23	15	4	56	100
Zinc, %	2	15	26	14	24	14	4	56	100
Iodine, %	2	21	24	14	23	13	3	58	100

eq., equivalents; MUFA, monounsaturated fatty acids; PUFA, polyunsaturated fatty acids; RAE, retinol activity equivalents; SAFA, saturated fatty acids.

Table 5. Mean (SD) intake and population proportion [24] of energy and nutrients on weekdays among 5 to 6-year-old children who eat three meals at preschool (n = 233). Each child had data for 1 to 4 days; the total number of days was 405.

	Breakfast, Outside Preschool	Breakfast, Preschool	Lunch, Preschool	Afternoon Snack, Preschool	Dinner, Outside Preschool	Evening Snack, Outside Preschool	Other Snack, Outside Preschool	Preschool Food, Total	Total, per Day
% of days that included the meal	27	100	100	100	95	88	50		
Energy, MJ	0.17 (0.35)	0.85 (0.28)	1.58 (0.61)	1.03 (0.42)	1.34 (0.65)	0.93 (0.54)	0.47 (0.58)	3.46 (0.94)	6.37 (1.25)
Protein, g	1 (3)	8 (3)	18 (8)	9 (4)	17 (9)	8 (5)	2 (4)	35 (11)	64 (16)
Carbohydrates, g	6 (10)	27 (10)	40 (14)	33 (15)	31 (17)	29 (18)	17 (22)	99 (27)	182 (42)
Sucrose, g	2 (4)	2 (3)	3 (3)	8 (7)	3 (5)	7 (6)	7 (11)	13 (9)	32 (17)
Added sugar, g	1 (4)	1 (3)	2 (3)	7 (7)	3 (6)	5 (6)	7 (13)	10 (9)	27 (19)
Fiber, g	0.5 (0.9)	3.2 (1.7)	4.2 (1.7)	2.7 (1.4)	2.3 (1.5)	2.9 (2.3)	1.0 (1.5)	10.1 (3.4)	16.7 (4.7)
Fat, g	1 (4)	6 (3)	15 (7)	8 (4)	13 (8)	7 (6)	3 (6)	29 (10)	54 (14)
SAFA, g	0.5 (1.7)	1.9 (1.3)	4.8 (2.5)	3.0 (2.0)	4.8 (3.4)	3.0 (2.6)	1.4 (2.4)	9.8 (4.0)	19.5 (6.2)
MUFA, g	0.4 (1.2)	2.1 (1.3)	5.6 (2.9)	2.8 (1.7)	4.8 (3.1)	2.0 (1.9)	1.1 (2.0)	10.5 (4)	18.8 (5.3)
PUFA, g	0.2 (0.6)	1.2 (0.8)	3.0 (1.8)	1.5 (0.9)	2.0 (1.6)	1.0 (1.1)	0.5 (1.0)	5.7 (2.4)	9.4 (3.1)
Vitamin A, μg RAE	9 (26)	73 (54)	212 (289)	105 (87)	167 (584)	73 (123)	20 (44)	389 (315)	659 (654)
Vitamin D, μg	0.2 (0.7)	2.5 (1.2)	3.1 (2.4)	2.6 (1.3)	1.9 (1.9)	1.5 (1.3)	0.3 (0.7)	8.2 (3.7)	12.1 (4.7)
Vitamin E, mg	0.2 (0.5)	1.0 (0.6)	2.2 (1.4)	1.3 (0.6)	1.5 (1.2)	0.9 (0.9)	0.4 (0.6)	4.5 (1.8)	7.5 (2.4)
Thiamine, mg	0.02 (0.06)	0.11 (0.06)	0.30 (0.17)	0.12 (0.05)	0.23 (0.14)	0.13 (0.10)	0.04 (0.06)	0.53 (0.21)	0.95 (0.28)
Riboflavin, mg	0.05 (0.11)	0.31 (0.14)	0.45 (0.19)	0.34 (0.15)	0.40 (0.27)	0.30 (0.21)	0.08 (0.13)	1.10 (0.37)	1.93 (0.59)
Niacin eq., mg	0.5 (1.3)	2.8 (1.1)	6.2 (3.5)	2.7 (1.2)	6.2 (3.2)	2.8 (1.9)	0.8 (1.3)	11.7 (4.3)	22.0 (6.3)
Vitamin B6, mg	0.0 (0.1)	0.2 (0.1)	0.4 (0.2)	0.2 (0.1)	0.3 (0.2)	0.2 (0.2)	0.1 (0.2)	0.7 (0.3)	1.3 (0.4)
Folate, μg	5 (10)	24 (14)	51 (39)	25 (11)	35 (43)	26 (18)	8 (11)	100 (48)	174 (67)
Vitamin B12, μg	0.1 (0.3)	0.6 (0.4)	1.3 (1.1)	0.7 (0.3)	1.5 (2.9)	0.6 (0.4)	0.1 (0.3)	2.5 (1.3)	4.8 (3.4)
Vitamin C, mg	3 (10)	9 (11)	16 (9)	11 (9)	14 (13)	15 (20)	7 (14)	35 (19)	74 (38)
Salt, g	0.1 (0.4)	1.2 (0.5)	1.8 (0.8)	0.7 (0.3)	1.4 (0.7)	0.7 (0.5)	0.2 (0.3)	3.6 (1.2)	6.0 (1.6)
Potassium, mg	74 (155)	381 (148)	935 (399)	410 (167)	661 (345)	403 (264)	136 (188)	1726 (557)	2999 (797)
Phosphorous, mg	32 (78)	217 (80)	333 (135)	217 (95)	280 (148)	196 (130)	50 (78)	767 (231)	1326 (347)
Calcium, mg	29 (74)	189 (89)	232 (100)	211 (114)	210 (142)	192 (141)	49 (85)	632 (228)	1113 (358)
Magnesium, mg	7 (14)	47 (17)	74 (28)	43 (18)	52 (26)	40 (28)	14 (19)	164 (46)	278 (65)
Iron, mg	0.2 (0.4)	1 3 (0.7)	2.2 (1.1)	1.0 (0.5)	1.9 (1.5)	1.1 (0.8)	0.4 (0.6)	4.6 (1.6)	8.2 (2.4)
Zinc, mg	0.2 (0.5)	1.4 (0.6)	2.4 (1.2)	1.3 (0.6)	2.3 (1.3)	1.3 (0.8)	0.3 (0.5)	5.0 (1.8)	9.1 (2.5)
Iodine, μg	5 (12)	45 (19)	53 (34)	31 (14)	52 (31)	28 (21)	7 (12)	128 (48)	220 (69)
Energy, %	3	13	25	16	21	15	7	54	100
Protein, %	2	13	28	14	27	13	4	55	100
Carbohydrates, %	3	15	22	18	17	16	9	54	100
Sucrose, %	5	7	9	24	11	22	22	39	100
Added sugar, %	5	6	6	26	10	21	27	37	100
Fiber, %	3	19	25	16	13	17	6	61	100
Fat, %	2	11	28	15	25	13	6	54	100
SAFA, %	3	10	25	15	25	15	7	50	100
MUFA, %	2	11	30	15	26	11	6	56	100
PUFA, %	2	13	32	16	21	10	5	61	100
Vitamin A, %	1	11	32	16	25	11	3	59	100
Vitamin D, %	2	20	26	21	16	12	2	68	100
Vitamin E, %	2	14	29	17	20	12	5	60	100
Thiamine, %	2	12	31	12	24	14	4	56	100
Riboflavin, %	3	16	23	17	21	16	4	57	100
Niacin eq., %	2	13	28	12	28	13	4	53	100
Vitamin B6, %	3	12	28	13	23	14	7	53	100
Folate, %	3	14	29	14	20	15	5	58	100
Vitamin B12, %	2	13	26	14	31	12	2	53	100
Vitamin C, %	5	12	21	14	19	20	9	48	100
Salt, %	2	19	29	12	23	11	3	60	100
Potassium, %	2	13	31	14	22	13	5	58	100
Phosphorous, %	2	16	25	16	21	15	4	58	100
Calcium, %	3	17	21	19	19	17	4	57	100
Magnesium, %	3	17	27	15	19	15	5	59	100
Iron, %	2	16	27	13	23	13	5	56	100
Zinc, %	2	15	26	14	25	14	4	55	100
Iodine, %	2	20	24	14	24	13	3	58	100

eq., equivalents; MUFA, monounsaturated fatty acids; PUFA, polyunsaturated fatty acids; RAE, retinol activity equivalents; SAFA, saturated fatty acids.

The mean proportions of energy from protein and saturated fatty acids in preschool meals were above those recommended for ECEC food services (Table 6). The different food groups are presented as sources of energy and nutrients in Supplementary Tables S3–S58. The main sources of energy were cereals and bakery products, milk and dairy products, and meat and meat dishes in both age groups, both at and outside preschool (Supplementary Tables S3 and S4). Lunch and dinner accounted for most of the protein and fat in the children's diet (Tables 4 and 5). Milk and dairy products, meat and meat dishes, and cereals and bakery products were the greatest sources of protein both at home and at preschool (Supplementary Tables S5 and S6). The 'margarine and fat spread' sub-group was the most important source of mono- and polyunsaturated fatty acids, but also of saturated fatty acids during preschool hours (Supplementary Tables S17–S22). The proportion of saturated fat from milk and dairy products was lower at preschool than outside preschool (Supplementary Tables S17 and S18). On average, dinner and lunch were the meals that contributed the highest amounts of saturated fatty acids.

The mean daily intake of fiber was 15.3 g and 16.7 g among the three- to four-year-olds and five- to six-year-olds, respectively. Of this, more than a third was contributed by cereals and bakery products consumed at preschool (Supplementary Tables S13 and S14). The mean percentage of energy from added sugar on Monday to Friday was 6.2 E% in the younger and 7.0 E% in the older age group (Table 6). Most of the sucrose and added sugar intake was outside preschool (Tables 4 and 5). The meals accounting for the most added sugar intake on weekdays were the afternoon snack at preschool, evening snack, and other snacks outside preschool. The main source of added sugar at preschool was fruit and berry soups (Supplementary Tables S11 and S12), which were eaten at the afternoon snack and breakfast. However, the mean percentage of energy from added sugar at preschool was only 4–5 E% (Table 6).

Table 6. Energy-yielding nutrient intakes [mean, (SD)] during preschool hours and the whole day (Monday to Friday) of children who eat three meals at preschool.

	Finnish Recommendation for Served Preschool Meals	3- to 4-Year-Olds (*n* = 324) Preschool	Total	5- to 6-Year-Olds (*n* = 233) Preschool	Total
Carbohydrates, E%	45–60	49 (6)	49 (5)	49 (5)	49 (5)
Sucrose, E%		6.1 (4)	8.1 (3.8)	6.2 (3.9)	8.5 (4.1)
Added sugar, E%	<10	4.5 (3.6)	6.2 (3.5)	4.8 (3.8)	7.0 (4.6)
Protein, E%	10–15	17 (3)	17 (2)	17 (3)	17 (3)
Fat, E%	30–40	30 (7)	31 (5)	31 (6)	31 (5)
Saturated fatty acids, E%	<10	10.1 (2.8)	11.4 (2.4)	10.3 (2.6)	11.3 (2.6)
Monounsaturated fatty acids, E%		11.0 (2.8)	10.9 (2.1)	11.1 (2.5)	10.9 (2.1)
Polyunsaturated fatty acids, E%		6.0 (1.8)	5.3 (1.3)	6.1 (1.7)	5.4 (1.4)
Fiber g/MJ		3.0 (0.8)	2.7 (0.7)	3.0 (0.7)	2.7 (0.7)

E%, percentage of the total energy.

3.3. Micronutrients

Preschool food was an important source of vitamins D and E ($\geq$60% of total intake in both age groups; Tables 4 and 5). Vitamin D fortified milk and margarine and fat spread were the main sources of vitamin D (Supplementary Tables S25 and S26). The sub-group 'margarine and fat spread' was the main source of vitamins A and E in preschool (Supplementary Tables S23, S24, S27, and S28). Calcium intake was distributed evenly between the five main meals of the day (Tables 4 and 5) and milk was its main source (Supplementary Tables S49 and S50). Milk was also the most important source of riboflavin (Supplementary Tables S31 and S32) and iodine (Supplementary Tables S57 and S58). Folate came from a large variety of food groups in the diet, but at preschool, breads other than white bread were important sources (Supplementary Tables S37 and S38). Fresh fruit was a more important source of vitamin C at home than at preschool (Supplementary Tables S41 and S42). Preschool food contributed 60% to the total salt intake in both age groups; the mean salt intake at preschool was 3.2 and 3.6 g/day in the younger and older age group, respectively (Tables 4 and 5). Meat and meat dishes, and cereals and bakery products were especially significant sources of salt (Supplementary Tables S43 and S44).

4. Discussion

We investigated the contribution of preschool meals to the weekdays' total energy and nutrient intake among Finnish preschoolers who eat three meals at preschool. We also examined the amounts of the foods consumed and the food sources of nutrients during preschool and outside preschool hours. We found that preschool meals contributed significant shares of some of the food groups that are considered part of a health-promoting diet [16] (fish, fat-free dairy, whole-grain products, and vegetable-oil-based spreadable fats). Preschool meals were also low in sugary foods. Preschool food provided on average 54% of the total energy on a weekday, and $\geq$60% of the total fiber, polyunsaturated fatty acids, and vitamins D and E. Salt intake was too high overall, and 60% of salt came from preschool food.

The results show that the most typical meal pattern of a Finnish preschool child consists of five meals per day: breakfast, lunch, afternoon snack, dinner, and evening snack. Small snacking also occurred outside these meals. Although lunch and dinner were the main meals, more than half of the total daily energy was consumed during the other meals. In a study of Dutch children, lunch and dinner together had a higher share of total energy than that in our study and other meals accounted for about 44% of the daily energy [8]. In our study, each of the three smaller meals (breakfast at preschool, afternoon snack at preschool and evening snack outside preschool) provided a similar share of energy. Common anecdotes on the importance of breakfast should not obscure the fact that based on energy intake, afternoon and evening snacks are as important as breakfast in the diet of Finnish preschoolers. Thus, breakfast, afternoon snack, and evening snack deserve equal attention regarding healthy food choices.

In our study, the total daily energy intake on weekdays for three- to four-year-olds was 5.6 MJ, which is comparable with the results of Goldbohm et al. [26] in the Netherlands, in which the mean daily total energy intake for three-year-old children attending day care was 5.8 MJ. We found that preschool meals did not cover two thirds of the daily energy, which is the target level set in the Finnish recommendation for ECEC food services [15]. The distribution of energy between day care and home among three-year-old children in the Netherlands was similar to that in our findings; their energy intake in day care was about 3.0 MJ/d and the daily total 5.9 MJ [8].

The distribution of the consumption of fish between home and ECEC has seldom been reported. Lehtisalo et al. [10] found more consumers of fish among Finnish children who attended ECEC than among children taken care of at home. In our study, the consumption of fish dishes at preschool was about twice that consumed at home. Our results concerning fresh fruit consumption contradict those of previous studies in the Netherlands [8] and Oklahoma, USA [9], which found higher consumption in ECEC than at home. Overall, there is room to increase fruit intake at Finnish preschools.

Our study supports previous findings that more low-fat dairy products [9,10] and more vegetable oil-based spreadable fats [10] are consumed in ECEC than at home. Despite this positive finding, the mean proportion of energy from saturated fatty acids exceeded the recommendation for ECEC food services (<10 E%). Meat and meat dishes, along with spreadable fats, were important sources of saturated fatty acids. An increased amount of vegetarian main courses, if well accepted by the children and if prepared without ingredients high in saturated fatty acids such as cheese, might be one strategy to improve the fatty acid profile as well as to increase vegetable consumption at preschools. However, it should be noted that about half of the saturated fatty acid intake (but less than half of the energy intake) occurred outside preschool.

Bread consumption (largely as whole-grain bread) and along with it, also margarine/fat spread consumption, were relatively high at preschool. This combination provided large shares of nutrients such as fiber; folate; unsaturated fatty acids; and vitamins A, D, and E. On the other hand, bread with margarine/fat spread also contributed significantly to the saturated fatty acid and salt intakes, both of which should be reduced. Margarines with 60% fat content generally contain 16–18 g of saturated fatty acids/100 g [27] and the development of products with an even lower saturated fatty acid content could be useful in reducing the saturated fatty acid intake. Since flour is not fortified in Finland, white bread was not a relevant source of total folate (including folic acid).

We found that protein intake was higher at preschool than recommended, and milk and dairy products and meat and meat dishes were important sources of protein. Finnish food-based dietary guidelines state that over the day, 4 dL of fluid milk products (e.g., milk, sourmilk, yogurt, Finnish cultured milk) and one slice of cheese is enough for preschool-aged children [16]. Our results show that on average, this is exceeded on weekdays. It might be possible to adjust the protein content and type (animal vs. plant protein) of preschool meals by reducing the amount of milk and adding more vegetarian dishes to the menu.

In our study, the percentage of energy from added sugar at preschool was well within the limits of the recommendation (<10 E%) [15]. Strategies to limit the use of added sugar in the food services at the participating preschools included, for example, sweetening plain yogurt with only fruit and berry purees. The main sources of added sugar outside preschool were sugar-sweetened dairy products, beverages, bakery products, and sweets and chocolate. At preschool, a considerably smaller amount of added sugar came from these food groups. In contrast to our results, some previous studies have found that sweet snacks are more often consumed in ECEC than at home [8,11]. When interpreting the results of our study, it is important to note that we did not include weekend days, which are likely to include more sugary products, in the analysis. We found that the mean density of fiber was 3 g/MJ at preschool in both age groups. In the Netherlands, three-year-olds on average ate a total of 13 g of fiber per day, of which 7.2 g was at day care [8], which is slightly lower than in our sample.

The total daily salt intake of two- to ten-year-old children should not exceed 3 to 4 g/day [16] and the intake at preschool should not exceed 2 to 2.6 g/day [15]. We found that the mean salt intake on weekdays far exceeded these recommendations. In Belgium, the total sodium intake of preschool children also greatly exceeded the acceptable range [28]. In Portugal, children eating preschool meals had a total intake of salt of about 6.3 g/day [29]. In our study, cereals and bakery products were the main source of salt at preschool. Meat and meat dishes were also an important source of salt both at and outside preschool. Preschool food services should reduce the sodium content in their porridge and main course recipes, and offer low-sodium bread.

A limitation of the study was the low participation rate in the DAGIS cross-sectional survey (24%) and the fact that the strict inclusion criteria further limited the sample used in the analyses for this paper. The data also includes siblings, meaning that when means were calculated, some families had a larger representation than others. The estimate of salt intake at home may be more prone to bias than that at preschool due to the fact that in the home dishes, salt content estimates were based on typical Finnish recipes in the database, whereas at preschool, the salt content of the dishes was, for most municipalities, based on recipes provided by the food services. A strength of this study was its comparatively large sample. Its methodological strengths included the use of a picture book that was specifically designed for use in children's portion size estimation. This has been used with similar accuracy by parents and ECEC personnel in a validity study [20]. Detailed information on the recipes and products used at preschools further aided the careful analysis of the diet.

Meal planning in ECEC food services may have an important influence on the formation of dietary habits and long-term effects on the health of children. Only a few previous studies have examined how different meals at ECEC and at home contribute to the diets of children. Although our study was a single-time cross-sectional study, the results are useful for the purposes of nutritional education, communication, and policy target setting for further developing the dietary quality of preschool meals. A long-term monitoring system of the actual dietary intake at preschools in Finland would be even more effective. As Lucas et al. [30] point out, such monitoring would allow the evaluation of how changes in policy and guidance actually affect children's intakes. As an example, possible changes in milk consumption should be accompanied by an analysis of their effects on the overall diet, as milk is an important source of a variety of nutrients in Finnish children's diets.

5. Conclusions

Finland provides preschool meals free of charge and the law requires the served food to be healthy. We found that Finnish children who attend full-time care eat preschool meals that contribute significant shares of favorable food groups and nutrients to their total weekday diet. Salt intake, however, was high at preschool and exceeded the recommendation. Thus, tackling salt intake is an important goal for guidance. In addition, fruit consumption and vegetarian food consumption at preschool could be increased. The intake of protein and saturated fatty acids also needs to be monitored.

Supplementary Materials: The following are available online at http://www.mdpi.com/2072-6643/11/7/1531/s1: Tables S1 and S2: Mean (SD) intake and population proportion of energy and nutrients on weekdays among 3- to 4-year-old/5- to 6-year-old children who eat three meals at preschool. Results for days when the child ate the meal. Tables S3–S58: Sources of energy and nutrients (mean and population proportion) in the diet on weekdays among Finnish 3- to 4-year-old/5- to 6-year-old preschool children who eat three meals at preschool. Main food groups and selected food groups are presented.

Author Contributions: Conceptualization, L.K. (Liisa Korkalo) and K.N.; Methodology, L.K. (Liisa Korkalo), E.S., K.N., H.V., M.E., R.L., R.K.; Formal analysis, L.K. (Liisa Korkalo); Investigation, E.S., H.V., K.N., R.L., R.K., and L.K. (Liisa Korkalo); Data curation, L.K. (Liisa Korkalo), E.S., R.L., H.V., K.N., and R.K. Writing—original draft preparation, L.K. (Liisa Korkalo) and K.N.; Writing—review and editing, E.S, H.V., R.L., E.R., L.K. (Leena Koivusilta), R.K., N.S. and M.E.; Supervision, M.E., L.K. (Leena Koivusilta), and E.R.; Funding acquisition, M.E., N.S., K.N., and E.R.

Funding: This study was funded by the Folkhälsan Research Center, the University of Helsinki, the Ministry of Education and Culture in Finland, the Ministry of Social Affairs and Health, the Academy of Finland (Grants: 285439, 287288, 288038, 315817), the Juho Vainio Foundation, the Signe and Ane Gyllenberg Foundation, the Finnish Cultural Foundation/South Ostrobothnia Regional Fund, the Päivikki and Sakari Sohlberg foundation, the Medicinska Föreningen Liv och Hälsa, the Finnish Foundation for Nutrition Research, and Finnish Food Research Foundation.

Acknowledgments: The authors thank the preschools and their personnel, as well as the families for their participation in the DAGIS study. We also thank the staff for collecting the data.

Conflicts of Interest: Liisa Korkalo is a board member of the company TwoDads. The authors declare no other conflict of interest.

References

1. Mikkilä, V.; Räsänen, L.; Raitakari, O.; Pietinen, P.; Viikari, J. Consistent dietary patterns identified from childhood to adulthood: The cardiovascular risk in Young Finns Study. *Br. J. Nutr.* **2005**, *93*, 923–931. [CrossRef] [PubMed]
2. Craigie, A.M.; Lake, A.A.; Kelly, S.A.; Adamson, A.J.; Mathers, J.C. Tracking of obesity-related behaviours from childhood to adulthood: A systematic review. *Maturitas* **2011**, *70*, 266–284. [CrossRef] [PubMed]
3. Daniels, S.R.; Arnett, D.K.; Eckel, R.H.; Gidding, S.S.; Hayman, L.L.; Kumanyika, S.; Robinson, T.N.; Scott, B.J.; St Jeor, S.; Williams, C.L. Overweight in children and adolescents: Pathophysiology, consequences, prevention, and treatment. *Circulation* **2005**, *111*, 1999–2012. [CrossRef] [PubMed]
4. Kaikkonen, J.E.; Mikkilä, V.; Raitakari, O.T. Role of childhood food patterns on adult cardiovascular disease risk. *Curr. Atheroscler. Rep.* **2014**, *16*, 443. [CrossRef] [PubMed]
5. Briley, M.E.; Jastrow, S.; Vickers, J.; Roberts-Gray, C. Dietary intake at child-care centers and away: Are parents and care providers working as partners or at cross-purposes? *J. Am. Diet. Assoc.* **1999**, *99*, 950–954. [CrossRef]
6. Sepp, H.; Lennernäs, M.; Pettersson, R.; Abrahamsson, L. Children's nutrient intake at preschool and at home. *Acta Paediatr.* **2001**, *90*, 483–491. [CrossRef] [PubMed]
7. Padget, A.; Briley, M.E. Dietary intakes at child-care centers in central Texas fail to meet Food Guide Pyramid recommendations. *J. Am. Diet. Assoc.* **2005**, *105*, 790–793. [CrossRef] [PubMed]
8. Gubbels, J.; Raaijmakers, L.; Gerards, S.; Kremers, S. Dietary intake by Dutch 1-to 3-year-old children at childcare and at home. *Nutrients* **2014**, *6*, 304–318. [CrossRef] [PubMed]
9. Sisson, S.B.; Kiger, A.C.; Anundson, K.C.; Rasbold, A.H.; Krampe, M.; Campbell, J.; DeGrace, B.; Hoffman, L. Differences in preschool-age children's dietary intake between meals consumed at childcare and at home. *Prev. Med. Rep.* **2017**, *6*, 33–37. [CrossRef] [PubMed]
10. Lehtisalo, J.; Erkkola, M.; Tapanainen, H.; Kronberg-Kippilä, C.; Veijola, R.; Knip, M.; Virtanen, S.M. Food consumption and nutrient intake in day care and at home in 3-year-old Finnish children. *Public Health Nutr.* **2010**, *13*, 957–964. [CrossRef] [PubMed]
11. Ziegler, P.; Briefel, R.; Ponza, M.; Novak, T.; Hendricks, K. Nutrient intakes and food patterns of toddlers' lunches and snacks: Influence of location. *J. Am. Diet. Assoc.* **2006**, *106*, S124–S134. [CrossRef] [PubMed]

12. National Institute of Health and Welfare. Tilastoraportti (Statistics Report) 32/2018. Varhaiskasvatus (Early Education) 2017. 2018. Available online: http://urn.fi/URN:NBN:fi-fe2018100937865 (accessed on 23 May 2019).
13. Act on Early Childhood Education and Care (540/2018). Available online: https://www.finlex.fi/fi/laki/ajantasa/2018/20180540 (accessed on 23 May 2019).
14. Finnish National Board of Education Regulation. National Core Curriculum for Early Childhood Education and Care. 2016. Available online: https://www.ellibs.com/fi/book/9789521363290/national-corecurriculum-for-early-childhood-education-and-care-2016 (accessed on 23 May 2019).
15. National Nutrition Council. *Health and Joy from Food—Meal Recommendations for Early Childhood Education and Care*; National Institute for Health and Welfare: Helsinki, Finland, 2018. Available online: http://urn.fi/URN:ISBN:978-952-343-033-4 (accessed on 23 May 2019).
16. National Nutrition Council. *Eating Together—Food Recommendations for Families with Children*; National Institute for Health and Welfare: Helsinki, Finland, 2016. Available online: http://urn.fi/URN:ISBN:978-952-302-626-1 (accessed on 23 May 2019).
17. Hasunen, K.; Kalavainen, M.; Keinonen, H.; Lagström, H.; Lyytikäinen, A.; Nurttila, A.; Peltola, T.; Talvia, S. *Lapsi, perhe ja ruoka. Nutrition recommendations for infants and young children*; Ministry of Social Affairs and Health: Helsinki, Finland, 2004. Available online: http://julkaisut.valtioneuvosto.fi/handle/10024/70144 (accessed on 23 May 2019).
18. Lehto, E.; Ray, C.; Vepsäläinen, H.; Korkalo, L.; Lehto, R.; Kaukonen, R.; Suhonen, E.; Nislin, M.; Nissinen, K.; Skaffari, E.; et al. Increased Health and Wellbeing in Preschools (DAGIS) Study—Differences in Children's Energy Balance-Related Behaviors (EBRBs) and in Long-Term Stress by Parental Educational Level. *Int. J. Environ. Res. Public Health* **2018**, *15*, E2313. [CrossRef] [PubMed]
19. Cole, T.J.; Lobstein, T. Extended international (IOTF) body mass index cut-offs for thinness, overweight and obesity. *Pediatr. Obes.* **2012**, *7*, 284–294. [CrossRef] [PubMed]
20. Nissinen, K.; Korkalo, L.; Vepsäläinen, H.; Mäkiranta, P.; Koivusilta, L.; Roos, E.; Erkkola, M. Accuracy in the estimation of children's food portion sizes against a food picture book by parents and early educators. *J. Nutr. Sci.* **2018**, *7*, e35. [CrossRef] [PubMed]
21. Nissinen, K.; Sillanpää, H.; Korkalo, L.; Roos, E.; Erkkola, M. *Annoskuvakirja Lasten Ruokamäärien Arvioinnin Avuksi (The Children's Food Picture Book)*; Helsingin Yliopisto, Seinäjoen Ammattikorkeakoulu, Samfundet Folkhälsan: Helsinki, Finland; Seinäjoki, Finland, 2015. Available online: http://rty.fi/wp-content/uploads/2013/09/annoskuvakirja.pdf (accessed on 23 May 2019).
22. Vásquez-Caicedo, A.; Bell, S.; Hartmann, B. Report on Collection of Rules on Use of Recipe Calculation Procedures including the Use of Yield and Retention Factors for Imputing Nutrient Values for Composite Foods. Available online: http://www.webcitation.org/78Kr2gJr7 (accessed on 23 May 2019).
23. Lehto, R.; Ray, C.; Vepsäläinen, H.; Korkalo, L.; Nissinen, K.; Skaffari, E.; Määttä, S.; Roos, E.; Erkkola, M. Early educators' practices and opinions in relation to pre-schoolers' dietary intake at pre-school: Case Finland. *Public Health Nutr.* **2019**, *22*, 1567–1575. [CrossRef] [PubMed]
24. Krebs-Smith, S.; Kott, P.; Guenther, P. Mean proportion and population proportion: Two answers to the same question? *J. Am. Diet. Assoc.* **1989**, *89*, 671–676. [PubMed]
25. REGULATION (EU) No 1308/2013 OF THE EUROPEAN PARLIAMENT AND OF THE COUNCIL of 17 December 2013 Establishing a Common Organisation of the Markets in Agricultural Products and Repealing Council Regulations (EEC) No 922/72, (EEC) No 234/79, (EC) No 1037/2001 and (EC) No 1234/2007. Available online: https://eur-lex.europa.eu/legal-content/EN/TXT/PDF/?uri=CELEX:32013R1308&rid=1 (accessed on 23 May 2019).
26. Goldbohm, R.; Rubingh, C.; Lanting, C.; Joosten, K. Food consumption and nutrient intake by children aged 10 to 48 months attending day care in the Netherlands. *Nutrients* **2016**, *8*, 428. [CrossRef] [PubMed]
27. National Institute for Health and Welfare. Fineli Food Composition Database. Available online: https://fineli.fi (accessed on 23 May 2019).
28. Huybrechts, I.; De Henauw, S. Energy and nutrient intakes by pre-school children in Flanders-Belgium. *Br. J. Nutr.* **2007**, *98*, 600–610. [CrossRef] [PubMed]

29. Moreira, T.; Severo, M.; Oliveira, A.; Ramos, E.; Rodrigues, S.; Lopes, C. Eating out of home and dietary adequacy in preschool children. *Br. J. Nutr.* **2015**, *114*, 297–305. [CrossRef] [PubMed]
30. Lucas, P.; Patterson, E.; Sacks, G.; Billich, N.; Evans, C. Preschool and school meal policies: An overview of what we know about regulation, implementation, and impact on diet in the UK, Sweden, and Australia. *Nutrients* **2017**, *9*, 736. [CrossRef] [PubMed]

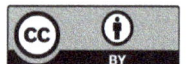

© 2019 by the authors. Licensee MDPI, Basel, Switzerland. This article is an open access article distributed under the terms and conditions of the Creative Commons Attribution (CC BY) license (http://creativecommons.org/licenses/by/4.0/).

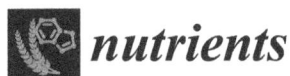

Article

Fruit, Vegetable, and Fibre Intake among Finnish Preschoolers in Relation to Preschool-Level Facilitators and Barriers to Healthy Nutrition

Reetta Lehto [1,2,*], Carola Ray [1,2], Liisa Korkalo [2], Henna Vepsäläinen [2], Kaija Nissinen [3], Leena Koivusilta [4], Eva Roos [1,2,5] and Maijaliisa Erkkola [2]

1. Folkhälsan Research Center, Topeliuksenkatu 20, 00250 Helsinki, Finland
2. Department of Food and Nutrition, University of Helsinki, 00014 Helsinki, Finland
3. School of Food and Agriculture, Seinäjoki University of Applied Sciences, 60101 Seinäjoki, Finland
4. Department of Social Research, University of Turku, 20014 Turku, Finland
5. Department of Public Health, Clinicum, University of Helsinki, 00014 Helsinki, Finland
* Correspondence: reetta.lehto@folkhalsan.fi

Received: 24 May 2019; Accepted: 24 June 2019; Published: 27 June 2019

Abstract: Preschool is a major factor affecting food consumption among young children in Finland, given that most preschoolers eat three meals a day in that setting. Thus, it is important to recognise the determinants of dietary intake at preschool. The aim of this study was to examine food-related factors at the preschool and manager level, and their association with the dietary intake of children in childcare. The study was a part of the cross-sectional DAGIS survey conducted in 2015 to 2016 in Finland. The managers of 58 preschools filled in a questionnaire related to food and nutrition at their preschools. Preschool personnel kept food records for the children (n = 585) on two preschool days. Multilevel linear and logistic regression analyses were conducted with age, gender, and municipality as covariates, preschool-level factors as independent variables, and children's vegetable (g/day) and fruit (yes vs. no) consumption and fibre intake (g/MJ) as outcome variables. Having many written food policies in the preschool was associated with a higher intake of vegetables (p = 0.01) and fibre (p = 0.03) among the children. Having at least two out of three cooperation-related challenges with the catering service was associated with a higher intake of fibre (p = 0.03) and lower odds of eating fruit (p = 0.01). Factors that are relatively distal from meal situations may have an effect, and should be taken into account in the promotion of healthy eating at preschool, but more studies are needed.

Keywords: childcare; dietary intake; children; environmental influences; manager

1. Introduction

In Finland and other Western countries, the majority of children under school age attend formal childcare [1], from here on referred to as preschools, where most of them eat several meals a day. Thus, food intake at preschools constitutes a significant proportion of the children's total dietary intake, and may have an impact on the formation of eating habits [2]. Recognising the factors that contribute to dietary intake at preschool would be beneficial given the increased prevalence of obesity among children [3] and the consequent need to promote a healthy diet at a young age.

According to socio-ecological models, the environment (in addition to personal characteristics) affects an individual's health behaviour on several levels [4] representing environmental factors ranging from the immediate surroundings, such as home, to more distal levels, such as the organisational and societal level. Each level has its various physical, social, and political factors. Preschool could be seen as one level that affects children's health behaviour. There has been an increasing amount of research on the preschool environment and children's food intake in recent years. Most of the factors under study relate directly to meal times, such as the (un)healthiness of the food served [5–7] and, to some extent, the feeding practices of the personnel [8–11]. Less attention has been given to other preschool-level factors that are more distal from meal times. These factors could be characterised as political (e.g., preschool-level rules and policies concerning food), sociocultural (preschool-level practices including the personnel's knowledge about nutrition), physical (such as whether the food is cooked on the premises), and managerial (e.g., the manager's perceptions and attitudes).

Associations have been found linking food-related policies and regulations with the food and beverages served in childcare establishments [12], as well as with children's dietary intake [13]. It appears that, in the US, healthier food is served to children in childcare centres that participate in the Child and Adult Care Food Program (CACFP) [14,15], which are more heavily regulated by the state and receive reimbursement for serving healthier food. There has been some qualitative research on preschool managers' views about the barriers to and facilitators of healthy food intake and healthy energy-balance-related behaviour at preschool, but these studies did not examine any associations with the children's food intake [16]. According to Van de Kolk [16], Dutch preschool managers mentioned physical (e.g., food availability), sociocultural (e.g., the personnel's feeding practices), economic (e.g., food costs), and political (existing policies and guidelines) factors as both facilitators of and barriers inhibiting healthy eating among children. Studies in other settings also refer to the importance of the person in charge: In Canada, Olstad et al. [17] concluded in their study of managers in recreational sports settings that nutritional knowledge, attitudes, and perceptions shape their decisions and actions regarding the adoption and implementation of dietary guidelines.

Most preschools in Finland are municipal (public). All food is provided, and children are not allowed to bring their own food with them. Preschools provide three meals a day: Breakfast (often porridge), a warm meal at lunchtime, and an afternoon snack. There are national recommendations concerning dietary requirements and feeding practices [18,19], but these are not binding. The food is cooked either at the premises of municipal or private catering services (central kitchens) or in the preschool's own kitchen (following the same menu as other municipal preschools). Either the municipality or the private catering service from which it buys its preschool meals is responsible for planning the menus and purchasing the food. Although the municipalities play a major role when it comes to food availability and mealtime practices, preschool managers may also influence food-related practices and policies.

Our aim in this study was to examine the association between preschool-level factors and the dietary intake of children during preschool hours. We focused on the following preschool factors: Food policies, the manager's concern about the children's consumption of fruit and vegetables, the manager's perceived influence on the supply of fruit and vegetables, cooperation challenges with the catering service as perceived by the manager, the lack of resources, and kitchen type (whether the preschool kitchen is used for cooking or heating up food, or for distribution). The dietary factors we studied included the children's fruit and vegetable consumption and their fibre intake.

2. Materials and Methods

This study is part of the cross-sectional survey "Increased Health and Wellbeing in Preschools" (DAGIS) conducted in Finnish preschools in 2015–2016 [20,21]. The aim of the whole survey was to examine health behaviour and stress regulation among preschool children aged between three and six years in relation to socioeconomic status and both the home and the preschool environments. The study was conducted in accordance with the Declaration of Helsinki, and the protocol was approved by the Ethics Committee of the University of Helsinki Ethical Review Board in the Humanities and Social and Behavioural Sciences in February 2015 (#6/2015). The cross-sectional survey was conducted in eight municipalities in Southern and Western Finland. A total of 169 municipal preschools were invited to participate. The eligibility criteria were: (a) The language of the preschool must be Finnish or Swedish; (b) it must be public (municipal), or the municipality should purchase early-education services from it; (c) it should function only during the daytime (excluding 24-hour preschools); (d) like all municipal preschools, it should charge income-dependent fees; e) it should have at least one group of approximately three-to-six-year-old children. Sixteen of the invited preschools were excluded because they did not meet the eligibility criteria. Of the remaining 153, 56% (86) agreed to participate. Families of the three-to-six-year-old children were invited to take part in the survey via the preschools. If the overall family-participation rate remained under 30%, the study was not conducted in that particular preschool. This was the case in 20 preschools, hence 66 were eligible to take part in the study. Of the 3592 families contacted in those preschools, 892 (27%) agreed to take part. Ultimately, we collected at least some research data from 864 children (24% of those invited), whom we consider the participants of the survey. The recruitment of the participants and the flow chart have been thoroughly described previously [21].

2.1. Preschool Factors

Preschool managers filled in a questionnaire covering policies, preschool-level practices, and their own views on factors related to the health behaviour of children at preschool. We received filled-in questionnaires from 53 preschool managers encompassing 58 preschools, as five managers filled in separate questionnaires for the two preschools for which they were responsible. We used seven manager-reported variables in the analyses, many of which were summed up from several questions/statements. The variables are grouped under the following headings: Policy factors, sociocultural factors, physical factors, and manager-related psychosocial factors. All the variables are presented in Table 1.

2.2. Policy Factors

The managers were asked if their preschool had written policies (preschool's own or municipal/national) concerning 18 different food/nutrition-related matters, such as using food as a reward or punishment, and birthday treats (see Table 1). The policies were summed up and the preschools were divided into tertiles according to the number of policies in place (Table 2).

2.3. Sociocultural Factors

The first sociocultural factor represents food education at the preschool. This variable combines three questions: (i) Has the preschool offered its personnel in-service training on children's nutrition during the last two years? (at least once vs. no); (ii) Have there been preschool theme weeks focusing on food/nutrition during the last two years? (at least once vs. no); (iii) Has the preschool ever used or does it currently use the Sapere method [22]? (yes/no). A positive response scored one point on each of these three actions, and the variable was categorised in three classes: 0, 1, and 2 or 3 points. The second sociocultural factor concerned challenges related to cooperation with the catering service. The managers were asked whether (i) a lack of cooperation with the catering-service personnel inhibited healthy nutrition, (ii) the limitations of the catering service inhibited healthy nutrition or food education, and (iii) communication between the preschool personnel and the catering personnel was fluent. The variable was categorised in three classes: 0, 1, and 2 or 3 barriers. The third sociocultural factor related to a lack of resources as a barrier to children's healthy nutrition at preschool, broken down into three resource types. The managers reported separately on whether a lack of planning time, a lack of personnel, and a lack of materials inhibited healthy nutrition (yes/no). The responses were then classified as indicating either at least one of these barriers or none of them.

2.4. Manager-Related Psychosocial Factors

We considered two psychosocial factors. The first was the manager's concern about the fruit and vegetable intake of the children, assessed from their responses to two questions. First, they were asked: "To what extent do you think there is generally a problem among three-six-year-old children concerning a low intake of vegetables/low intake of fruit?". The responses were given on a five-point Likert scale (1–5) ranging from "not a problem" to "a very big problem," summed and divided into three groups based on the distribution of the answers (Table 2). Second, they were asked if they had any influence in terms of the fruit and vegetable content of preschool meals. The question was asked separately for all meals. The answers were combined in a single dichotomous variable, since the same managers answered similarly to all questions (yes to all questions vs. no to all questions).

2.5. Physical Factors

The managers were asked what type of kitchen facilities the preschool had: (a) Cooking, (b) distribution, (c) heating, (d) other, what? and (e) there is no kitchen. The responses were categorised as cooking/heating vs. all other alternatives to distinguish the kitchens in which at least some cooking was done. The managers who responded other, what? ($n = 3$) were categorized in the right group based on their open answers following the question.

2.6. Children's Dietary Intake

The children's food intake while at preschool was measured using a two-day pre-coded food record that was kept by the personnel and covered the food and drink consumed as well as the amounts. Breakfast, lunch, and the afternoon snack had predefined templates grouping food commonly consumed at each meal to make the record-keeping easier. The personnel estimated portion sizes in household measures, or with the help of a validated Children's Food Picture Book [23,24] that is specifically designed to facilitate the estimation of portion sizes among children. Five of the eight municipalities supplied complete recipes for the food obtained from the preschool catering service, one municipality supplied some recipes, and two did not give any. When no recipe was available, recipes from other catering services were used. The food-record data were entered into the dietary-calculation software AivoDiet, version 2.2.0.0 (Aivo Finland Oy, Turku, Finland) for the computation of the children's food consumption and nutrient intake. The program uses the Finnish national food composition database, Fineli [25].

In this study, we used fruit consumption (yes vs. no), vegetable consumption (g/day), and fibre density (g/MJ) as the relevant dietary factors representing a healthy dietary intake. The Finnish child-nutrition recommendation for vegetables and fruit combined is a minimum of five handfuls (about 250 g), and for fibre density, 3 g/MJ a day [19]. A dichotomous variable was used for fruit consumption because a large proportion (37%) of the children did not eat any fruit during the two days of food record-keeping. Vegetable consumption included raw and cooked vegetables eaten as such, but not vegetables included in main dishes. Potatoes were not considered vegetables. We used the data from children who had eaten all the preschool meals (breakfast, lunch, and afternoon snack) on at least one of the two days when the food record was being kept. Both vegetable consumption per day and fibre density per day were calculated so that if the child had eaten the same meal (e.g., lunch) on both days, the mean intake was used. For example, if a child had eaten lunch and an afternoon snack on both days, but breakfast on only one day, the mean daily intake was calculated as the sum of the one breakfast and the mean intake of the two lunches and snacks.

Table 1. Description of the preschool-level variables *.

Variable	Questions/Statements	Response Options	Categorization
Policy factors	Does the preschool have its own or municipal/national policies related to the following: a. Members of staff encourage children to eat fruit and vegetables b. Using food as a reward or punishment c. Planned food education for the children d. Staff training on children's nutrition e. Family guidance on children's nutrition f. Food served on festive days g. Food served on birthdays h. Snacks children bring from home i. Products sold for fund-raising j. Special diets k. Ethical and religious diets l. Target portion sizes for vegetables m. Tasting rules n. Thirst-quenching drinks o. Taking children's individual preferences into account p. Staff taking meals with the children q. Staff eating food bought from home in the presence of the children r. Where the staff had their coffee break	a. No policies b. Oral policy c. Own written policy d. Municipal or national policy	
Written food policies			1 point for each written policy (c or d)

Table 1. Cont.

Variable	Questions/Statements	Response Options	Categorization
Sociocultural factors			
	1. Has the preschool had in-service training for its personnel on child nutrition during the last 2 years?	a. No b. Once c. Twice or more	a = 0 points, b or c = 1 point
Food education	2. Has the preschool had theme weeks about nutrition/food education during the last 2 years?	a. No b. Once c. Twice or more	a = 0 points, b or c = 1 point
	3. Is the Sapere method familiar to you?	a. The method has been used in the preschool b. The method is currently being used in the preschool c. The method is familiar, but it has not been used in the preschool d. The method is not familiar	a or b = 1 point, c or d = 0 points
	Is the following a barrier to healthy nutrition? Lack of cooperation with the catering service.	Yes/no	Yes = 1 point No = 0 points
	Is the following a barrier to the promotion of healthy nutrition/food education in your preschool? Limitations of the catering service or food supplier.	Yes/no	Yes = 1 point No = 0 points
Cooperation challenges with the catering service	How would you describe the communication between the early educators and the catering service staff?	a. Fluent b. There are some challenges.	a = 0 points b = 1 point
Lack of resources as a barrier to healthy nutrition	Is the following a barrier to healthy nutrition? A. Lack of planning time. B. Lack of materials. C. Lack of staff	Yes/no	1 point for each barrier (scale 0–3)

110

Table 1. *Cont.*

Variable	Questions/Statements	Response Options	Categorization
Manager-related psychosocial factors			
Concern about children's fruit and vegetable consumption	To what extent do you think the following matters are generally a problem among 3 to 6-year-old children? A. Low intake of vegetables and B. Low intake of fruit and berries	1 not a problem 2 hardly a problem 3 a problem to some extent 4 quite a big problem 5 a very big problem	Sum of a and b (scale 2–10)
Perceived influence over fruit and vegetable supply	Can the manager influence the supply of fruit and vegetables for different meals?	Yes/no (separate questions for each meal)	Yes to all questions vs. no to all questions
Physical factors			
Kitchen type	What type of kitchen facilities do you have in your preschool?	a. Cooking b. Distribution c. Heating d. Other, what? e. There is no kitchen	a and c combined vs. all others

* The questionnaire was available in Finnish and Swedish. The authors did the English translation.

Table 2. Descriptive results on the preschool-level factors.

Policy factors	
Number of written food policies (scale 0–18)	%
4 or less points	35
5–9 points	36
10 or more points	29
Sociocultural factors	
Food education (scale 0–3)	
0 points	45
1 point	34
2 or 3 points	22
Perceived cooperation challenges with the catering service (scale 0–3)	
No challenges	54
1 challenge	24
2 or 3 challenges	22
Lack of resources as a barrier to healthy nutrition	
no barriers	81
1–3 barriers	19
Manager-related psychosocial factors	
Concern about children's fruit and vegetable consumption (scale 2–10)	
5 or less points	19
6 points	44
7 or more points	36
Perceived influence over fruit and vegetable supply	
yes	19
no	81
Physical factors	
Kitchen type	
Cooking or heating kitchen	37
Other	63

2.7. Statistical Analyses

First, we checked the distributions of vegetable consumption and fibre density. Unlike fibre density, vegetable consumption was not normally distributed and thus we used square root transformation. We subjected the associations between the preschool-level factors and children's dietary intake to multi-level linear and logistic regression analysis with preschool as the random effect: The manager was included in the models as a new random effect, but the result was not statistically significant. We used two models: A crude model with no adjustments and a model adjusting for the child's age, gender, and municipality (as a dummy variable). Results of the linear regression analyses are expressed as beta coefficients (beta) and those of logistic regression analyses as odds ratios (OR). Furthermore, a 95% confidence interval (CI) is used with both. In one municipality, there were only three children who met the inclusion criteria of having three meals at preschool and they were all from the same preschool: We deleted these children from the analyses due to the lack of variation. IBM Statistics SPSS version 25.0 (SPSS Inc., Chicago, IL, USA) and statistical software Mplus version 7.4 [26] were used for the analyses.

3. Results

Table 2 shows the descriptive results for the preschool variables. Most managers did not report a lack of resources or cooperation challenges with the catering service. Four out of five indicated that they could not influence the content of fruit and vegetables in the preschool meals, and most of them reported having less than half of the food policies. Table 3 gives the characteristics of the children and the preschool managers. All preschool managers were women. Less than half of the children were girls and children's mean age was 4.7 years. Table 4 describes the dietary intake of the children. Food records were kept for 822 children, but the 586 children (72% of them) who had eaten all three meals at preschool on at least one of the days the food record was kept constitute the participants of this study. These children did not differ from the others in terms of age, gender, or socioeconomic background. Of them, 63% had eaten fruit, and on average, they consumed 39 g of raw and cooked vegetables and 9 g of dietary fibre during a preschool day.

Table 3. Characteristics of the children and of the preschool managers.

	% or Mean (SD)
Child-level characteristics (*n* = 586)	
Age, years	4.7 (0.9)
Gender, girls	47%
Preschool manager's characteristics (*n* = 53)	
Gender, women	100%
Age, years	48.4 (7.7)
Educational level	
Bachelor of educational science/Early education teacher	60%
Other	40%
Work experience as a manager, years	13.7 (11.8)

Table 4. Children's dietary intake at preschool.

Children's Dietary Intake at Preschool (Breakfast, Lunch, and Afternoon Snack) (*n* = 586)	
Energy (kJ)	3229 (910)
Fibre g	9.4 (3.1)
Fibre density g/MJ	3.0 (0.8)
Vegetables (g), raw and cooked	38.5 (28.3)
Fruit consumption, proportion of fruit eaters	63%

Having at least 10 of the 18 food policies in place (i.e., being in the highest tertile of the number of food policies), compared to less than five (i.e., the lowest tertile), was associated with higher vegetable consumption (beta coefficient 0.89, 95% CI 0.20–1.58) and a higher fibre intake (beta coefficient 0.24, 95% CI 0.02–0.46) among the children (Table 5). Among the sociocultural factors, associations were found regarding cooperation-related challenges with the catering service: Having at least two of the three types of challenge, compared to having none, was associated with a higher fibre intake among the children (beta coefficient 0.22, 95% CI 0.03–0.42) and a lower likelihood of eating fruit at preschool (OR 0.28, 95% CI 0.11–0.76). Neither the other sociocultural factors, such as food education, nor manager-related psychosocial factors, such as perceived influence over fruit and vegetable supply, were associated with the children's intake of fruit, vegetables, or fibre.

Table 5. Linear and logistic multi-level regression analyses of preschool-level factors and children's fruit and vegetable consumption, and fibre intake at preschool.

		Fruit Consumption (Yes vs. No) [a]						Vegetable Consumption (g/day, Square–Root Modified) [b]						Fiber Density (g/MJ) [b]					
		Model 1			Model 2			Model 1			Model 2			Model 1			Model 2		
		OR	95% CI	p	OR	95% CI	p	beta	95% CI	p	beta	95% CI	p	beta	95% CI	p	beta	95% CI	p
Policy factors																			
Written food policies	1st tertile (0–4)	1			1			0			0			0			0		
	2nd tertile (5–9)	1.18	(0.40–3.51)	0.76	1.19	(0.48–2.94)	0.70	0.57	(−0.28–1.41)	0.19	0.70	(−0.02–1.41)	0.06	−0.07	(−0.30–0.15)	0.53	−0.02	(−0.21–0.16)	0.82
	3rd tertile (10–18)	1.47	(0.36–5.89)	0.59	0.44	(0.10–1.91)	0.27	0.73	(0.00–1.45)	0.05	0.89	(0.20–1.58)	0.01	0.03	(−0.19–0.24)	0.80	0.24	(0.02–0.46)	0.03
Sociocultural factors																			
Food education	Low (0 points)	1			1			0			0			0			0		
	Medium (1 point)	0.75	(0.24–2.31)	0.61	0.62	(0.25–1.52)	0.30	0.20	(−0.48–0.89)	0.56	−0.09	(−0.71–0.53)	0.77	0.05	(−0.16–0.25)	0.66	−0.03	(−0.23–0.17)	0.77
	High (2 or 3 points)	0.70	(0.20–2.41)	0.58	1.44	(0.45–4.58)	0.53	0.10	(−0.88–1.07)	0.84	0.00	(−1.10–1.10)	0.99	0.00	(−0.24–0.24)	0.99	−0.11	(−0.30–0.09)	0.29
Cooperation challenges with the catering service	0	1			1			0			0			0			0		
	1	0.70	(0.23–2.10)	0.53	1.24	(0.50–3.11)	0.64	−0.41	(−1.20–0.39)	0.32	−0.15	(−0.87–0.57)	0.69	−0.02	(−0.26–0.22)	0.87	0.05	(−0.17–0.27)	0.64
	2–3	0.28	(0.10–0.83)	0.02	0.28	(0.11–0.76)	0.01	0.32	(−0.35–0.99)	0.35	0.48	(−0.23–1.18)	0.18	0.15	(−0.04–0.34)	0.12	0.22	(0.03–0.42)	0.03
Lack of resources as a barrier to healthy nutrition	No barriers	1			1			0			0			0			0		
	1–3 barriers	0.24	(0.07–0.82)	0.02	0.44	(0.17–1.13)	0.09	−0.13	(−1.21–0.95)	0.82	0.13	(−0.97–1.22)	0.82	−0.09	(−0.34–0.16)	0.47	−0.06	(−0.31–0.19)	0.65
Manager-related psychosocial factors																			
Concern about fruit and vegetable consumption	Low	1			1			0			0			0			0		
	Medium	0.45	(0.14–1.44)	0.18	0.37	(0.12–1.19)	0.10	−0.91	(−0.21–0.49)	0.55	−0.47	(−1.17–0.24)	0.20	0.01	(−0.20–0.22)	0.91	−0.12	(−0.35–0.10)	0.28
	High	1.48	(0.47–4.63)	0.5	1.05	(0.29–3.82)	0.94	−0.28	(−1.06–0.49)	0.47	−0.13	(−1.04–0.78)	0.78	−0.14	(−0.36–0.09)	0.23	−0.18	(−0.42–0.06)	0.14
Perceived influence over fruit and vegetable supply	No	1			1			0			0			0			0		
	Yes	2.95	(0.87–10.00)	0.08	1.83	(0.54–6.16)	0.33	1.01	(0.08–1.95)	0.03	0.68	(−0.55–1.91)	0.28	0.12	(−0.17–0.40)	0.42	−0.08	(−0.38–0.22)	0.6
Physical factors																			
Kitchen type	Other	1.00			1			0			0			0			0		
	Cooking/heating	0.29	(0.11–0.76)	0.01	0.58	(0.24–1.44)	0.24	0.04	(−0.69–0.77)	0.91	0.33	(−0.68–1.34)	0.52	0.13	(−0.04–0.31)	0.14	0.17	(−0.04–0.38)	0.12

Model 1: no adjustments; Model 2: adjusted for child's age, gender and municipality; [a] logistic regression; [b] linear regression.

4. Discussion

We examined the extent to which certain preschool-level factors other than food availability and mealtime practices are associated with the intake of fruit, vegetables, and fibre among three- to six-year-old Finnish preschoolers. A larger number of food-related policies was associated with a higher consumption of vegetables and a higher intake of fibre. A higher number of manager-perceived challenges related to cooperation with the catering service was associated with lower odds of children eating fruit, and also with a higher fibre intake. However, kitchen type, food education, and a lack of resources were not associated with dietary intake. Apart from food policies, the preschool-level factors we used have seldom been studied, and to our knowledge, this is the first study to report on their associations with the food intake of children.

Some previous studies have reported an association between food policies and children's dietary intake [12,13]. Himberg-Sundet et al. found that having their own written guidelines concerning the food and beverages that preschools offer to children was associated with a higher consumption of vegetables. According to the managers, these guidelines were developed largely in line with national recommendations. In our study, too, having written policies (its own or municipal/national) was associated with higher vegetable consumption and fibre intake in the preschool. Treating all policies as equal is misleading, however, given the variation in their type, content, and the extent to which they are enforced [27]. Some countries have laws concerning specific foods and beverages used in childcare establishments, and law changes have been found effective in changing the supply of beverages, for example [12]. National recommendations on preschool food and feeding practices are not binding in Finland, however, and compliance is not monitored nationally. In addition, given that neither the managers nor the preschools decide what kind of food and beverages will be served to children in Finnish preschools, most of the policies we studied concerned food education and feeding practices. In other studies that have examined food policies, the policies included have mostly concerned foods that should or should not be served to the children [12,13,27]. It would be useful in future analyses to investigate any association between the content of the policies and/or the extent to which the policies are enforced and the children's dietary intake.

Compliance with national or municipal policies may vary depending on the manager's or the personnel's own interests in promoting healthy nutrition among children [17], and on the environmental context, resources, or social influences [28]. As we do not know the content of the policies nor the extent of compliance with them in preschools, we cannot hypothesise how they contribute to higher vegetable consumption and fibre intake. As cross-sectional associations, the associations which were found might also not be causal.

Perceived challenges related to cooperation with the catering service were related to both lower odds of eating fruit and a higher intake of fibre. To our knowledge, this is the first study to examine and find associations between cooperation-related conflict between preschools and catering services with children's food intake. Byrd-Williams et al. [29] investigated perceived barriers to healthy nutrition at preschool among managers and other personnel and found that, to some extent, the limitations of the food-service provider and a lack of support from its personnel constituted such barriers. Moreover, the preschool personnel reported more barriers than the managers did [29]. The managers mentioned a similar number of barriers as our informants did [30].

The surprising finding of an association between a higher level of challenges related to the catering service and a higher intake of fibre could be attributable to the sources of dietary fibre. Nissinen et al. [30] examined nutrient intake and sources at preschool and at home among participants of the DAGIS survey, and found that the major source of dietary fibre at preschool was cereals (~64%), whereas only 19% came from fruit and vegetables and vegetable dishes. In fact, crispbread, which is commonly available as part of every preschool lunch, accounted for 21% of dietary-fibre intake: Eating a lot of crispbread could mean that other parts of the meal are not eaten, and it is usually discouraged. It would be worth finding out whether there are other differences in food intake, concerning the main dish for example, depending on the perceived challenges with the catering service. Given that challenges were also associated with a lower likelihood of children eating fruit, further investigation focusing on cooperation between the preschool and the catering service would be warranted.

Our examination of environmental factors and their associations with children's food intake was limited to one socioecological level (preschool) and it examined only single associations at a time. As food intake is affected by a web of factors, it would be interesting in future studies to focus on interactions within and between levels, as well as on mediation from a more distal level to food intake via factors in the immediate surroundings. In addition, as cross-sectional studies cannot verify causality, longitudinal studies, and especially intervention studies, on preschool environments' effects on children's food intake are warranted. Finally, we examined a limited number of preschool-level factors, and acknowledge the need to investigate numerous political, economic, sociocultural, and physical aspects, including the personal characteristics and interests of managers.

The major strength of our study is its focus on hitherto rather neglected associations between a variety of preschool-level factors and children's fruit and vegetable consumption and fibre intake at preschool. Another strength is the rigorous data on food intake gathered from the children by means of food records kept by the personnel and recipes obtained from catering services. Having conducted a validation study, Nissinen et al. [24] found that the preschool personnel's assessments of children's portion sizes from the Children's Food Picture Book achieved a similar level of accuracy as the parents' assessments. One limitation, however, is the low participation rate of the children, despite the relatively large number of children on whom we had food data for. Having more preschools involved would have been advantageous in terms of giving more power to the analyses. Another limitation is that the vegetable consumption variable did not include vegetables in main dishes, but in Finnish preschools, vegetables are mainly eaten separately as salad or raw vegetables. We are aware that if vegetables in main dishes would have been included, the intake of vegetables might have been a bit higher. It should also be noted that the dichotomous fruit intake variable (eaters vs. non-eaters) might rather describe the supply of fruit at preschool and not the children's willingness to eat it, and thus the results on fruit consumption should be interpreted with caution. Fruit was served on average 2.5 times a week (data not shown), and it is therefore possible that none was served on the two days on which records were kept for some children. Another limitation is that, given the lack of ready-made questionnaires that suited our purposes, we had to formulate the questions we used to assess the preschool-level factors largely by ourselves, and they have not been validated.

5. Conclusions

We examined the extent to which preschool-level factors other than food availability and mealtime practices are associated with the intake of vegetables, fruit, and fibre among three- to six-year-old Finnish preschoolers. Written food policies and manager-perceived cooperation-related challenges with the catering service were associated with the children's dietary intake at preschool. These findings demonstrate that preschool factors not directly related to food availability or feeding practices can still be associated with dietary intake, and these factors could be relevant in the promotion of healthy food intake at preschools. There is clearly a need for more studies focusing on such issues.

Author Contributions: Conceptualization, R.L., C.R. and M.E.; methodology, R.L., C.R. and M.E.; formal analysis, R.L.; investigation, R.L., K.N., L.K. (Liisa Korkalo) and H.V.; resources, E.R.; data curation, R.L., L.K. (Liisa Korkalo) and H.V.; writing—original draft preparation, R.L.; writing—review and editing, R.L., C.R., M.E., L.K. (Liisa Korkalo), H.V., K.N., L.K. (Leena Koivusilta) and E.R.; visualization, R.L.; supervision, C.R., M.E., L.K. (Leena Koivusilta) and E.R.; project administration, E.R., M.E. and C.R.; funding acquisition, R.L., E.R., C.R., M.E. and K.N.

Funding: This research was funded by Folkhälsan Research Center, University of Helsinki, The Ministry of Education and Culture in Finland, The Ministry of Social Affairs and Health, The Academy of Finland (Grants: 285439, 287288, 288038), The Juho Vainio Foundation, The Signe and Ane Gyllenberg Foundation, The Finnish Cultural Foundation/South Ostrobothnia Regional Fund, The Päivikki and Sakari Sohlberg Foundation, Medicinska Föreningen Liv och Hälsa, Finnish Foundation for Nutrition Research, and Finnish Food Research Foundation.

Acknowledgments: We thank Rejane Figueiredo for helping with the statistical analyses. We also want to thank all families and preschools participating in the study.

Conflicts of Interest: Liisa Korkalo is a board member of the company TwoDads. The authors declare no other conflict of interest. The funders had no role in the design of the study; in the collection, analyses, or interpretation of data; in the writing of the manuscript; or in the decision to publish the results.

References

1. Organisation for Economic Co-operation and Development. *Starting Strong 2017: Key OECD Indicators on Early Childhood Education and Care*; Starting Strong, OECD Publishing: Paris, France, 2017. Available online: https://www.oecd.org/education/starting-strong-2017-9789264276116-en.htm (accessed on 23 May 2019).
2. Larson, N.; Ward, D.S.; Neelon, S.B.; Story, M. What Role can Child-Care Settings Play in Obesity Prevention? A Review of the Evidence and Call for Research Efforts. *J. Am. Diet. Assoc.* **2011**, *111*, 1343–1362. [CrossRef] [PubMed]
3. NCD Risk Factor Collaboration (NCD-RisC). Worldwide Trends in Body-Mass Index, Underweight, Overweight, and Obesity from 1975 to 2016: A Pooled Analysis of 2416 Population-Based Measurement Studies in 128.9 Million Children, Adolescents, and Adults. *Lancet* **2017**, *390*, 2627–2642. [CrossRef]
4. Sallis, J.F.; Owen, N.; Fisher, E.B. Ecological models of health behavior. In *Health Behavior and Health Education: Theory, Research, and Practice*, 4th ed.; Glanz, K., Rimer, B.K., Viswanath, K., Eds.; Jossey-Bass: San Francisco, CA, USA, 2008; pp. 465–482.
5. Copeland, K.A.; Benjamin Neelon, S.E.; Howald, A.E.; Wosje, K.S. Nutritional Quality of Meals Compared to Snacks in Child Care. *Child. Obes.* **2013**, *9*, 223–232. [CrossRef] [PubMed]
6. Gerritsen, S.; Dean, B.; Morton, S.M.B.; Wall, C.R. Do Childcare Menus Meet Nutrition Guidelines? Quantity, Variety and Quality of Food Provided in New Zealand Early Childhood Education Services. *Aust. N. Z. J. Public Health* **2017**, *41*, 345–351. [CrossRef] [PubMed]
7. Ward, S.; Belanger, M.; Donovan, D.; Vatanparast, H.; Engler-Stringer, R.; Leis, A.; Carrier, N. Lunch is Ready but Not Healthy: An Analysis of Lunches Served in Childcare Centres in Two Canadian Provinces. *Can. J. Public Health* **2017**, *108*, e342–e347. [CrossRef] [PubMed]
8. Gubbels, J.S.; Kremers, S.P.; Stafleu, A.; Dagnelie, P.C.; de Vries, N.K.; Thijs, C. Child-Care Environment and Dietary Intake of 2- and 3-Year-Old Children. *J. Hum. Nutr. Diet.* **2010**, *23*, 97–101. [CrossRef] [PubMed]
9. Gubbels, J.S.; Gerards, S.M.; Kremers, S.P. Use of Food Practices by Childcare Staff and the Association with Dietary Intake of Children at Childcare. *Nutrients* **2015**, *7*, 2161–2175. [CrossRef]
10. Ward, S.; Blanger, M.; Donovan, D.; Vatanparast, H.; Muhajarine, N.; Engler-Stringer, R.; Leis, A.; Humbert, M.L.; Carrier, N. Association between Childcare Educators' Practices and Preschoolers' Physical Activity and Dietary Intake: A Cross-Sectional Analysis. *BMJ Open* **2017**, *7*, e013657. [CrossRef]
11. Lehto, R.; Ray, C.; Vepsalainen, H.; Korkalo, L.; Nissinen, K.; Skaffari, E.; Maatta, S.; Roos, E.; Erkkola, M. Early Educators' Practices and Opinions in Relation to Preschoolers' Dietary Intake at Pre-School: Case Finland. *Public Health Nutr.* **2019**, *22*, 1567–1575. [CrossRef]
12. Ritchie, L.D.; Sharma, S.; Gildengorin, G.; Yoshida, S.; Braff-Guajardo, E.; Crawford, P. Policy Improves what Beverages are Served to Young Children in Child Care. *J. Acad. Nutr. Diet.* **2015**, *115*, 724–730. [CrossRef]
13. Himberg-Sundet, A.; Kristiansen, A.L.; Bjelland, M.; Moser, T.; Holthe, A.; Andersen, L.F.; Lien, N. Is the Environment in Kindergarten Associated with the Vegetables Served and Eaten? the BRA Study. *Scand. J. Public Health* **2018**. [CrossRef] [PubMed]
14. Ritchie, L.D.; Boyle, M.; Chandran, K.; Spector, P.; Whaley, S.E.; James, P.; Samuels, S.; Hecht, K.; Crawford, P. Participation in the Child and Adult Care Food Program is Associated with More Nutritious Foods and Beverages in Child Care. *Child. Obes.* **2012**, *8*, 224–229. [CrossRef] [PubMed]
15. Liu, S.T.; Graffagino, C.L.; Leser, K.A.; Trombetta, A.L.; Pirie, P.L. Obesity Prevention Practices and Policies in Child Care Settings Enrolled and Not Enrolled in the Child and Adult Care Food Program. *Matern. Child Health J.* **2016**, *20*, 1933–1939. [CrossRef]
16. Van de Kolk, I.; Goossens, A.J.M.; Gerards, S.M.P.L.; Kremers, S.P.J.; Manders, R.M.P.; Gubbels, J.S. Healthy Nutrition and Physical Activity in Childcare: Views from Childcare Managers, Childcare Workers and Parents on Influential Factors. *Int. J. Environ. Res. Public Health* **2018**, *15*, 2909. [CrossRef] [PubMed]

17. Olstad, D.L.; Raine, K.D.; McCargar, L.J. Adopting and implementing nutrition guidelines in recreational facilities: Public and private sector roles. A multiple case study. *BMC Public Health* **2012**, *12*, 376. [CrossRef] [PubMed]
18. Valtion ravitsemusneuvottelukunta. *Terveyttä Ja Iloa Ruoasta-Varhaiskasvatuksen Ruokailusuositus [Health and Joy from Food-Food Recommendations for Early Childhood Education and Care]*; National Institute for Health and Welfare: Helsinki, Finland, 2018.
19. Terveyden ja hyvinvoinnin laitos, Valtion ravitsemusneuvottelukunta. *Syödään Yhdessä-Ruokasuositukset Lapsiperheille [Eating together-Food Recommendations for Families with Children]*; National Institute for Health and Welfare: Tampere, Finland, 2016.
20. Maatta, S.; Lehto, R.; Nislin, M.; Ray, C.; Erkkola, M.; Sajaniemi, N.; Roos, E. DAGIS research group. Increased Health and Well-being in Preschools (DAGIS): Rationale and Design for a Randomized Controlled Trial. *BMC Public Health* **2015**, *15*, 402. [CrossRef]
21. Lehto, E.; Ray, C.; Vepsalainen, H.; Korkalo, L.; Lehto, R.; Kaukonen, R.; Suhonen, E.; Nislin, M.; Nissinen, K.; Skaffari, E.; et al. Increased Health and Wellbeing in Preschools (DAGIS) Study-Differences in Children's Energy Balance-Related Behaviors (EBRBs) and in Long-Term Stress by Parental Educational Level. *Int. J. Environ. Res. Public Health* **2018**, *15*, 2313. [CrossRef] [PubMed]
22. Learning about Taste at School. Available online: https://www.sapere-association.com/ (accessed on 20 May 2019).
23. Nissinen, K.; Sillanpää, H.; Korkalo, L.; Roos, E.; Erkkola, M. *Annoskuvakirja Lasten Ruokamäärien Arvioinnin Avuksi [the Children's Food Picture Book]*; Helsingin yliopisto, Seinäjoen ammattikorkeakoulu, Samfundet Folkhälsan: Helsinki, Finland, 2015.
24. Nissinen, K.; Korkalo, L.; Vepsalainen, H.; Makiranta, P.; Koivusilta, L.; Roos, E.; Erkkola, M. Accuracy in the Estimation of Children's Food Portion Sizes Against a Food Picture Book by Parents and Early Educators. *J. Nutr. Sci.* **2018**, *7*, e35. [CrossRef]
25. National Institute for Health and Welfare, Nutrition Unit. Fineli-Finnish National Food Composition Database 2017. Release 18. Available online: http://www.fineli.fi/ (accessed on 20 May 2019).
26. Muthén, L.K.; Muthén, B.O. *Mplus User's Guide*, 8th ed.; Muthén & Muthén: Los Angeles, CA, USA, 1998–2012.
27. Lucas, P.J.; Patterson, E.; Sacks, G.; Billich, N.; Evans, C.E.L. Preschool and School Meal Policies: An Overview of what we Know about Regulation, Implementation, and Impact on Diet in the UK, Sweden, and Australia. *Nutrients* **2017**, *9*, 736. [CrossRef]
28. Seward, K.; Finch, M.; Yoong, S.L.; Wyse, R.; Jones, J.; Grady, A.; Wiggers, J.; Nathan, N.; Conte, K.; Wolfenden, L. Factors that Influence the Implementation of Dietary Guidelines regarding Food Provision in Centre Based Childcare Services: A Systematic Review. *Prev. Med.* **2017**, *105*, 197–205. [CrossRef]
29. Byrd-Williams, C.; Dooley, E.E.; Sharma, S.V.; Chuang, R.J.; Butte, N.; Hoelscher, D.M. Best Practices and Barriers to Obesity Prevention in Head Start: Differences between Director and Teacher Perceptions. *Prev. Chronic Dis.* **2017**, *14*, E139. [CrossRef] [PubMed]
30. Korkalo, L.; Nissinen, K.; Skaffari, E.; Vepsäläinen, H.; Lehto, R.; Kaukonen, R.; Koivusilta, L.; Sajaniemi, N.; Roos, E.; Erkkola, M. The Contribution of Preschool Meals to the Diet of Finnish Preschoolers. *Nutrients* **2019**, submitted for publication.

© 2019 by the authors. Licensee MDPI, Basel, Switzerland. This article is an open access article distributed under the terms and conditions of the Creative Commons Attribution (CC BY) license (http://creativecommons.org/licenses/by/4.0/).

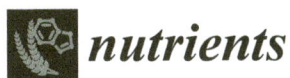

Article

Perceived Barriers to Fruit and Vegetable Gardens in Early Years Settings in England: Results from a Cross-Sectional Survey of Nurseries

Sara E. Benjamin-Neelon [1,2,*], Amelie A. Hecht [3], Thomas Burgoine [2] and Jean Adams [2]

1. Department of Health, Behavior and Society, 615 North Wolfe Street, Johns Hopkins University, Baltimore, MD 21205, USA
2. UKCRC Centre for Diet and Activity Research (CEDAR), MRC Epidemiology Unit, University of Cambridge School of Clinical Medicine, Box 285, Institute of Metabolic Science, Cambridge Biomedical Campus, Cambridge CB2 0QQ, UK; tb464@medschl.cam.ac.uk (T.B.); jma79@medschl.cam.ac.uk (J.A.)
3. Department of Health Policy and Management, 624 North Broadway, Johns Hopkins University, Baltimore, MD 21205, USA; ahecht3@jhu.edu
* Correspondence: sara.neelon@jhu.edu

Received: 4 November 2019; Accepted: 27 November 2019; Published: 3 December 2019

Abstract: Garden-based interventions may increase child intake of fruits and vegetables and offset food costs, but few have been conducted in early care and education (ECE). This study assessed whether nurseries were interested in and perceived any barriers to growing fruits and vegetables. Surveys were mailed to a cross-sectional sample of nurseries in 2012–2013 throughout England. Nurseries were stratified based on socioeconomic status as most, middle, or least deprived areas. We fit logistic regression models to assess the odds of nurseries interested in growing fruits and vegetables and perceiving any barriers, by deprivation tertile. A total of 851 surveys were returned (54% response). Most nurseries (81%) were interested in growing fruits and vegetables. After adjustment, there was no difference in interest in the middle (OR 1.55; CI 0.84, 2.78; $p = 0.16$) or most (OR 1.05; CI 0.62, 1.78; $p = 0.87$) deprived areas, compared to the least deprived. Nurseries reported barriers to growing fruits and vegetables, including space (42%), expertise (26%), and time (16%). Those in the most deprived areas were more likely to report space as a barrier (OR 2.02; 95% CI 1.12, 3.66; $p = 0.02$). Nurseries in the most deprived areas may need creative solutions for growing fruits and vegetables in small spaces.

Keywords: Child Care; Early Care and Education; Gardens; Produce

1. Introduction

Recent studies demonstrate that young children in high-income countries like the United States (US) and the United Kingdom (UK) consume insufficient servings of fruits and vegetables [1–3]. Children from low socioeconomic status families are particularly at risk for poor dietary intake [4–6], and interventions to increase fruit and vegetable consumption could be tailored to reach this vulnerable population [7]. Traditionally, the family has been the primary influence on young children's dietary intake. Parent preferences and parents modeling healthy behaviors have been shown to be important determinants [8]. However, a growing number of parents share caregiving and feeding responsibilities with early care and education (ECE) providers [9,10], and these providers can impact children's dietary intake [11]. In high-income countries, nearly 80% of children ages 3–6 years and 25% of children ages 0–3 years spend time in some form of non-parental child care [12]. Children may consume one-half to two-thirds of their daily calories in these settings [13], including most of their carbohydrates and servings of fruit [14].

There is ample evidence that young children consume inadequate amounts of fruits and vegetables in ECE. A previous study of children in the US found they consumed one-third of a serving of fruit and one-quarter of a serving of vegetables per day in ECE—far fewer than the recommended national guidelines [15]. Moreover, nearly 50% of vegetables consumed in ECE were fried potatoes, and only 8% were the more nutrient-dense dark green or brightly colored vegetables [15]. Other studies of young children in the US and the Netherlands have found similar results [14,16–18]. In the UK, limited data suggest that children are also served insufficient quantities of fruits and vegetables. In one study in Northern England, about half of nurseries (one type of ECE setting) reported serving either a fruit or vegetable with lunch daily [19]. In our prior work, we found that 92% of nurseries reported serving a fruit and 70% reported serving a vegetable to children each day [20]. Although somewhat promising, this still falls below the recommended amount [21].

Studies show that exposure to fruits and vegetables by age 5 years is vital to establishing habitual consumption later in life [22–24]. Encouraging children to try and accept novel foods has been more effective in younger children than with older children, and repeated exposure has yielded positive results in ECE setting [23,25–28]. Interventions that engage children in food preparation, encourage hands-on experiences, and include home-grown foods have increased child fruit and vegetable consumption beyond that of an intervention that merely increases availability [11,29–35]. Thus, interventions that include growing fruits and vegetables, for example, have the potential to increase child intake, but only a handful have been conducted in ECE [36]. The ECE setting is perhaps ideal because preschool-aged children may be more likely to try new foods like vegetables with both repeated exposure and eating in a group setting [25,27,28,37].

Further, gardens may help offset costs associated with the purchasing of fruits and vegetables. School gardens in high-income countries have focused on promoting experiential learning and exposing children to fruits and vegetables to increase familiarity and consumption [38–40]. An added benefit for ECE, however, is the potential to serve children what is grown. Generally, ECE programs tend to be smaller and there are often fewer children to feed, compared to schools. This may help offset food costs for fruits and vegetables served to children in ECE [41], in addition to other benefits.

The aims of this study were to assess whether nurseries were interested in growing their own fruits and vegetables and perceived any barriers to doing so. We further assessed whether responses to these questions differed by socioeconomic status. We hypothesized that nurseries in the most deprived areas of England would be more interested in growing their own fruits and vegetables as a means to offset food costs, but would report cost to establishing the garden as the primary barrier.

2. Materials and Methods

2.1. Study Design and Sample

For the cross-sectional Nutrition in Nurseries study, we mailed surveys to a stratified random sample of 2000 nurseries throughout England in 2012–2013. We obtained a list of registered nurseries in England from Ofsted, the organization responsible for regulating ECE programs in England. Ofsted defines nurseries to include any ECE setting that provides care for children on a regular basis that is not located on domestic premises. Thus, nurseries may include preschools or child care centers but not childminders or family child care homes (i.e., care on domestic premises). To stratify, we first used nursery addresses to geocode them at the postcode level, using geographic information system (GIS) (Arc GIS 10, ESRI Inc., Redlands, CA, USA) software. We used the geocoded data to categorize nurseries within lower super output areas (LSOA)—small administrative boundaries containing approximately 1,500 residents. Next, we stratified nurseries based on LSOA tertile of the index of multiple deprivation (IMD). IMD data were for 2010, which were the most recent scores available at the time of the survey. The IMD is published by the Department for Communities and Local Government in England and is a measure of income, employment, health and disability, education, barriers to housing, and crime. Expecting a lower response rate, we oversampled nurseries in the most deprived tertile. We mailed 1000 surveys to nurseries in the most deprived LSOAs, 500 to the middle and 500 to the least-deprived LSOAs. Additional information about the Nutrition in Nurseries study has been reported elsewhere [20].

2.2. Survey

A primary goal of the Nutrition in Nurseries study was to evaluate the nutritional quality of meals and snacks served in nurseries and assess consistency with mandatory and voluntary nutrition standards [20]. Secondarily, we assessed manager interest in growing fruits and vegetables at the nursery and perceived barriers to doing so in order to inform potential development and implementation of a future gardening intervention. We designed the survey to be completed by nursery managers in approximately 20 min. The survey assessed a number of factors related to nutrition and healthy food provision within the nursery. The final survey included 23 questions about food practices and the nutrition environment within the nursery; 16 demographic questions about children in the nursery and the manager; and two questions assessing the amount of time spent completing the survey. We used three existing surveys developed to assess nutrition and healthy eating practices in US-based ECE [42–44], modifying the questions for use in England. The first showed moderate to high validity and reliability [42]; the second demonstrated moderate to high reliability, but was not tested for validity [43]; and the third, to our knowledge, was not evaluated for either, though the authors note that it was based in part on the previous two surveys [44]. The survey was then reviewed by nutrition experts, parents of preschool-aged children, and nursery care providers in England prior to the launch of the study. We included a human subjects fact sheet with the mailed survey stating that completion constituted consent to participate in the study. Thus, all subjects gave their informed consent for inclusion before they participated in the study. The study was conducted in accordance with the Declaration of Helsinki, and the protocol was approved by the Ethics Committee of the University of Cambridge Psychology Research (Project identification code: Pre.2012.49).

We asked managers to report whether or not they were interested in growing their own fruits and vegetables at the nursery. If interested, we asked whether they were already growing fruits and vegetables at the nursery. We also asked whether managers perceived any barriers to establishing fruit and vegetable gardens. We then provided a list of potential barriers (e.g., time or expertise) developed by the research team and also allowed for write-in responses. We categorized these responses as cost, external threats (e.g., pests or vandalism would be a problem), ownership/shared use (e.g., the nursery did not have the authority to use the outdoor space for gardening), and seasonality or growing conditions (e.g., the nursery was closed during peak growing season or the soil was not suitable for growing fruits and vegetables).

2.3. Analysis

We fit binary logistic regression models to assess the odds of interest in growing fruits and vegetables and perceiving any barriers to growing fruits and vegetables, by deprivation tertile with the least deprived tertile as the referent group. We adjusted for covariates that were of a priori interest based on prior studies [20,45], including nursery type (based in a workplace, run by a non-profit, or part of a corporate chain), total number of children enrolled, years in operation, and manager education (less than a 2-year degree or a 2-year degree or higher). Further, we included an indicator for urbanicity when we examined space as a barrier, as location in an urban versus rural area may explain any potential association. We present results in terms of odds ratios, 95% confidence intervals (CI), and two-sided p-values. We conducted all analyses using Stata version 14.1 (StataCorp LP, College Station, TX, USA) at a significance level of < 0.05.

3. Results

A total of 851 of nurseries returned a completed survey, resulting in a 54% response rate after accounting for surveys returned undelivered and nurseries that had closed for business, did not care for children regularly, or did not provide meals and snacks to children. The response rate was similar across all deprivation tertiles. Of the 851 surveys returned, 846 provided complete data for this analysis (five were missing information required to geocode nurseries). Nurseries had been in operation for a mean and standard deviation (SD) of 17.1 (12.3) years and over half (58%) of nursery managers had a 2-year degree or higher (Table 1). Nurseries were based in a workplace (43%), run by a non-profit (25%), or part of a corporate chain (33%). Nurseries had a mean (SD) of 49.9 (37.3) children enrolled (range 2–310); nearly all (97%) nursery managers were women.

Table 1. Demographic characteristics of nurseries and managers, by deprivation tertile, in England, 2012–2013.

	Total Sample ($n = 846$)	Least Deprived ($n = 229$)	Middle Deprived ($n = 219$)	Most Deprived ($n = 398$)
Nursery Characteristics	Number (%)			
Facility Type				
Based in workplace	312 (43)	86 (43)	82 (41)	144 (44)
Run by non-profit	180 (25)	57 (29)	50 (25)	73 (22)
Part of corporation or chain	238 (33)	57 (29)	68 (34)	113 (34)
Located in urban area	691 (82)	152 (66)	157 (72)	382 (96)
	Mean (SD)			
Years in operation	17.1 (12.3)	19.0 (12.8)	17.9 (11.6)	15.5 (12.2)
Number of children enrolled	49.9 (37.3)	46.9 (33.9)	46.4 (37.9)	53.6 (38.5)
Number of full-time staff	8.5 (7.3)	7.9 (7.4)	7.8 (7.6)	9.1 (7.0)
Number of classrooms	2.5 (1.8)	2.3 (1.6)	2.6 (1.9)	2.7 (1.8)
Manager Characteristics	Number (%)			
Gender, female	797 (97)	219 (97)	205 (96)	373 (96)
Education				
Less than 2-year degree	331 (42)	89 (42)	97 (47)	145 (39)
2-year degree or higher	459 (58)	122 (58)	109 (53)	228 (61)
	Mean (SD)			
Age, years	43.0 (11.1)	43.3 (10.8)	42.9 (11.6)	42.9 (11.1)
Years worked in child care field	17.2 (9.3)	16.5 (9.1)	17.1 (9.3)	17.7 (9.5)
Years worked in nursery	9.9 (7.4)	9.5 (7.3)	10.3 (7.3)	9.9 (7.4)

Most nurseries (81%) were interested in growing their own fruits and vegetables (Table 2). Seventeen nurseries did not respond to the question and were therefore not included as not interested or interested in Table 2 below. Of those interested, 40% of nurseries were already growing some fruits or vegetables. Among all nurseries, a small percentage (18%) were not interested in growing fruits or vegetables.

In adjusted analyses, interest in growing fruits and vegetables did not differ by deprivation tertile (interest was not associated with deprivation in the middle (OR 1.55; 95% CI 0.84, 2.87; $p = 0.16$) or most deprived (OR 1.05; 95% CI 0.62, 1.78; $p = 0.87$) tertile, compared to nurseries in the least deprived tertile). Nursery managers reported a number of perceived barriers to growing fruits and vegetables, including space (42%), expertise (26%), and time (16%). However, 24% reported no barriers. Nurseries already growing, compared to those who were interested but not yet growing, were significantly more likely to report no barriers (OR 2.90; CI 1.87, 4.50; $p \leq 0.001$) and significantly less likely to report space (OR 0.36; CI 0.24, 0.55; $p \leq 0.001$), expertise (OR 0.30; CI 0.19, 0.49; $p \leq 0.001$), or time (OR 0.58; CI 0.34, 1.0; $p = 0.049$) as a barrier. There were no significant differences between groups regarding likelihood of reporting cost, external threats, ownership/shared use, or seasonality/growing conditions as barriers.

Of nurseries that were interested but not yet growing, those in the most deprived areas were more likely to report space as a barrier (OR 2.02; 95% CI 1.12, 3.66; $p = 0.02$) (Table 3). However, adjusting for urban location did not substantially change the results (OR 2.19; 95% CI 1.18, 4.06; $p = 0.01$). There were no other differences in perceived barriers by deprivation tertile.

Table 2. Interest in and perceived barriers to growing fruits and vegetables.

	Total Sample ($n = 846$)	Not Interested in Growing ($n = 154$ [a])	Interested in Growing ($n = 675$ [a])	
			Already ($n = 268$)	Not yet ($n = 407$)
		Number (%)		
Deprivation Level				
Least deprived	229 (27)	45 (29)	74 (28)	107 (26)
Middle deprived	219 (26)	33 (21)	75 (28)	106 (26)
Most deprived	398 (47)	76 (49)	119 (44)	194 (47)
Barriers				
Space	281 (42)	N/A	74 (28)	207 (51)
Expertise	178 (26)	N/A	41 (15)	137 (34)
Time	106 (16)	N/A	29 (11)	77 (19)
Cost	9 (1)	N/A	1 (0)	8 (2)
Ownership/shared use	24 (4)	N/A	5 (12)	19 (5)
Seasonality/growing conditions	19 (3)	N/A	9 (3)	10 (3)
External threats	11 (2)	N/A	3 (1)	8 (2)
No barriers	165 (25)	N/A	93 (35)	72 (18)

[a] 17 nurseries did not respond and were therefore not included as not interested or interested.

Table 3. Adjusted [a] odds ratios and 95% confidence intervals (CI) of perceived barriers to growing for nurseries interested in growing [b] ($n = 407$).

	Odds Ratio (95% CI)	p-Value
Time		
Least deprived	Ref	Ref
Middle deprived	1.71 (0.71, 4.14)	0.23
Most deprived	1.24 (0.55, 2.83)	0.60
Expertise		
Least deprived	Ref	Ref
Middle deprived	1.26 (0.64, 2.49)	0.51
Most deprived	1.68 (0.91, 3.11)	0.10
Space		
Least deprived	Ref	Ref
Middle deprived	1.43 (0.75, 2.71)	0.28
Most deprived	2.02 (1.12, 3.66)	0.02
Cost		
Least deprived	Ref	Ref
Middle deprived	1.22 (0.19, 7.82)	0.84
Most deprived	0.49 (0.07, 3.75)	0.50

Table 3. Cont.

	Odds Ratio (95% CI)	p-Value
External Threats		
Least deprived	Ref	Ref
Middle deprived	0.44 (0.04, 5.01)	0.51
Most deprived	0.98 (0.17, 5.69)	0.98
Ownership/Shared Use		
Least deprived	Ref	Ref
Middle deprived	1.32 (0.35, 4.95)	0.68
Most deprived	0.71 (0.18, 2.81)	0.62
Seasonality/Growing Conditions		
Least deprived	Ref	Ref
Middle deprived	0.72 (0.13, 3.99)	0.71
Most deprived	0.22 (0.02, 2.25)	0.20
No Barriers		
Least deprived	Ref	Ref
Middle deprived	0.54 (0.24, 1.22)	0.14
Most deprived	0.51 (0.25, 1.06)	0.07

[a] Adjusted for type of facility, total number of children enrolled, years in operation, and manager education.
[b] Among nurseries interested but not yet growing fruits and vegetables.

4. Discussion

In this cross-sectional survey of nursery managers throughout England, we found that the majority were interested in growing their own fruits and vegetables and interest did not vary based on area deprivation level. This finding was contrary to our hypothesis. We expected nursery managers in the most deprived areas to be more interested in growing fruits and vegetables, in part to offset food costs. We also assessed barriers and hypothesized that costs associated with establishing gardens would be the primary barrier reported. Instead, very few nurseries reported cost as a barrier to growing fruits and vegetables and space was the most commonly reported barrier.

Most nursery managers in our study expressed interest in growing fruits and vegetables. Gardens in ECE may expose children to fruits and vegetables through experiential learning, which may ultimately encourage greater consumption. In a recent qualitative study in the US, ECE providers reported that the ECE environment had the potential to exert a strong influence over children and was an ideal setting for introducing less familiar foods [46]. In another qualitative study in the Netherlands, managers believed it was vital to encourage healthy eating for the children in their care [47]. Managers emphasized the importance of making healthy foods, like fruits and vegetables, readily available in the ECE environment [47].

Moreover, child care providers in the US believed that fruit and vegetable gardens could help increase children's willingness to try new foods [46]. A handful of prior gardening interventions have been conducted in ECE settings [48–50]. One observed a modest increase in vegetable but not fruit intake in children [48], another found the intervention itself to be well received but did not measure dietary intake [51], and a third did not find any improvement in child fruit and vegetable intake [49]. These prior studies were limited, however, by a small sample size, lack of a control or comparison group, or self-reported outcomes [32,50–52]. Larger intervention studies with more robust study designs and rigorous outcome measures are needed to fully assess the potential impact of fruit and vegetable gardens in ECE. Our study provides some justification for a future garden-based intervention in ECE in England, although we focused on perceived barriers rather than motivators to start a garden.

We also found that space was the most common barrier reported among nurseries. Although this was not what we expected, this finding provides information that can be used to tailor a future gardening intervention. While having enough space to grow sufficient amounts of produce can be challenging, there are solutions to help overcome this challenge. In our prior study where we established gardens in ECE programs in the US [49], we used creative solutions to establish gardens in small spaces. There are numerous resources available for gardening in small or restricted areas that can apply to nurseries with insufficient space (e.g., hanging tomatoes pots) to address this barrier.

We expected nurseries to report cost as a primary barrier to establishing gardens. In a review of gardening interventions with older children, schools reported financial challenges as a substantial impediment to growing fruits and vegetables [53]. To overcome this barrier, schools solicited donations from local businesses, held fundraising events, and applied for small grants to offset costs [53]. In a prior qualitative study in ECE, providers expressed concern about having adequate financial resources to grow fruits and vegetables sufficient to feed children [16]. Despite these prior findings, most nursery managers in our study did not express concern about costs associated with establishing fruit and vegetable gardens.

Food costs have been reported as a barrier to serving more fruits and vegetables during meals and snacks in previous studies in ECE. Growing fruit and vegetables as a way to reduce food costs may be a viable option for some ECE programs. Monsivais et al. found that increasing food expenditures in ECE settings would increase the total servings of fruits and vegetables available to children [41]. A recent intervention in US-based Head Start centers established a fruit and vegetable delivery program with local farms to provide additional low-cost fruits and vegetables to children [54]. Head Start serves mainly low-income children, and this study highlights the need to help offset costs associated with fruits and vegetables in this setting.

However, in order to reduce food costs, gardens need to yield sufficient produce to help feed all children in care. In our prior ECE garden study, we planned for one additional serving of fruits and vegetables per week for each child [49]. Although this may not have a large impact on food costs, it could make a meaningful difference, especially over the long term if gardens are sustained. However, most of the prior gardening interventions designed for children 5 years and younger required only a modest amount of growing (e.g., seedlings in small paper cups) and did not result in full-scale gardens that would produce enough servings of fruits and vegetables for child consumption [52,55]. Thus, the majority of the existing gardening programs aimed to expose children to growing fruits and vegetables but were not designed to provide enough to help offset food costs. If a goal is to decrease costs associated with purchasing fruits and vegetables, then it is important to establish gardens that will yield sufficient produce to feed rather than just expose children.

There are some limitations to this study. First, we obtained nursery manager opinions only, although we did encourage managers to speak with teachers at the nursery prior to completing the survey. However, interest in and perceived barriers to growing fruits and vegetables are likely reflective of the nursery manager and not the entire nursery staff. Responses may have differed if we had surveyed teachers (perhaps the ones more likely to care for the gardens) rather than managers. Generalizability is also limited by the response rate, even though responses were similar across deprivation tertiles in our sample. Despite this, our results may not be generalizable to other nurseries in England. However, our response rate is nearly identical to that of a similar survey of 211 ECE programs in New Zealand (54% versus 55%) [56]. Further, we used surveys rather than qualitative interviews or focus groups because we were interested in assessing a wide range of nurseries across England and quantitatively exploring associations rather than the range of perceptions present. However, while IMD provides information on the area where the nursery is located, it does not necessarily reflect the socioeconomic status of the children in care (i.e., some children may not live close to the nursery). Therefore, the deprivation results apply to nurseries as a business located in their specific geographic area, but not necessarily to the children within the nurseries. Finally, we asked nursery managers if they were interested in growing fruits and vegetables at the nursery. However, we did not assess motivators to starting a garden. Also, the question of interest was not specific enough to assess interest in growing sufficient amounts of fruits and vegetables to help offset food costs at the nursery.

5. Conclusions

As more interventions target ECE programs, gardens have the potential to yield enough produce to serve the harvested fruits and vegetables with meals and snacks. This may have a small but meaningful impact if children eat what they grow. We found that most nurseries were interested in growing fruits and vegetables. This speaks to the potential for uptake of a future wide-scale garden-based intervention in England. Findings from this cross-sectional survey of nurseries may be used to further underpin further research examining the impact of gardens on children's fruit and vegetable intake (e.g., a large scale cluster randomized controlled trial). A productive garden has the potential to supplement the supply of produce available for meals and snacks in ECE programs. Our prior pilot intervention found that children exposed to gardens in ECE increased their intake of vegetables [49]. Children from low socioeconomic status families are particularly at risk for poorer dietary intake [4–6]. Growing fruits and vegetables in ECE programs in the most deprived areas of England—those that serve children from low-income families—may help offset food costs. Gardens can help ensure that the most vulnerable children are exposed to a variety of fruits and vegetables early in childhood, which could help establish healthy consumption habits later in life.

Author Contributions: S.E.B.-N. formulated the research question, designed and implemented the study, and drafted the article. A.A.H. and T.B. assisted with the research question, conducted the analysis, and reviewed and approved the final manuscript. J.A. provided critical feedback on the analysis and reviewed and approved the final manuscript.

Funding: This work was undertaken by the Centre for Diet and Activity Research (CEDAR), a UK Clinical Research Collaboration (UKCRC) Public Health Research Centre of Excellence. Funding from the British Heart Foundation, Cancer Research UK, Economic and Social Research Council, Medical Research Council, the National Institute for Health Research, and the Wellcome Trust, under the auspices of the UK Clinical Research Collaboration, is gratefully acknowledged. The funders had no role in the design, execution, interpretation, or writing of the study.

Conflicts of Interest: The authors declare no conflict of interest.

References

1. Fox, M.K.; Gearan, E.; Cannon, J.; Briefel, R.; Deming, D.M.; Eldridge, A.L.; Reidy, K.C. Usual food intakes of 2-and 3-year old US children are not consistent with dietary guidelines. *BMC Nutr.* **2016**, *2*, 67. [CrossRef]
2. Fox, M.K.; Condon, E.; Briefel, R.R.; Reidy, K.C.; Deming, D.M. Food consumption patterns of young preschoolers: Are they starting off on the right path? *J. Acad. Nutr. Diet.* **2010**, *110*, S52–S59. [CrossRef] [PubMed]
3. Hess, J.; Slavin, J. Snacking for a cause: Nutritional insufficiencies and excesses of US children, a critical review of food consumption patterns and macronutrient and micronutrient intake of US children. *Nutrients* **2014**, *6*, 4750–4759. [CrossRef] [PubMed]
4. Mello, J.A.; Gans, K.M.; Risica, P.M.; Kirtania, U.; Strolla, L.O.; Fournier, L. How is food insecurity associated with dietary behaviors? An analysis with low-income, ethnically diverse participants in a nutrition intervention study. *J. Acad. Nutr. Diet.* **2010**, *110*, 1906–1911. [CrossRef]
5. Kendall, A.; Olson, C.M.; Frongillo, E.A., Jr. Relationship of Hunger and Food Insecurity to Food Availability and Consumption. *J. Acad. Nutr. Diet.* **1996**, *96*, 1019–1024. [CrossRef]
6. Dunn, R.; Sharkey, J.; Lotade-Manje, J.; Bouhlal, Y.; Nayga, R. Socio-economic status, racial composition and the affordability of fresh fruits and vegetables in neighborhoods of a large rural region in Texas. *Nutrition* **2011**, *10*, 6. [CrossRef]
7. de Jong, E.; Visscher, T.L.; HiraSing, R.A.; Seidell, J.C.; Renders, C.M. Home environmental determinants of children's fruit and vegetable consumption across different SES backgrounds. *Pediatr. Obes.* **2015**, *10*, 134–140. [CrossRef]
8. Larsen, J.K.; Hermans, R.C.; Sleddens, E.F.; Engels, R.C.; Fisher, J.O.; Kremers, S.P. How parental dietary behavior and food parenting practices affect children's dietary behavior. Interacting sources of influence? *Appetite* **2015**, *89*, 246–257. [CrossRef]

9. Bernard, K.; Peloso, E.; Laurenceau, J.P.; Zhang, Z.; Dozier, M. Examining change in cortisol patterns during the 10-week transition to a new child-care setting. *Child Dev.* **2015**, *86*, 456–471. [CrossRef]
10. Ziegler, P.; Briefel, R.; Ponza, M.; Novak, T.; Hendricks, K. Nutrient intakes and food patterns of toddlers' lunches and snacks: Influence of location. *J. Am. Diet. Assoc.* **2006**, *106*, S124–S134. [CrossRef]
11. Gubbels, J.S.; Gerards, S.M.; Kremers, S.P. Use of food practices by childcare staff and the association with dietary intake of children at childcare. *Nutrients* **2015**, *7*, 2161–2175. [CrossRef] [PubMed]
12. The child care transition, Innocenti Report Card 8, 2008. Florence, Italy, 2008. Available online: https://www.unicef-irc.org/publications/pdf/rc8_eng.pdf (accessed on 16 July 2019).
13. Kharofa, R.Y.; Kalkwarf, H.J.; Khoury, J.C.; Copeland, K.A. Are mealtime best practice guidelines for child care centers associated with energy, vegetable, and fruit intake? *J. Child. Obes.* **2016**, *12*, 52–58. [CrossRef] [PubMed]
14. Gubbels, J.S.; Raaijmakers, L.G.; Gerards, S.M.; Kremers, S.P. Dietary intake by Dutch 1- to 3-year-old children at childcare and at home. *Nutrients* **2014**, *6*, 304–318. [CrossRef] [PubMed]
15. Ball, S.C.; Benjamin, S.E.; Ward, D.S. Dietary intakes in North Carolina child-care centers: Are children meeting current recommendations? *J Acad. Nutr. Diet.* **2008**, *108*, 718–721. [CrossRef] [PubMed]
16. Benjamin Neelon, S.E.; Vaughn, A.; Ball, S.C.; McWilliams, C.; Ward, D.S. Nutrition practices and mealtime environments of North Carolina child care centers. *J. Child. Obes. (Print)* **2012**, *8*, 216–223. [CrossRef] [PubMed]
17. Benjamin-Neelon, S.E.; Vaughn, A.E.; Tovar, A.; Ostbye, T.; Mazzucca, S.; Ward, D.S. The family child care home environment and children's diet quality. *Appetite* **2018**, *126*, 108–113. [CrossRef]
18. Gubbels, J.S.; Kremers, S.P.; Stafleu, A.; Dagnelie, P.C.; de Vries, N.K.; Thijs, C. Child-care environment and dietary intake of 2- and 3-year-old children. *J. Hum. Nutr. Diet.* **2010**, *23*, 97–101. [CrossRef]
19. Moore, H.; Nelson, P.; Marshall, J.; Cooper, M.; Zambas, H.; Brewster, K.; Atkin, K. Laying foundations for health: Food provision for under 5s in day care. *Appetite* **2005**, *44*, 207–213. [CrossRef]
20. Neelon, S.E.; Burgoine, T.; Hesketh, K.R.; Monsivais, P. Nutrition practices of nurseries in England. Comparison with national guidelines. *Appetite* **2015**, *85*, 22–29. [CrossRef]
21. School Food Trust. Voluntary Food and Drink Guidelines for for Early Years Settings in England—A Practical Guilde. London, England, 2012. Available online: https://www.eyalliance.org.uk/sites/default/files/voluntary_food_and_drink_guidelines_for_ey_settings.pdf (accessed on 16 July 2019).
22. Nicklaus, S.; Remy, E. Early origins of overeating: Tracking between early food habits and later eating patterns. *Curr. Obes. Rep.* **2013**, *2*, 179–184. [CrossRef]
23. Howard, A.J.; Mallan, K.M.; Byrne, R.; Magarey, A.; Daniels, L.A. Toddlers' food preferences. The impact of novel food exposure, maternal preferences and food neophobia. *Appetite* **2012**, *59*, 818–825. [CrossRef] [PubMed]
24. Harris, G.; Coulthard, H. Early eating behaviours and food acceptance revisited: Breastfeeding and introduction of complementary foods as predictive of food acceptance. *Curr. Obes. Rep.* **2016**, *5*, 113–120. [CrossRef] [PubMed]
25. Noradilah, M.; Zahara, A. Acceptance of a test vegetable after repeated exposures amoung preschoolers. *Mal. J. Nutr.* **2012**, *18*, 67–75.
26. O'Connell, M.L.; Henderson, K.E.; Luedicke, J.; Schwartz, M.B. Repeated exposure in a natural setting: A preschool intervention to increase vegetable consumption. *J. Acad. Nutr. Diet.* **2012**, *112*, 230–234. [CrossRef]
27. Johnson, S.L. Developmental and environmental influences on young children's vegetable preferences andconsumption. *Adv. Nutr.* **2016**, *7*, 220s–231s. [CrossRef]
28. Nekitsing, C.; Blundell-Birtill, P.; Cockroft, J.E.; Hetherington, M.M. Systematic review and meta-analysis of strategies to increase vegetable consumption in preschool children aged 2-5 years. *Appetite* **2018**, *127*, 138–154. [CrossRef]
29. Scherr, R.E.; Linnell, J.D.; Dharmar, M.; Beccarelli, L.M.; Bergman, J.J.; Briggs, M.; Brian, K.M.; Feenstra, G.; Hillhouse, J.C.; Keen, C.L.; et al. A Multicomponent, school-based intervention, the Shaping Healthy Choices Program, improves nutrition-related outcomes. *J. Nutr. Educ. Behav.* **2017**, *49*, 368–379.e1. [CrossRef]
30. Burt, K.G.; Burgermaster, M.; Jacquez, R. Predictors of school garden integration: Factors critical to gardening success in New York City. *Health Educ. Behav.* **2018**, *45*, 849–854. [CrossRef]
31. Evans, A.; Ranjit, N.; Rutledge, R.; Medina, J.L.; Jennings, R.; Smiley, A.; Stigler, M.; Hoelscher, D. Exposure to multiple components of a garden-based intervention for middle school students increases fruit and vegetable consumption. *Health. Promot. Chronic Dis. Prev. Can.* 2012. [CrossRef]

32. Castro, D.C.; Samuels, M.; Harman, A.E. Growing healthy kids: A community garden-based obesity prevention program. *Am. J. Prev. Med.* **2013**, *44*, S193–S199. [CrossRef]
33. Duncan, M.J.; Eyre, E.; Bryant, E.; Clarke, N.; Birch, S.; Staples, V.; Sheffield, D. The impact of a school-based gardening intervention on intentions and behaviour related to fruit and vegetable consumption in children. *J. Ment. Health Clin. Psychol.* **2015**, *20*, 765–773. [CrossRef] [PubMed]
34. Savoie-Roskos, M.R.; Wengreen, H.; Durward, C. Increasing fruit and vegetable intake among children and youth through gardening-based interventions: A systematic review. *J. Acad. Nutr. Diet* **2017**, *117*, 240–250. [CrossRef] [PubMed]
35. Parmer, S.M.; Salisbury-Glennon, J.; Shannon, D.; Struempler, B. School gardens: An experiential learning approach for a nutrition education program to increase fruit and vegetable knowledge, preference, and consumption among second-grade students. *J. Nutr. Educ. Behav.* **2009**, *41*, 212–217. [CrossRef] [PubMed]
36. Hodder, R.K.; Stacey, F.G.; O'Brien, K.M.; Wyse, R.J.; Clinton-McHarg, T.; Tzelepis, F.; James, E.L.; Bartlem, K.M.; Nathan, N.K.; Sutherland, R.; et al. Interventions for increasing fruit and vegetable consumption in children aged five years and under. *Cochrane Database Syst. Rev.* **2018**, *1*, Cd008552. [CrossRef]
37. Lumeng, J.C.; Hillman, K.H. Eating in larger groups increases food consumption. *Ar. Arch. Dis. Child.* **2007**, *92*, 384–387. [CrossRef]
38. Huys, N.; De Cocker, K.; De Craemer, M.; Roesbeke, M.; Cardon, G.; De Lepeleere, S. School gardens: A qualitative study on implementation practices. *Int. J. Environ. Res. Public. Health* **2017**, *14*. [CrossRef]
39. Robinson-O'Brien, R.; Story, M.; Heim, S. Impact of garden-based youth nutrition intervention programs: A review. *J. Acad. Nutr. Diet.* **2009**, *109*, 273–280. [CrossRef]
40. Davis, J.N.; Spaniol, M.R.; Somerset, S. Sustenance and sustainability: Maximizing the impact of school gardens on health outcomes. *Ethiop J. Public. Health. Nutr.* **2015**, *18*, 2358–2367. [CrossRef]
41. Monsivais, P.; Rehm, C.D. Potential nutritional and economic effects of replacing juice with fruit in the diets of children in the United States. *Arch. Pediatr. Adolesc. Med.* **2012**, *166*, 459–464. [CrossRef]
42. Benjamin, S.E.; Neelon, B.; Ball, S.C.; Bangdiwala, S.I.; Ammerman, A.S.; Ward, D.S. Reliability and validity of a nutrition and physical activity environmental self-assessment for child care. *nt J. Behav. Nutr. Phys. Act.* **2007**, *4*, 29. [CrossRef]
43. Ward, D.; Hales, D.; Haverly, K.; Marks, J.; Benjamin, S.; Ball, S.; Trost, S. An instrument to assess the obesogenic environment of child care centers. *Am. J. Health Econ.* **2008**, *32*, 380–386. [CrossRef]
44. Whitaker, R.C.; Gooze, R.A.; Hughes, C.C.; Finkelstein, D.M. A national survey of obesity prevention practices in Head Start. *Arch. Pediatr. Adolesc. Med.* **2009**, *163*, 1144–1150. [CrossRef] [PubMed]
45. Benjamin Neelon, S.E.; Mayhew, M.; O'Neill, J.R.; Neelon, B.; Li, F.; Pate, R.R. Comparative evaluation of a South Carolina policy to improve nutrition in child care. *J. Acad. Nutr. Diet.* **2016**, *116*, 949–956. [CrossRef] [PubMed]
46. Davis, K.L.; Brann, L.S. Examining the benefits and barriers of instructionalgardening programs to increase fruit and vegetable intake among preschool-age children. *Eur. J. Environ. Public Health* **2017**, *2017*, 2506864. [CrossRef]
47. van de Kolk, I.; Goossens, A.J.M.; Gerards, S.; Kremers, S.P.J.; Manders, R.M.P.; Gubbels, J.S. Healthy nutrition andphysical activity in childcare: Views from childcare managers, childcare workers andparents on influential factors. *Int J. Environ. Res. Public Health* **2018**, *15*. [CrossRef]
48. Lee, R.E.; Parker, N.H.; Soltero, E.G.; Ledoux, T.A.; Mama, S.K.; McNeill, L. Sustainability via Active Garden Education (SAGE): Results from two feasibility pilot studies. *BMC Public Health* **2017**, *17*, 242. [CrossRef]
49. Namenek Brouwer, R.J.; Benjamin Neelon, S.E. Watch me grow: A garden-based pilot intervention to increase vegetable and fruit intake in preschoolers. *BMC Public Health* **2013**, *13*, 363. [CrossRef]
50. Soltero, E.G.; Parker, N.H.; Mama Dr, P.S.; Ledoux, T.A.; Lee, R.E. Lessons learned from implementing of garden education program in early child care. *Health Promot. Chronic Dis. Prev. Can.* 2019. [CrossRef]
51. Sharma, S.V.; Hedberg, A.M.; Skala, K.A.; Chuang, R.-J.; Lewis, T. Feasibility and acceptability of a gardening-based nutrition education program in preschoolers from low-income, minority populations. *J. Early Child Res.* **2015**, *13*, 93–110. [CrossRef]
52. Kos, M.; Jerman, J. Preschool children learning about the origin of food, on local farms and in the preschool garden. *J. Clin. Nutr. Food Sci.* **2012**, *42*, 324–331. [CrossRef]

53. Ohly, H.; Gentry, S.; Wigglesworth, R.; Bethel, A.; Lovell, R.; Garside, R. A systematic review of the health and well-being impacts of school gardening: Synthesis of quantitative and qualitative evidence. *BMC Public Health* **2016**, *16*, 286. [CrossRef]
54. Hoffman, J.A.; Agrawal, T.; Wirth, C.; Watts, C.; Adeduntan, G.; Myles, L.; Castaneda-Sceppa, C. Farm to family: Increasing access to affordable fruits and vegetables among urban Head Start families. *J. Hunger Environ. Nutr.* **2012**, *7*, 165–177. [CrossRef]
55. Farfan-Ramirez, L.; Diemoz, L.; Gong, E.J.; Lagura, M.A. Curriculum intervention in preschool children: Nutrition Matters! *J. Nutr. Educ. Behav.* **2011**, *43*, S162–S165. [CrossRef] [PubMed]
56. Dawson, A.; Richards, R.; Collins, C.; Reeder, A.I.; Gray, A. Edible gardens in early childhood education settings in Aotearoa, New Zealand. *Health Promot J. Austr.* **2013**, *24*, 214–218. [CrossRef] [PubMed]

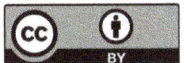

© 2019 by the authors. Licensee MDPI, Basel, Switzerland. This article is an open access article distributed under the terms and conditions of the Creative Commons Attribution (CC BY) license (http://creativecommons.org/licenses/by/4.0/).

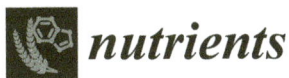

Article

Opportunities and Challenges Arising from Holiday Clubs Tackling Children's Hunger in the UK: Pilot Club Leader Perspectives

Clare E. Holley *, Carolynne Mason and Emma Haycraft

School of Sport, Exercise and Health Sciences, Loughborough University, Epinal Way, LE11 3TU Loughborough, UK; C.L.J.Mason@lboro.ac.uk (C.M.); E.Haycraft@lboro.ac.uk (E.H.)
* Correspondence: C.Holley@lboro.ac.uk; Tel.: +44-(0)-1509-226376

Received: 7 May 2019; Accepted: 28 May 2019; Published: 30 May 2019

Abstract: With the school holidays being recognised as a high-risk time for children to experience food insecurity, there is a growing prevalence of school holiday initiatives that include free food. However, information is lacking into what constitutes effective practice in their delivery, and how this can be evaluated. This paper provides insight from individuals who implemented a pilot of a national project which provided free food for children at UK community summer holiday sports clubs in 2016. Focus groups were conducted with all 15 leaders of the holiday clubs that participated in the pilot to understand: (1) what opportunities are provided by community holiday sports clubs which include free food; (2) what challenges arose as a result of offering free food within a broader community holiday club sports offer. Results indicate that offering free food at such clubs creates multiple opportunities for attending children, including: experiencing social interactions around food; enhancing food experiences and food confidence; and promoting positive behaviour. However, free food provision is associated with challenges including resource constraints and tensions around project aims. Future work should determine whether holiday clubs can positively impact children's wellbeing and healthy eating.

Keywords: child; food poverty; food insecurity; holiday hunger; intervention; evaluation

1. Introduction

Food insecurity has been defined as "limited or uncertain availability of nutritionally adequate and safe foods or limited or uncertain ability to acquire acceptable foods in socially acceptable ways (e.g., without resorting to emergency food supplies, scavenging, stealing or other coping strategies)" [1]. While food insecurity in UK children has not been measured to date, a recent UNICEF report indicates that food insecurity is prevalent in the UK, with 20% of children aged under 15 years old living with a respondent who is moderately or severely food insecure and 10% living with a respondent who is severely food insecure [2]. Research asserts that children who experience food insecurity are less likely to eat fruits, vegetables and brown bread, and are more likely to consume unhealthy foods such as chips and hamburgers [3]. Children who experience food insecurity are also likely to experience holiday hunger; the phenomenon by which children (particularly those who rely on free school meals during term-time) fall into a nutritional and calorie deficit in the school holidays [4,5].

Holiday hunger is likely to have a detrimental effect on school children's educational performance, health and wellbeing. Although there are common issues with measurement of changes in educational attainment, gaps in attainment between US children in high and low poverty schools which increase across the summer have been reported [6], with summer learning loss also being evidenced among low socioeconomic status (SES) school children in the UK [7]. Moreover, food insecurity is associated with poorer health status and emotional wellbeing [8]. For example, 6-year-old to 11-year-old children from food insecure families demonstrate difficulty getting on with other children and are more likely to have seen a psychologist [9].

While free food services are increasingly in demand in the UK [10], there can be an associated social stigma that can inhibit families from utilising them [11]. However, free food provision integrated within holiday clubs presents an opportunity to encourage more individuals to attend these clubs while removing the social stigma associated with attending other free food services [12]. Creating holiday food provision within local communities therefore not only facilitates social support, which has a well-established relationship with health and wellbeing [13], but also ensures that the provision is accessible. This will likely maximise both the utility and the uptake of such provision. Tackling holiday hunger can lessen the nutritional deficit experienced by a significant proportion of UK children [14]. The disparity in educational attainment, health and wellbeing associated with food insecurity may also be reduced, while utilising this opportunity to engage the population in physical activity and other community-based activities.

Despite there being an increasing number of holiday clubs across the UK attempting to tackle holiday hunger, there is incredibly limited research into the operational aspects and effectiveness of these clubs [5], and there is no published literature on similar projects in other countries of the developed world [15]. Previous qualitative research suggests that holiday breakfast clubs in the north-west of England and Northern Ireland may have positive social, nutritional, educational and financial impacts for those attending [12,16]. In further qualitative research, school holiday club staff asserted that holiday food provision is needed and that clubs can provide access to food and other activities including social and informal learning opportunities [17]. However, free food provision at community holiday sports clubs has not previously been examined and an in-depth analysis of the challenges that food provision presents is yet to be conducted.

Holiday clubs typically develop organically and are context specific and therefore operate without a fixed format, which presents challenges for robust evaluation work. Moreover, food insecurity is a multi-faceted issue, with multiple consequences, and there is variance in which aspects are targeted by holiday clubs. A recent systematic review has suggested that the evidence base regarding food insecurity interventions is mixed, has methodological limitations and that evaluations may be missing key areas of impact [15]. With this in mind, more information is needed on how the effectiveness of holiday projects which include free food can be evaluated, and how any potential impact can be assessed in future evaluation work.

The current study sought to distil learning from the experiences of the 15 leaders who organised and delivered the holiday clubs which participated in the StreetGames Fit and Fed programme pilot (community holiday sports clubs including free food provision). The study sought to address two research questions: *(1) what opportunities are provided by holiday sports clubs which offer free food in disadvantaged communities; (2) what challenges arose as a result of offering free food within holiday sports clubs in disadvantaged communities.* Exploration of these questions was undertaken with the goal of informing further research to support the future success of the Fit and Fed project, and other holiday clubs that incorporate sport and food.

2. Methods

2.1. Ethics

The study was conducted in accordance with the Declaration of Helsinki, and Ethical clearance was obtained for this study from the Loughborough University Institutional Review Board.

2.2. Participants

Participants were the 15 leaders who organised and ran the pilot holiday clubs that were delivered through the Fit and Fed project over the school summer holiday period in 2016. These clubs took place across multiple counties within the UK, with the majority of these clubs (77%) taking place in the top 20% of deprived neighbourhoods in England and Wales as categorised by the English and Welsh indices of deprivation [18,19].

2.3. The Fit and Fed Programme

Fit and Fed is a national project run by the charity StreetGames. StreetGames utilises doorstep sport to achieve positive change in the lives of children from disadvantaged communities [20]. In response to large numbers of children who attend their neighbourhood youth sport opportunities experiencing holiday hunger, StreetGames developed the Fit and Fed project to provide free meals to children within disadvantaged community holiday sports clubs across the UK. The programme aims to tackle three main inequalities—holiday hunger, isolation, and inactivity—by providing food alongside the opportunity to participate in sporting activities and physical activity. Clubs do not operate under a fixed format, but rather implement their activities in the format appropriate for their club and the available resources. In its initial (pilot) year, the Fit and Fed project comprised 33 holiday clubs overseen by 15 holiday club leaders. The research team are entirely independent from StreetGames and the Fit and Fed project.

2.4. Recruitment

After the school summer holiday in 2016, the 15 pilot club leaders were invited to participate in a feedback day to share their experiences of the pilot and ideas for the future progression of the programme. All leaders of pilot clubs attended the feedback day. One element of this feedback day was focus groups to capture club leaders' insights based on their diverse pilot experiences.

2.5. Focus Groups

Written informed consent was obtained from participants before the onset of the focus group, with individuals informed of their right to withdraw at any point. Focus groups were conducted to create dynamic discussions between participants. In order to ensure sustained discussion at the same time as allowing space for all members to participate, the participants were split into two focus groups [21]. Group one had seven participants and lasted for 33 min and group two had eight participants and lasted for 44 min.

The focus groups were digitally recorded. They were facilitated by the lead author (CH) who posed a series of questions compiled by the research team. The questions were derived from discussions within the research team as well as a review of the literature.

2.6. Descriptive Information about the Holiday Clubs

After participating in the focus groups, pilot club leaders completed a questionnaire to provide information on the number, gender and age of children attending their clubs, the frequency and duration of the club sessions and the food provided.

2.7. Analysis

Focus group recordings were transcribed verbatim and a thematic analysis was undertaken, following Braun and Clarke's guidance [22]. As this is an exploratory study, coding was undertaken both with an inductive and deductive approach, where data were coded with research questions in mind in order to generate the resultant themes. The research questions were: *(1) what opportunities are provided by holiday sports clubs which offer free food in disadvantaged communities; (2) what challenges arose as a result of offering free food within holiday sports clubs in disadvantaged communities?* First, the lead author fully immersed themselves in the data. Second, sections of the transcripts recognised as meaningful in relation to the study aims were identified and manually labelled with an appropriate code. Once both transcripts had been coded, the third step of grouping codes according to a common theme was undertaken. This resulted in a set of related themes with distinct conceptual meaning.

Research team members were involved in a discussion of the coded items to facilitate the creation of themes. Two of these members (C.M., E.H.) had not read the full transcripts of the focus groups and as such were judged to be suitable unbiased consultants. The reliability of the analysis was confirmed by a second, independent researcher (BAJ) who performed an analysis on 20% of the transcripts. The second coder used their own coding scheme, corroborated the themes that were identified by the primary researcher, and did not identify any further themes. This method of assessing reliability of the analysis is recognised as appropriate for a thematic analysis and has been widely used in previous research [23].

3. Results

3.1. Descriptive Information about the Holiday Clubs

Descriptive information about the frequency and duration of the holiday clubs is presented in Table 1. There was variability in the number of weeks that the clubs ran for, the number of sessions offered per week, and the duration of these sessions. Most clubs ran for five or more weeks, with some running once a week and some running every day. The profile of the child attendees also varied between clubs. However, 85% of attendees across clubs were aged 13 years or under, and slightly more attendees were male than female.

Table 1. Descriptive information on the frequency and duration of the Fit and Fed pilot clubs ($n = 15$).

Holiday Club Information	Mean	Min	Max	SD
Number of weeks ran for	4.53	1.00	6.00	1.55
Number of sessions per week	2.63	1.00	5.00	1.23
Session duration (hours)	4.30	2.00	6.00	1.27
Percentage of male attendees	65.95	40.43	95.00	13.48

SD = standard deviation.

Group leaders reported on the foods offered during the holiday club sessions across the summer (Table 2). All clubs provided sandwiches, while almost half provided a hot meal. Most clubs provided some form of fruit, while almost half provided a form of salad or vegetable. In addition, 53% of clubs offered a cooking or food related activity for the children to engage in, alongside food provision.

Table 2. Descriptive information on the number and percentage of Fit and Fed pilot clubs ($n = 14$ due to missing data) serving different types of food.

Food	n of Clubs Which Served Food	%
Sandwich/wrap	14	92.9
Hot meal	6	42.9
Crisps	5	35.7
Biscuits	7	46.7
Fruit	13	92.9
Salad/Vegetable	6	42.9

3.2. Thematic Analysis

Pilot club leaders' insights from the project were explored in relation to two research questions: (1) what opportunities are provided by holiday sports clubs which offer free food in disadvantaged communities; (2) what challenges arose as a result of offering free food within holiday sports clubs in disadvantaged communities? For each of the two research questions, several themes were identified. These are discussed in detail in the following sections.

3.3. Research Question One: What Opportunities are Provided by Holiday Sports Clubs That Offer Free Food in Disadvantaged Communities?

The comments of the pilot club leaders revealed a number of different opportunities arising from the inclusion of the food offer at community holiday sports clubs. These opportunities were: promoting engagement, alleviating food scarcity, enhancing children's food experiences, increasing 'food confidence', promoting social experiences with food and promoting positive behaviours.

3.3.1. Opportunity 1: Promoting Engagement

Almost all pilot club leaders identified that providing free food promoted children's engagement with the holiday clubs. Leaders perceived that free food was a motivator for attendance at the sports clubs: *"the last session where we provided food was the busiest one"*, *"I think some people attended ours just for the free food"*; and that the provision of food increased the number of children attending their clubs: *"I think the food was a massive attraction and the numbers [of attendees] were better than [for previous] stuff we'd put on"*. These comments indicate that providing food can be an important incentive to encourage participation in projects that may deliver a range of positive health outcomes for children. Furthermore, providing universal free food for all attendees at the holiday clubs promoted engagement and removed the potential for the stigma associated with projects which seek to solely alleviate food insecurity: *"We were just a sports academy so that was it, other than Fit and Fed it was just a sports academy, there was no stigmatisation on anything else"*.

3.3.2. Opportunity 2: Alleviating Food Scarcity

Pilot club leaders perceived the inclusion of the food offer to be important for addressing food scarcity related specifically to the school holiday period (holiday hunger). Pilot club leaders reported that parents face additional financial pressure in the school holidays: *"it costs more to live during the school holidays, and they're preparing to go back to school in September; maybe school uniform is too small, got to get new ... "*. These discussions suggested that families were forced to make decisions about how to prioritise their spending to afford the necessities. Some pilot club leaders also commented that food scarcity decreased the amount of food that parents allowed themselves to eat to provide food for their children: *"I see mums that don't eat, because they don't want to take the food out of the kids' mouths, because that's the only food that they're gonna get"*.

3.3.3. Opportunity 3: Enhancing Children's Food Experiences

In addition to restrictions on the quantity of food available, pilot club leaders were concerned about the quality of food that was available to families within the targeted communities as a result of lack of money and a lack of access to more nutritionally appropriate (expensive) food: *"there's no transport, there's no finance – it's difficult"*. It was recognised by pilot club leaders that financial issues impacted parents food provision, with them reporting that children and families opted to buy foods with lower nutritional value which were often cheaper and more readily available than healthy foods: *"some of the chicken places charge £1! For chicken and chips! A parent is going to look at that and go, do you know what, I've got a £1 for that but I can't go shopping and spend £5 to do a meal"*.

Pilot club leaders perceived there to be opportunities for the holiday clubs to enhance children's experiences with food, but in doing so they demonstrated some stereotyped views on children's prior food experiences. Pilot club leaders made assumptions around what they perceived to be evidence of a restricted diet: *"some kids don't even know what tomatoes and cucumbers are!"*, *"The kids in Blackpool didn't even know you could get red apples, because mum and dad just always buy green. 'What's that?!' 'It's an apple.' 'Don't be so stupid, it's red!'"*. Moreover, pilot club leaders reported witnessing child attendees choosing foods which were perceived to be 'unhealthy' when given a free rein: *"They'd come back with a two-litre bottle of something blue or like loads of bags of crisps and loads of sweets"*.

3.3.4. Opportunity 4: Increasing 'Food Confidence'

Related to the opportunity to alleviate food scarcity is the opportunity to increase 'food confidence'. Pilot club leaders indicated that some attendees were very reluctant to try new foods that were not familiar to them, and they attributed this to children having a lack of confidence to try new foods: *"You're all talking about the nutritional thing, we didn't even do that. It was food confidence for us, it was some of these kids thinking 'what's that?!'"*. Some club leaders adopted innovative strategies to try and address this lack of food confidence by developing games and activities to encourage children to try different foods, with fruit and vegetable consumption being particularly targeted. Strategies included use of a smoothie bike where participants' pedal power enabled the ingredients to be converted into smoothies: *"they were making these green smoothies with like spinach, banana, and they were tasting them like 'well actually, that's really nice, have that!'"*. Pilot club leaders also described how getting children involved in food preparation encouraged them to try foods they would not otherwise: *"it worked so well [using a bike powered blender] because where the kids ... wouldn't have eaten a banana, chuck it in milkshake, and because they'd done the pedalling themselves, they enjoyed it"*. The way in which food was prepared and delivered was noted as impacting on participants' willingness to try new foods. For example: *"some of the coaches were saying to me that fruit was better received if it was chopped up to small bite sized pieces than it was if you gave them a whole apple"*. One pilot club leader suggested that this approach mirrored supermarket moves to sell prepared fruit which they sell at a premium price. Other strategies included quizzes and 'bush tucker trials' (eating challenges that appear in the popular television programme 'I'm a celebrity ... get me out of here').

3.3.5. Opportunity 5: Promoting Social Experiences with Food

Pilot club leaders discussed several ways in which they provided opportunities to promote children's social experiences with food. Some of the projects, particularly those that adopted a multi-partner delivery model which was accompanied by greater resourcing, deliberately engaged children in the preparation of the food that was eaten. This approach was seen as having the advantage of being an effective way of engaging parents and other family members in both cooking and the physical activity which was offered at clubs: *"I think it brought everyone into a whole new element because who doesn't like to prep food, cook food and eat food? So, we called our project [name of project] ... we had babies coming in, parents with the rest of the family coming in"*.

A number of pilot club leaders mentioned the significance of sitting around the table when eating and this was something that was clearly considered to be both important and impactful by some club leaders: *"We always had a dessert as well because ... it was a way of keeping them at the table and having that kind of meal environment"*. This is an interesting finding as this indicates again that pilot club leaders aspired to do more than just ensure children were not going hungry during the school holidays. Pilot club leaders described attempts to create a meal which they clearly associated as being a valuable and positive experience for participants and something that some leaders assumed may not happen at home for these children.

3.3.6. Opportunity 6: Promoting Positive Behaviours

Some pilot club leaders indicated that for some of the attendees at Fit and Fed, the provision of food impacted positively on children's behaviour: *"there were changes in the behaviour of the young people because they were then fed, and obviously ... they're not then as lethargic, they've got their energy to talk and do things"*. Furthermore, pilot club leaders described improvements in both children's mood as a result of being fed: *"a hungry child is an angry child"*; and also in their concentration: *"because they haven't got to worry where their next meal is coming from they can concentrate more"*. Pilot club leaders also described changes in mood as altering the perceptions that other people may have of the young attendees: *"they'll probably have been told oh you know 'moody young kid', 'moody teenager', 'always causing* trouble again', whereas there's an actual reason for it, and those are the things that we can eradicate, and they can now be seen in a whole different light".

3.4. Research Question Two: What Challenges Arose as a Result of Offering Free Food Within Holiday Sports Clubs in Disadvantaged Communities?

The focus clubs uncovered five different overarching challenges arising from including free food at the holiday clubs. These challenges were: food provision, other resource constraints, the age of participants, staff attitudes and nutritional understanding and peer pressure.

3.4.1. Challenge 1: Food Provision

The discussions with pilot club leaders indicated considerable variation in the food that was provided at the different Fit and Fed projects. The availability of food was determined by a range of different factors but was perhaps most heavily influenced by the financial resources available: "we didn't have the funding to be able to go and get a lot of these things [foods], I mean we kept it basic". Issues with obtaining food supplies from big companies were also evident: "we went to [name of supermarket] and they wanted nothing to do with it"; and similarly, from food banks, who had insufficient supplies: "we weren't getting there early enough so all the other projects were getting the good stuff". Lastly, the available facilities dictated the kinds of food that clubs could provide and led to compromises: "We didn't have a cooker though, so we just sort of made sandwiches".

3.4.2. Challenge 2: Other Resource Constraints

Pilot club leaders also described challenges related to other resources including a lack of staff: "if we'd got 40 kids turning up and we've only got two [sport] coaches then we've got a safeguarding issue on our hands". Limited capacity and ensuring the health and safety of children and children at the facilities was also identified as a challenge: "if it was bad weather ... we could literally have no more than 30 odd kids in there, so we were a bit restricted".

3.4.3. Challenge 3: Age of Participants

The majority of the club leaders in the pilot stated that they had predominantly engaged younger children (5–11) despite some staff suggesting that older children may have a greater need for a food offer: "we work with what we class as the forgotten group, the 11–14 year olds, because if you're younger than that someone will help you out, and if you're older than 14 where we're from you're already making money".

3.4.4. Challenge 4: Staff Attitudes and Nutritional Understanding

It was clear from the focus groups that staff had varying attitudes towards what constituted healthy eating, what children should be eating, and how they should be encouraged to eat healthily. Fruit and vegetables were generally perceived as foods to be encouraged by all staff: "We tried to build it into every meal so ... we had a main meal and a dessert so [in] one or the other there'd be either fruit or veg in both. Usually in every meal". Some staff were much more positive about participants accessing food high in sugar (e.g., desserts, sweets) than other staff: "We always had a dessert as well.", "One of our most popular meals was the ice cream, little cones, because they came up for seconds", "We do give the kids treats like that as well as the fruit".

Some pilot club leaders were traditional in their attempts to encourage children to eat healthy food as they discouraged participants from actions which limited the food that was eaten. These staff expected participants to eat the food they were provided with and were reluctant to adapt the food on offer to tailor for individual preferences: "They were requesting 'can I have that without salad?', [and we were saying to them] 'No, you can't!'". Furthermore, some pilot club leaders were adamant that the food on offer needed to be 'healthy', while for other club leaders the need to tackle 'food shortage' was of primary importance: "The most important thing is that they're full, and the second most important thing is well if we can make things better then that's great". This tension was not easily reconciled: "We knew that *parents and children wanted those normal, everyday nice foods, and part of us, our heartstrings were saying you know if these kids haven't had a meal then they should have something they can enjoy as well that is not too radical for them, but on the other hand we should be promoting healthy eating".*

3.4.5. Challenge 5: Peer Pressure

Pilot club leaders highlighted that children's eating behaviour was influenced by peers. This peer influence could be positive: *"they would kind of serve each other smoothies and they really liked that"*, but it could also be a challenge: *"we'd got them sandwiches, and they sat and picked all of the salad out of it, put it in the bin, closed the sandwich again . . . I am talking every single one of them would sit there and take the [salad] out".*

4. Discussion

This study aimed to distil learning from the experiences of 15 pilot club leaders who provided free food for children attending community holiday sports clubs across the UK. It utilised the insights of leaders of the clubs who participated in the pilot project to determine: *(1) what opportunities are provided by holiday sports clubs which offer free food in disadvantaged communities; (2) what challenges arose as a result of offering free food within holiday sports clubs in disadvantaged communities.*

Pilot club leaders reported that providing free food as part of their holiday clubs promoted attendees' engagement with the clubs. Children's participation in sport can have multiple positive outcomes [24], with recreational sport developing children's self-confidence, communication and teamwork skills, and willingness to challenge themselves [25]. Moreover, club leaders identified that embedding food provision within these sport contexts reduced the stigma of attending a free food initiative, supporting assertions made in previous research and highlighting the strength of this approach [12]. With UK government funding for holiday clubs being contingent on providing daily physical activity alongside free food [26], such opportunities for positive outcomes and reduced stigma are increasingly prevalent.

Pilot club leaders reported opportunities for increasing food confidence, as well as enhancing children's food experiences. This belief was rooted in a perception that participants had access to both a limited quantity and a limited range of food during the school holidays. Staff also reported that these issues were compounded by participants lacking food confidence and therefore self-limiting the food they chose to eat, as well as by the social influences on children's food choices - notably the influence of peers. As diets low in fruit and vegetables are associated with an increased risk of numerous non-communicable diseases [27], holiday clubs that provide opportunities to diversify children's diets and improve eating behaviours have the potential to prevent the development of disease and ill health. With this in mind, future research is needed to evidence whether holiday clubs do improve children's food confidence and eating behaviours.

Although comments from club leaders identified opportunities to enhance children's food experiences and food confidence, not all clubs capitalised on this opportunity. Food provision was a significant challenge for clubs, and while most (93%) clubs offered fruit, just 43% offered vegetables. While it is important that children experiencing food insecurity are given energy-dense foods which will help to attenuate their calorie deficit, the nutritional deficit they experience should also be tackled by such community interventions if potential health benefits are to be realised. This would require implementing a minimum standard of food which provides child attendees with the most appropriate foods in terms of both macro- and micro-nutrients, in order to achieve maximal health benefits. While this was beyond the reach of the clubs who participated in this pilot, this is a new requirement of the Department for Education's recently pledged funding for holiday clubs across the UK, where all food provided at clubs (including snacks) must meet the school food standards [26]. Future work should seek to determine how the challenges of providing nutritionally balanced foods within holiday club contexts can be overcome.

A further opportunity described by pilot club leaders was promoting social experiences with food, with some clubs able to engage children in food preparation and/or enjoy shared mealtimes around a table. Previous research has suggested that involving children in cooking can increase children's consumption of vegetables as well as meals, highlighting the potential of this opportunity [28–30], and the impact of this should be explored in future research. Moreover, shared mealtimes are associated with children having a reduced risk of substance abuse and paediatric obesity, promoting language development and higher academic achievement [31] and better psychological wellbeing [32], highlighting the value of these new experiences. With this in mind, wellbeing may be one appropriate indicator of intervention success in future research.

Some pilot club leaders outlined opportunities for the provision of free food to promote positive behaviours. Food insecurity has been associated with increased odds of substance abuse and behavioural, anxiety, and mood disorders during the previous year [33]. Moreover, Maslow's hierarchy of needs suggests that children are unable to perform higher order behaviours, such as respect for self and others, until lower order needs, such as hunger, are satisfied [34]. Here, hunger shows a prepotency over behaving in a socially acceptable way. In line with one leader's statement that "a hungry child is an angry child", it therefore seems plausible that short-term alleviation of food insecurity could be related to improvements in children's moods. This suggests that by tackling holiday hunger, projects may have the potential to reduce the likelihood of antisocial behaviour among some attendees who have a propensity towards these behaviours. Further work is needed to explore this.

Pilot club leaders widely reported that resources were a challenge for community holiday clubs and that these restricted the food provision and the number of children each club could accommodate. This is also supported by the descriptive information gathered from the clubs. The number of weeks that the clubs ran for and the frequency of sessions they offered varied greatly in accordance with resource constraints as a lack of resources unfortunately appears to be common. However, with the UK government's Department for Education (DfE) pledging £9 million in funding for holiday clubs for children in disadvantaged communities, there is optimism that these resource issues can be minimised for many clubs.

This paper has focused primarily on understanding what happens when free food is offered alongside physical and social activities to create a broader provision for children. Such provision potentially offers better value for money in that multiple outcomes can be achieved simultaneously. However, this model creates challenges in terms of evaluating the effectiveness of the project because the aims are complex and inter-linked.

It was clear from the experiences discussed in the focus groups that there was considerable diversity in terms of what the projects sought to achieve within their clubs and also considerable variation in how the clubs undertook the Fit and Fed pilot project. They varied in terms of inter alia partners involved, settings, delivery approach/activities, age range of participants, reach and aims of the club. Such variation raises questions about what constitutes effectiveness and how this can best be measured, including whether success of community projects should be measured according to local community aims, or the aims of broader public health programmes. Indeed, whilst many of the clubs included in this study met the DfE's minimum standards required for 2019 publicly funded UK holiday clubs, it also underlines the complexities of achieving (and assessing) the UK government's aspiration of locally coordinated free holiday activities and healthy food for disadvantaged children.

While most projects aimed to ensure that children did not experience 'holiday hunger', they adopted different ways of addressing the issue of food scarcity. Indeed, most projects were concerned with much broader food aims related to the quality of participants' food experiences. In addition to tackling food scarcity, most projects also attempted to promote 'healthy' eating, but again, there was considerable variation in terms of what was considered as 'healthy' eating and how this outcome could best be achieved. Moreover, some projects promoted intake of food regardless of nutritional composition, which may exacerbate unhealthy eating behaviours in some children.

The novel contribution of this paper includes highlighting the challenges that exist regarding developing a robust evidence base for projects that are not uniformly implemented, where evaluation of impact needs to be aligned with the overarching aims of these projects. The aspirations for including a food offer within clubs were not clearly articulated by many clubs. Developing a more robust evidence base will require not only the articulation of these intended outcomes, but also a more advanced understanding of how these outcomes can best be delivered for which children. Having unpacked the insights of holiday club leaders on the opportunities provided by holiday clubs, this paper provides novel insight into previously unexplored areas of potential impact across a range of outcomes associated with child wellbeing and healthy eating, including dietary variety, dietary intake, food choice and willingness to try new foods.

This study provides an important account of pilot club leaders' perceptions of the opportunities that community projects which offer free meals during the school holidays can provide. By gathering qualitative data, a detailed picture of the potential impact of these projects was developed. While the qualitative methods employed here have clear strengths, it must be acknowledged that the evidence collected for this study is experiential and future research should seek to further explore the assertions made in these focus groups. For example, club leaders may have held stereotyped perceptions of the child attendees and, in turn, the opportunities created for these children by the holiday clubs. Future research is also needed which explores the views of children and families who engage in these projects, as those with the best knowledge of their own experiences [35]. The limited data gathered in this study prevents conclusions being drawn about the efficacy of a particular format of a successful club, or what a club must offer in order to be successful or what constitutes success for holiday hunger clubs. However, it does provide valuable insight into potential areas of impact to be explored in future research.

5. Conclusion

This study provides valuable insight into the opportunities presented by adding a free food provision to community holiday clubs, as well as the challenges this creates. With holiday hunger becoming a more prominent issue, projects that provide greater value for money by seeking to address a range of complex inter-related outcomes may be preferential to other models of intervention. However, progress in securing a strong evidence base about what works, why and for whom regarding holiday hunger is only in its infancy. Future research should seek to evaluate these projects according to these newly identified areas of potential impact around children's wellbeing and healthy eating. Future research should also assess the appropriateness and benefits of recently introduced minimum standards for UK government projects of this nature, to ensure that projects are able to maximise the opportunities and benefits they provide for children and their families.

Author Contributions: C.E.H. contributed to the data collection, design, analysis and write up of this paper; C.M. contributed to the analysis and write up of the manuscript; E.H. contributed to the design, analysis and write up of the manuscript. All authors read and approved the final manuscript.

Funding: This research received no external funding.

Acknowledgments: We thank Jane Ashworth OBE for access to the participants in this research and for her insights and information about the run of the Fit and Fed project. Thank you also to Bethany A. Jones for her valuable contribution as a second coder.

Conflicts of Interest: The authors declare no conflict of interest.

References

1. Taylor, A.; Loopstra, A. Too Poor to Eat: Food Insecurity in the UK. Available online: https://foodfoundation.org.uk/wp-content/uploads/2016/07/FoodInsecurityBriefing-May-2016-FINAL.pdf (accessed on 1 March 2017).
2. Pereira, A.; Handa, S.; Holmqvist, G. *Prevalence and Correlates of Food Insecurity among Children across the Globe*; Publisher: Florence, Italy, 2017.
3. Molcho, M.; Gabhainn, S.; Kelly, C. Food poverty and health among schoolchildren in Ireland: Findings from the Health Behaviour in School-aged Children (HBSC) study. *Public Health Nutr.* **2007**, *10*, 364–370. [CrossRef] [PubMed]

4. Kellogg's, Y. Isolation and Hunger: The Reality of the School Holidays for Struggling Families. Available online: https://www.kelloggs.co.uk/content/dam/europe/kelloggs_gb/pdf/HOLIDAY+HUNGER+REPORT.pdf (accessed on 1 March 2017).
5. Lambie-Mumford, H.; Sims, L. 'Feeding Hungry Children': The Growth of Charitable Breakfast Clubs and Holiday Hunger Projects in the UK. *Child. Soc.* **2018**, *32*, 244–254. [CrossRef]
6. von Hippel, P.; Hamrock, C. Do test score gaps grow before, during, or between the school years? Measurement artifacts and what we can know in spite of them. *Sociol. Sci.* **2019**, *6*, 43–80. [CrossRef]
7. Shinwell, J.; Defeyter, M.A. Investigation of Summer Learning Loss in the UK-Implications for Holiday Club Provision. *Front. Public Health* **2017**, *5*, 270. [CrossRef] [PubMed]
8. Ashiabi, G. Household food insecurity and children's school engagement. *J. Child. Poverty* **2005**, *11*, 3–17. [CrossRef]
9. Alaimo, K.; Olson, C.M.; Frongillo, E.A., Jr. Food Insufficiency and American School-Aged Children's Cognitive, Academic, and Psychosocial Development. *Pediatrics* **2001**, *108*, 44–53.
10. Trussell Trust. Mid Year Stats April–September 2018. Available online: https://www.trusselltrust.org/news-and-blog/latest-stats/mid-year-stats/ (accessed on 6 December 2018).
11. Holford, A. Take-up of Free School Meals: Price Effects and Peer Effects. *Economica* **2015**, *82*, 976–993. [CrossRef]
12. Defeyter, M.A.; Graham, P.L.; Prince, K. A Qualitative Evaluation of Holiday Breakfast Clubs in the UK: Views of Adult Attendees, Children, and Staff. *Front. Public Health* **2015**, *3*, 199. [CrossRef]
13. Berkman, L.F.; Syme, S.L. Social networks, host resistance, and mortality: A nine-year follow-up study of Alameda County residents. *Am. J. Epidemiol.* **1979**, *109*, 186–204. [CrossRef]
14. Public Health England & Food Standards Agency. National Diet and Nutrition Survey: Results from Years 1, 2, 3 and 4 (Combined) of the Rolling Programme (2008/2009–2011/2012). Available online: https://www.gov.uk/government/uploads/system/uploads/attachment_data/file/310995/NDNS_Y1_to_4_UK_report.pdf (accessed on 1 March 2017).
15. Holley, C.E.; Mason, C. A Systematic Review of the Evaluation of Interventions to Tackle Children's Food Insecurity. *Curr. Nutr. Rep.* **2019**, *8*, 1–17.
16. Graham, P.; Russo, R.; Blackledge, J. Breakfast and beyond: The dietary, social and practical impacts of a universal free school breakfast scheme in the North West of England, UK. *Int. J. Sociol. Agric. Food* **2014**, *21*, 261–274.
17. Graham, P.L.; Crilley, E.; Stretesky, P.B.; Long, M.A.; Palmer, K.J.; Steinbock, E.; Defeyter, M.A. School Holiday Food Provision in the UK: A Qualitative Investigation of Needs, Benefits, and Potential for Development. *Front. Public Health* **2016**, *4*, 172. [CrossRef]
18. Smith, T.; Noble, M.; Noble, S.; Wright, G.; McLennan, D.; Plunkett, E. *The English Indices of Deprivation 2015*; Department for Communities and Local Government: London, UK, 2015.
19. Statistics for Wales. The Welsh Indices of Deprivation 2014. Available online: https://gweddill.gov.wales/docs/statistics/2015/150812-wimd-2014-revised-en.pdf (accessed on 2 April 2019).
20. Mason, C. Physical activity opportunities for young people: A case study of StreetGames. In *Routledge Handbook of Physical Activity Policy and Practice*; Piggin, J., Mansfield, L., Weed, M., Eds.; Routledge: London, UK; New York, NY, USA, 2017; pp. 371–383.
21. Morgan, D. *Qualitative Research Methods: Focus Groups as Qualitative Research*, 2nd ed.; SAGE Publications Ltd.: Thousand Oaks, CA, USA, 1997. [CrossRef]
22. Braun, V.; Clarke, V. Using thematic analysis in psychology. *Qual. Res. Psychol.* **2006**, *3*, 77–101. [CrossRef]
23. Yardley, L. Demonstrating validity in qualitative psychology. In *Qualitative Psychology a Practical Guide to Research Methods*; Smith, J.A., Ed.; Sage: London, UK, 2008; pp. 235–251.
24. Holt, N.; Neely, K. Positive youth development through sport: A review. *Rev. Iberoam. Psicol. Ejerc.* **2011**, *6*, 229–316.
25. Armour, K.; Sandford, R. Positive youth development through an outdoor physical activity programme: Evidence from a four-year evaluation. *Educ. Rev.* **2013**, *65*, 85–108. [CrossRef]
26. Department for Education. Grants to Fund Local Coordination of Free Holiday Activities and Healthy Food for Disadvantaged Children During 2019 Summer Holidays Specification of Requirements. Available online: https://www.contractsfinder.service.gov.uk/Notice/1283df8a-1bac-4644-bd27-8027ce2bd867 (accessed on 2 April 2019).

27. Mwatsama, M.; Stewart, L. *Food Poverty and Health: Briefing Statement*; Royal Colleges of Physicians of the United Kingdom: London, UK, 2005.
28. Cunningham-Sabo, L.; Lohse, B. Cooking with Kids positively affects fourth graders' vegetable preferences and attitudes and self-efficacy for food and cooking. *Child. Obes.* **2013**, *9*, 549–556. [CrossRef]
29. Allirot, X.; da Quinta, N.; Chokupermal, K.; Urdaneta, E. Involving children in cooking activities: A potential strategy for directing food choices toward novel foods containing vegetables. *Appetite* **2016**, *103*, 275–285. [CrossRef]
30. van der Horst, K.; Ferrage, A.; Rytz, A. Involving children in meal preparation. Effects on food intake. *Appetite* **2014**, *79*, 18–24. [CrossRef]
31. Fiese, B.H.; Schwartz, M. Reclaiming the Family Table: Mealtimes and Child Health and Wellbeing. Social Policy Report. *Soc. Res. Child Dev.* **2008**, 22. [CrossRef]
32. White, H.J.; Haycraft, E.; Meyer, C. Family mealtimes and eating psychopathology: The role of anxiety and depression among adolescent girls and boys. *Appetite* **2014**, *75*, 173–179. [CrossRef]
33. McLaughlin, K.A.; Green, J.G.; Alegría, M.; Costello, J.E.; Gruber, M.J.; Sampson, N.A.; Kessler, R.C. Food insecurity and mental disorders in a national sample of U.S. adolescents. *J. Am. Acad. Child Adolesc. Psychiatry* **2012**, *51*, 1293–1303. [CrossRef]
34. Maslow, A. A theory of human motivation. *Psychol. Rev.* **1943**, *50*, 370–396. [CrossRef]
35. Fram, M.S.; Ritchie, L.D.; Rosen, N.; Frongillo, E.A. Child experience of food insecurity is associated with child diet and physical activity. *J. Nutr.* **2015**, *145*, 499–504. [CrossRef]

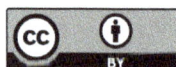

© 2019 by the authors. Licensee MDPI, Basel, Switzerland. This article is an open access article distributed under the terms and conditions of the Creative Commons Attribution (CC BY) license (http://creativecommons.org/licenses/by/4.0/).

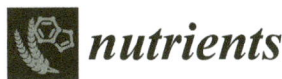

Article

Unravelling the Effects of the Healthy Primary School of the Future: For Whom and Where Is It Effective?

Nina Bartelink [1,2,3,*], Patricia van Assema [1,2], Stef Kremers [2], Hans Savelberg [4], Dorus Gevers [2] and Maria Jansen [3,5]

1. Department of Health Promotion, Care and Public Health Research Institute (CAPHRI), Maastricht University, P.O. Box 616 6200 MD Maastricht, The Netherlands
2. Department of Health Promotion, School of Nutrition and Translational Research in Metabolism (NUTRIM), Maastricht University, P.O. Box 616, 6200 MD Maastricht, The Netherlands
3. Academic Collaborative Centre for Public Health Limburg, Public Health Services, P.O. Box 33, 6400 AA Heerlen, The Netherlands
4. Department of Nutritional and Movement Sciences, Nutrition and Translational Research Institute Maastricht (NUTRIM), Maastricht University, P.O. Box 616, 6200 MD Maastricht, The Netherlands
5. Department of Health Services Research, Care and Public Health Research Institute (CAPHRI), Maastricht University, P.O. Box 616, 6200 MD Maastricht, The Netherlands
* Correspondence: n.bartelink@maastrichtuniversity.nl

Received: 13 June 2019; Accepted: 4 September 2019; Published: 5 September 2019

Abstract: The 'Healthy Primary School of the Future' (HPSF) aims to integrate health and well-being within the whole school system. This study examined the two-year effects of HPSF on children's dietary and physical activity (PA) behaviours at school and at home and investigated whether child characteristics or the home context moderated these effects. This study (n = 1676 children) has a quasi-experimental design with four intervention schools, i.e., two full HPSF (focus: nutrition and PA), two partial HPSF (focus: PA), and four control schools. Measurements consisted of accelerometry (Actigraph GT3X+) and questionnaires. Favourable effects on children's dietary and PA behaviours at school were found in the full HPSF; in the partial HPSF, only on PA behaviours. Children in the full HPSF did not compensate at home for the improved health behaviours at school, while in the partial HPSF, the children became less active at home. In both the full and partial HPSF, less favourable effects at school were found for younger children. At home, less favourable effects were found for children with a lower socioeconomic status. Overall, the effect of the full HPSF on children's dietary and PA behaviours was larger and more equally beneficial for all children than that of the partial HPSF.

Keywords: intervention effects; microsystems; nutrition; parenting practices; physical activity; school health promotion

1. Introduction

Dietary and physical activity (PA) habits are formed at a young age [1], whereby unhealthy habits can already lead to overweight and obesity [2]. Schools can play an important role in promoting healthy behaviours in children, since a significant proportion of a child's day is spent there, and schools reach all children [3–5]. However, the school is one of the microsystems that interact to shape a child's health and well-being [6,7]. This means that the impact of changes in the school may also interact with the child's behaviour in other microsystems, e.g., the home context. This could lead to a transfer of improved health behaviours to the home context. However, compensatory behaviours might also occur: improvements in children's health behaviours at school (extra PA or healthier dietary behaviours) may be compensated at home by, e.g., a decrease in PA or unhealthier dietary behaviours [8,9]. This school–home interaction might also cause different effects for children due to their home context.

For example, a school-based intervention may be of greater benefit to those children with a high socioeconomic status (SES) background than to children with a low SES background, which leads to increased health inequities [10]. Moreover, parents can have different nutrition- and PA-related practices at home, e.g., parental behaviours and rules, which may also moderate the effects of school interventions on children's health behaviours [6,7,11,12].

Additionally, not only might the home context moderate the effects of school health promotion efforts, child characteristics might also occur as an effect modifier [6]. Several reviews have stated that even though the intention of school health promotion efforts is to reach all children, specific subgroups of children often benefit more than others. The review by Stewart-Brown et al. [13] found gender-specific results in several studies: some school-based interventions showed larger improvements on PA and dietary behaviours in girls and others in boys. Age-specific effects were also found, with some interventions being more effective in older children and others in younger children [13]. The review by Cook-Cotton et al. indicated that overweight children may respond more slowly or less well to school-based interventions than other children [11].

The 'Healthy Primary School of the Future' (HPSF) is a Dutch initiative that aims to improve the health and well-being of all children in the school by sustainably integrating health and well-being within the whole school system [14,15]. The initiative is based on the principles of the Health Promoting School (HPS) framework, which includes a whole school approach, the participation of teachers, children and parents, and partnerships in the local community [16]. HPSF is being investigated in an overall study among four intervention and four control schools by a multi-disciplinary research group [14,15]. The overall study includes, among others, an extensive process evaluation and several effect evaluations. One of the effect evaluations found favourable intervention effects on children's health behaviours in the two intervention schools that focused on both healthy nutrition and PA [17]. The two intervention schools that focused only on PA found no effects, also not on children's PA behaviours. Since these results only presented overall effects, it is not known whether the effects occurred at school only or also at home. Nor is it known whether specific subgroups of children could be identified who benefitted more from HPSF in terms of PA and dietary behaviours [18].

The aim of the current study was to unravel the intervention effects of HPSF on children's health behaviours. Two main research questions were formulated: (1) What is the effect of HPSF on children's dietary and PA behaviours at school and at home? (2) Did child characteristics or the home context moderate the effects of HPSF on children's dietary and PA behaviours?

2. Methods

2.1. Study Design

The current study is part of the overall study that investigates HPSF [15] and uses a longitudinal quasi-experimental design with four intervention schools and four control schools. All eight participating schools are situated in the Parkstad region in the southern part of the Netherlands. This region has a low average SES, and unhealthy behaviours and overweight are higher in prevalence compared with the rest of the Netherlands [19]. Inclusion criteria for the schools were being a member of the educational board 'Movare', since they were one of the initiators of HPSF, and a minimum of 140 children in the study years two till five, to be able to study the effects of HPSF with enough statistical power. Ethical approval (14-N-142) for the overall study was given by the Medical Ethics Committee Zuyderland located in Heerlen (Parkstad, the Netherlands). A detailed description of the overall study and the recruitment of the eight schools is reported in Willeboordse et al. [15].

2.2. The Healthy Primary School of the Future

Three cooperating organizations, i.e., the regional educational board 'Movare', the regional public health services and Maastricht University, developed the HPSF initiative [15]. In line with the HPS framework [16], the initiative intends to establish a co-creation movement in schools for the development and implementation of health-promoting changes in different aspects of the school system, i.e., the school's physical and social environment, school's health policy, education, and school routines. In addition to the HPS framework, the aim was to create some form of positive disruption in the school by initiating two changes top–down: (1) a free healthy lunch each day and (2) daily structured PA and cultural sessions after lunch, both implemented by external pedagogical employees provided by childcare organizations. These changes are adapted bottom–up and should lead to momentum for more bottom–up processes to create additional health-promoting changes in school [14]. Two of the four intervention schools decided to implement both changes and are referred to as the 'full HPSF'. These schools also implemented additional health-promoting changes: they improved their health policy, e.g., policy regarding the consumption of water in school, they provided water bottles to all children, and have implemented an educational lunch once a week. The other two intervention schools only implemented the structured PA and cultural sessions and are referred to as the 'partial HPSF'. These schools did not implement any additional health-promoting changes. Each school selected one teacher as school coordinator, who managed HPSF in their school and all four schools involved teachers and parents in the adoption decision and the process of adapting the changes into the school context. Implementation started in all the schools in November 2015. Overarching the four schools, the HPSF initiative was led by a project leader from Movare and an executive board with representatives of the three collaborating organizations, including the project leader. A project team was created with representatives of all partners involved: the four schools, Movare, regional Public Health Services, Maastricht University, the Limburg provincial authorities, childcare organizations, a caterer, and sports and leisure organizations.

2.3. Study Population

All children (aged 4 to 12) and their parents in the eight schools ($n = 2326$ at T0) were invited to participate in this study. This included children from study years one to eight. Recruitment was done via information brochures for parents. The research team visited the classrooms to inform children about this study and encouraged them to ask their parents to participate [15]. Parents had to sign an informed consent form to participate in all measurements for themselves and their child(ren). The group of children included in this study were: at baseline (T0,) children from study years one to seven; at T1, children from study years two to eight; and at T2, children from study years three to eight. Children who joined this study at T1 or T2 were included even though no baseline data were available. Children who switched to other schools between 2015 and 2017 were excluded.

2.4. Measures

Data were gathered annually during one week of measurements, conducted between September and November 2015 (T0, previous to the start of HPSF in November 2015), 2016 (T1) and 2017 (T2). Inter-rater variability was minimised by training researchers according to a strict protocol. The data collection and data processing were identical to the evaluation of the overall effects on children's dietary and PA behaviours [17].

Potential Effect Modifiers

Child characteristics: Children's study year and gender were collected via the database of the educational board Movare. Children's weight status was assessed by measurements of their height and weight. BMI was determined and age- and gender-specific BMI cut-off points were used to define children's weight status, i.e., non-overweight versus overweight (including obesity) [20].

Children's socioeconomic background: A digital questionnaire for parents was used to obtain information about, among other things, children's SES. This was calculated as the mean of standardised scores on maternal education level, paternal educational level, and household income (adjusted for household size) [21]. The mean scores were categorised into low, middle and high SES scores based on tertiles.

Patterns of health-promoting parenting practices at home: The digital questionnaire for parents was also used to assess parents' nutrition-related practices (n = 9) and PA-related practices (n = 14), e.g., modelling behaviour and encouragement. The questions were based on previous work by Gevers et al. [22,23] and O'Connor et al. [24]. Each item described a practice by giving a statement, followed by some examples. Participants responded on a Likert scale from 1 (completely disagree) to 5 (completely agree). Two cluster analyses similar to Gevers et al. were conducted: one for the nutrition-related parenting practices and one for the PA-related parenting practices [22]. Detailed information of the results of each clustering is described in Supplementary file 1. Clustering of the nutrition-related parenting practices showed similar clusters of parents compared to the study by Gevers et al. [22]. The names of the clusters were: Cluster 1 (n = 226; 36.9%) "High involvement and supportive"; Cluster 2 (n = 102; 16.7%) "Low covert control and non-rewarding"; Cluster 3 (n = 78; 12.7%) "Low involvement and indulgent"; and Cluster 4 (n = 206; 33.7%) "High covert control and rewarding". Clustering of the PA-related parenting practices also resulted in four clusters. The names of the clusters were: Cluster 1 (n = 220; 35.0%) "High involvement and supportive"; Cluster 2 (n = 133; 21.2%) "Moderate involvement, indulgent of child's sedentary activities"; Cluster 3 (n = 17; 2.7%) "Low involvement and indulgent"; and Cluster 4 (n = 258; 41.1%) "Moderate involvement, supportive of child's sedentary activities".

2.5. Outcomes

Children's PA levels—accelerometry: At the beginning of the measurement week, all participating children from study years two to eight received an accelerometer for seven days (Actigraph GT3X+, 30 Hz, 10 s epoch). The monitor was attached to the hip with an elastic band and had to be worn all day except while sleeping or during activities in which water was involved (e.g., swimming, bathing and showering). The accelerometry data were processed using ActiLife version 6.13.3. Wear time validation was assessed using Choi's classification criteria [25]. Minimal wear time was defined as 480 min per day between 06:00 and 23:00 [26]. The first day of measurement was excluded to prevent reactivity [27]. Measurements containing at least three weekdays (after excluding the first measurement day) and one weekend day were used in the analyses [28]. The activity levels, classified using Evenson's cut-off points, were in counts per minute (CPM) [29]: sedentary behaviour (SB; $\leq$100 CPM), light PA (LPA; 101–2295 CPM), and moderate to vigorous PA (MVPA; $\geq$2296 CPM).

Children's dietary behaviours—a parent-reported questionnaire: A digital questionnaire for parents was used to obtain information about their children's dietary behaviours. All parents of participating children (study years one to eight) received the questionnaire. Twelve questions from the Local and National Youth Health Monitor were used to assess children's dietary behaviours [30,31]. Parents were asked about the number of days during the past week their child had breakfast, ate warm vegetables, salads or raw vegetables, fruits, consumed water and sugar-sweetened beverages (soft, sports, and energy drinks), and ate the following four snack types: chocolate, salted snacks, cookies, and soft ice-creams. A total score for healthy dietary behaviours (in mean days/week) was calculated by the mean number of days children consumed breakfast, fruits, vegetables (warm and cold), and water. A total score for unhealthy dietary behaviours (in mean days/week) was calculated by the mean number of days children consumed sugar-sweetened beverages and the four different snack types.

Children's dietary behaviours—two child-reported questionnaires: The first child questionnaire (for children of study years four to eight) was filled out by writing during class hours in the presence of at least one member of the research team. The questionnaire was used to assess, among other things, children's school water consumption (0 (almost) never; —1 sometimes (1–3 days per week); —2 often (4–6 days per week); —3 every day) and their breakfast intake. Breakfast questions consisted of recall questions (7 items) with yes/no answer options regarding the consumption of healthy food items, i.e., bread, cereals, butter, cheese, fruits, milk/yoghurt, and water, during breakfast that day. The items bread and cereals were combined into the food type grains, and milk/yoghurt and cheese were combined into the food type dairy. To give an indication about how healthy the children's breakfast was that day, the six different food types consumed were summed, and a dichotomous variable was created to study whether children consumed at least two of the food types during breakfast. The second questionnaire (for children of study years three to eight) was used to assess the children's lunch intake. The questions (except for an extra question regarding vegetable consumption during lunch) and the processing of the data were similar to those for the breakfast intake.

2.6. Analyses

Data were analysed using IBM SPSS Statistics for Windows (version 23.0. Armonk, NY, USA: IBM Corp). Missing data, including missing data at baseline, were imputed using a multiple imputation method with fully conditional specification (FCS) and 10 iterations, generating 50 complete datasets. Linear mixed-model analyses (continuous outcomes) and generalised estimating equations (binary outcomes) were used (see Bartelink et al. [17]) for the overall outcomes and school- and home-specific outcomes. Since measurements were repeated within participants, we used a two-level model with measurements as the first level and participants as the second level. The fixed part of the model consisted of group (full HPSF, partial HPSF, control), time (T0, T1, T2) and the interaction terms of group with time. We were not able to include class as a level in the model, because commonly more than one division of a class existed, e.g., 4a or 4b, and children often did not have fixed class divisions for all years. To obtain children's setting-specific PA behaviours, the overall accelerometry data were divided by filters on wear time during school hours (school-specific PA) and wear time outside of school hours (home-specific PA). Regarding children's dietary behaviour, the two total scores (healthy and unhealthy dietary behaviours) were used as overall outcomes; children's lunch intake and their school water consumption as school-specific outcomes; and children's breakfast intake as home-specific outcomes. All analyses were adjusted for gender, study year at baseline, ethnicity, SES, and children's BMI z-score at baseline. A two-sided p-value ≤0.05 was considered statistically significant. Standardised effect sizes (ES) were calculated, which were defined as estimated mean difference after two years divided by the square root of the residual variance at baseline (pooled over the intervention groups). Binary outcomes resulted in odds ratios (ORs). To investigate whether the intervention effects were similar for all children, the following potential effect modifiers were considered: gender (boys/girls), study year at baseline (lower (1–4)/higher (5–8) grades), baseline weight status (non-overweight/overweight), SES (low/middle/high), and the patterns of nutrition-related parenting practices (four clusters) and PA-related parenting practices (four clusters). To assess potential effect modification, the interaction term group*time*effect modifier, with all corresponding two-way interactions, was added to the model [17]. When this interaction term was significant (here, we used a significance level of 0.10 to deal with the fact that the power of a test for interaction is relatively low [32] and we did not want to miss any effect modification), the intervention effects were reported for all categories of the effect modifier separately.

3. Results

Of all the children ($n = 2326$) invited to participate in this study, 60.3% joined this study at baseline (n = 1403). Because of this study's dynamic population, a total of 1974 children and their parents participated in this study within the two-year follow-up period (data collected at least at one time point). Due to the selection used for the current study, i.e., children were eligible for the current research only when they were in study years one to seven at baseline and did not switch schools, 1676 children were included in the analyses. See Supplementary file 2 for characteristics of the study sample.

3.1. Intervention Effects

3.1.1. Intervention Effects at School

Both the full and partial HPSF resulted in significant favourable intervention effects on children's PA behaviours at school (Table 1). The time children spent in MVPA at school had increased significantly more in the full HPSF (ES = 0.34) and partial HPSF (ES = 0.29) compared to the children in the control schools. Favourable trends were found for both sedentary time (full HPSF: ES = −0.20; partial HPSF ES = −0.17) and light PA at school (full HPSF: ES = 0.11; partial HPSF ES = 0.09). Regarding children's dietary behaviours at school, several favourable significant intervention effects were found in the full HPSF compared to the control schools: more children increased their water consumption at school (ES = 1.14) and ate at least two food types during lunch (OR = 2.98). In the partial HPSF, no significant intervention effects were found on children's dietary behaviours at school.

Table 1. Intervention effects of Healthy Primary School of the Future (HPSF) at school and at home.

	Full HPSF vs. Control			Partial HPSF vs. Control		
	B (95% C.I.)	p	ES	B (95% C.I.)	p	ES
Overall PA and Dietary Behaviours *						
Sedentary (% per day)	−1.29 (−2.39−−0.19)	0.02	−0.23	−0.17 (−1.25−0.90)	0.76	−0.03
Light PA (% per day)	0.94 (0.07−1.81)	0.03	0.22	−0.03 (−0.88−0.82)	0.95	−0.01
MVPA (% per day)	0.36 (−0.10−0.82)	0.12	0.15	0.19 (−0.26−0.64)	0.41	0.08
Healthy dietary behaviours (mean days/week)	0.19 (0.01−0.37)	0.04	0.19	−0.02 (−0.20−0.16)	0.86	−0.02
Unhealthy dietary behaviours (mean days/week)	−0.07 (−0.21−0.07)	0.31	−0.11	0.00 (−0.14−0.15)	0.96	0.01
PA and dietary behaviours at school						
Sedentary (% per day at school)	−1.51 (−2.96−−0.06)	0.05	−0.20	−1.22 (−0.26−0.19)	0.10	−0.17
Light PA (% per day at school)	0.70 (−0.51−1.92)	0.29	0.11	0.54 (−0.67−1.74)	0.39	0.09
MVPA (% per day at school)	0.76 (0.29−1.24)	<0.01	0.34	0.67 (0.22−1.12)	<0.01	0.29
Minimal two food types during lunch ** (% yes)	2.98 (1.59−5.61)	<0.01	na	0.62 (0.36−1.05)	0.08	na
School water consumption (0−3)	1.17 (0.95−1.38)	<0.01	1.14	−0.02 (−0.23−0.20)	0.86	−0.02
PA and dietary behaviours at home						
Sedentary (% per day at home)	−0.47 (−1.92−0.99)	0.53	−0.06	1.33 (−0.07−2.72)	0.06	0.18
Light PA (% per day at home)	0.33 (−0.74−1.41)	0.55	0.06	−1.24 (−2.27−−0.21)	0.02	−0.23
MVPA (% per day at home)	0.16 (−0.50−0.82)	0.63	0.05	−0.08 (−0.71−0.54)	0.79	−0.02
Minimal two food types during breakfast ** (% yes)	0.95 (0.58−1.57)	0.85	na	1.16 (0.71−1.89)	0.54	na

* For convenience purposes, this table also includes the results from the previously conducted study on overall effects of HPSF on children's PA and dietary behaviours [17]. The number of children was not always the same in the analyses due to differences in the methods of and response to the measurements. The number of children in each statistical test is reported in the previously conducted study. ** Binary outcome, B-value is presented as odds ratio. Significance level: $p < 0.05$. Abbreviations: HPSF: Healthy Primary School of the Future; CI: confidence interval; p: p-value; ES: effect size; PA: physical activity; MVPA: moderate-to-vigorous physical activity; na: not applicable.

3.1.2. Intervention Effects at Home

The results showed no statistically significant favourable or adverse (compensatory) intervention effects of the full HPSF on children's PA and dietary behaviours at home (Table 1). In the partial HPSF, an adverse intervention effect was found at home for children's PA behaviours: the time children spent in light PA at home had decreased significantly more compared to children of the control schools. No significant favourable or adverse intervention effect was found for their dietary behaviours at home.

3.2. Effect Modifiers

3.2.1. Moderators of Overall Intervention Effects

Fewer moderators of intervention effects on children's dietary and PA behaviours were found in the full HPSF compared to the partial HPSF (1 vs. 4 significant moderators; Table 2). In the full HPSF, no moderators of children's dietary behaviours were found and one moderator of effects on children's PA behaviours was found. Gender moderated the effect on MVPA, as boys had increased their time in MVPA significantly more compared to boys in the control schools (ES = 0.34); this effect was not found in girls (ES = 0.02). In the partial HPSF, study year and SES were found to be significant moderators. Study year moderated the intervention effects on the time children spent sedentary and in light PA, with a favourable trend found in older children and an adverse trend in younger children. SES moderated the effects on the time spent in MVPA and unhealthy dietary behaviours. Each SES tertile showed a different trend, with a lack of consistency. In both the full and partial HPSF, no moderation was found by children's weight status and parenting practices.

Table 2. Effect modifiers of HPSF on overall intervention effects.

	Full HPSF vs. Control			Partial HPSF vs. Control		
	B (95% C.I.)	p	ES	B (95% C.I.)	p	ES
Gender						
Sedentary (% per day)	0.27 (−1.89–2.43)	0.81		−0.01 (−2.15–2.12)	0.99	
Light PA (% per day)	−1.03 (−2.73–0.68)	0.24		0.21 (−1.49–1.90)	0.81	
MVPA (% per day)	0.77 (−0.13–1.67)	**0.09**		−0.20 (−1.09–0.69)	0.66	
Boys	0.81 (0.13–1.49)	**0.02**	0.34	0.09 (−0.57–0.74)	0.80	0.04
Girls	0.04 (−0.57–0.65)	0.89	0.02	0.29 (−0.32–0.90)	0.36	0.12
Healthy dietary behaviours (mean days/week)	−0.16 (−0.52–0.20)	0.37		0.29 (−0.07–0.65)	0.11	
Unhealthy dietary behaviours (mean days/week)	0.16 (−0.12–0.45)	0.26		0.18 (−0.11–0.46)	0.23	
Study year						
Sedentary (% per day)	0.02 (−2.22–2.26)	0.98		2.18 (−0.07–4.42)	**0.06**	
Study years 1–4	−1.25 (−2.72–0.21)	0.09	−0.21	0.81 (−0.59–2.20)	0.26	0.13
Study years 5–8	−1.28 (−3.00–0.45)	0.15	−0.21	−1.37 (−3.14–0.40)	0.14	−0.23
Light PA (% per day)	−0.04 (−1.77–1.70)	0.97		−1.61 (−2.53–0.69)	0.08	
Study years 1–4	0.85 (−0.33–2.02)	0.16	0.18	−0.73 (−1.63–0.17)	0.20	−0.16
Study years 5–8	0.88 (−0.48–2.25)	0.21	0.19	0.88 (0.15–1.61)	0.23	0.19
MVPA (% per day)	0.01 (−0.92–0.93)	0.99		−0.56 (−1.51–0.38)	0.24	
Healthy dietary behaviours (mean days/week)	−0.11 (−0.49–0.27)	0.58		0.01 (−0.38–0.39)	0.97	
Unhealthy dietary behaviours (mean days/week)	−0.04 (−0.34–0.26)	0.81		0.12 (−0.18–0.43)	0.43	
Weight status						
Sedentary (% per day)	0.93 (−2.05–3.92)	0.54		0.82 (−1.86–3.49)	0.55	
Light PA (% per day)	−0.74 (−3.06–1.58)	0.53		−0.94 (−3.05–1.17)	0.38	
MVPA (% per day)	−0.19 (−1.45–1.07)	0.76		0.10 (−1.04–1.24)	0.86	
Healthy dietary behaviours (mean days/week)	−0.18 (−0.72–0.36)	0.50		−0.16 (−0.63–0.30)	0.49	
Unhealthy dietary behaviours (mean days/week)	−0.13 (−0.55–0.28)	0.53		0.07 (−0.30–0.43)	0.73	

Table 2. Cont.

	Full HPSF vs. Control			Partial HPSF vs. Control		
	B (95% C.I.)	p	ES	B (95% C.I.)	p	ES
Gender						
SES *						
Sedentary (% per day)		≥0.52			≥0.40	
Light PA (% per day)		≥0.57			≥0.87	
MVPA (% per day)		≥0.67			**≥0.05**	
Lowest tertile	0.29 (−0.61–1.19)	0.52	0.12	−0.51 (−1.36–0.33)	0.24	−0.21
Middle tertile	0.25 (−0.62–1.11)	0.57	0.10	0.72 (−0.11–1.55)	0.09	0.30
Highest tertile	0.50 (−0.26–1.25)	0.20	0.21	−0.21 (−0.56–0.97)	0.60	0.09
Healthy dietary behaviours (mean days/week)		≥0.26			≥0.43	
Unhealthy dietary behaviours (mean days/week)		≥0.13			**≥0.01**	
Lowest tertile	0.05 (−0.23–0.32)	0.73	0.07	0.04 (−0.21–0.30)	0.75	0.06
Middle tertile	0.05 (−0.21–0.30)	0.73	0.07	0.23 (−0.02–0.48)	0.07	0.35
Highest tertile	−0.22 (−0.44–−0.01)	0.06	−0.33	−0.24 (−0.48–0.00)	0.05	−0.36
PA-related parental practices *						
Sedentary (% per day)		≥0.26			≥0.62	
Light PA (% per day)		≥0.41			≥0.53	
MVPA (% per day)		≥0.30			≥0.20	
Nutrition-related parental practices *						
Healthy dietary behaviours (mean days/week)		≥0.45			≥0.66	
Unhealthy dietary behaviours (mean days/week)		≥0.69			≥0.10	

* The subgroups of SES and parenting practices are more than two (SES: low/middle/high; Parenting practices: four different clusters). To investigate the potential moderation, pairwise comparisons were conducted. The lowest p-value of the interaction terms was presented in the table (≥p-value). A complete overview of all interaction terms of each pairwise comparison is presented in Supplementary file 3. Analyses were conducted by linear mixed model analyses (continuous outcomes) or generalised estimating equations (binary outcomes), adjusted for baseline, gender, study year at T0, SES, ethnicity, and BMI z-score at T0. Significance level for the interaction term: $p < 0.10$. Significance level for each specific category of the subgroups with a significant interaction term (highlighted in green): $p < 0.05$. Abbreviations: HPSF: Healthy Primary School of the Future; CI: confidence interval; p: p-value; ES: effect size; PA: physical activity; MVPA: moderate-to-vigorous physical activity.

3.2.2. Moderators of Intervention Effects at School

Fewer moderators of intervention effects at school were found in the full HPSF compared to the partial HPSF (2 vs. 4 significant moderators; Table 3). In both the full and partial HPSF, intervention effects at school were moderated by study year. In the full HPSF, study year moderated the effects on sedentary time and light PA. In the partial HPSF, study year moderated the effect on sedentary time, light PA and school water consumption. Consistently throughout the subgroup analyses, it was found that in older children, the effects were more favourable than in younger children. No other moderations were found in the full HPSF. In the partial HPSF, school water consumption was significantly moderated by gender. An adverse significant intervention effect was found for girls (ES = −0.36), and a trend in a favourable direction was found for boys (ES = 0.26).

Table 3. Effect modifiers of HPSF on intervention effects at school.

	Full HPSF vs. Control			Partial HPSF vs. Control		
	B (95% C.I.)	p	ES	B (95% C.I.)	p	ES
	Gender					
Sedentary (% per day at school)	−0.06 (−1.52–1.40)	0.97		−1.33 (−4.03–1.38)	0.35	
Light PA (% per day at school)	0.15 (−2.07–2.36)	0.90		1.36 (−1.01–3.73)	0.26	
MVPA (% per day at school)	−0.06 (−0.94–0.81)	0.89		−0.03 (−0.94–0.84)	0.94	
Minimal two food types during lunch ** (% yes)	1.15 (.32–4.10)	0.83		1.04 (0.35–3.07)	0.94	
School water consumption (0–3)	−0.14 (−0.57–0.28)	0.51		−0.63 (−1.06−−0.20)	<0.01	
Boys	1.24 (0.94–1.53)	<0.01	1.21	0.26 (−0.03–0.55)	0.08	0.26
Girls	1.09 (0.78–1.40)	<0.01	1.07	−0.37 (−0.68−−0.05)	<0.01	−0.36
	Study year					
Sedentary (% per day at school)	3.11 (1.63–4.59)	0.04		2.58 (1.10–4.05)	0.08	
Study years 1–4	−0.07 (−1.91–1.77)	0.94	−0.01	−0.01 (−0.92–0.90)	0.99	0.00
Study years 5–8	−3.18 (−5.30−−1.06)	<0.01	−0.40	−2.59 (−3.78−−1.40)	0.03	−0.32
Light PA (% per day at school)	−2.47 (−0.373−−1.20)	0.05		−2.75 (−4.01−−1.50)	0.03	
Study years 1–4	−0.53 (−2.09–1.02)	0.52	−0.08	−0.61 (−1.67–0.46)	0.44	−0.09
Study years 5–8	1.93 (0.56–3.30)	0.06	0.29	2.15 (1.13–3.16)	0.03	0.32
MVPA (% per day at school)	−0.68 (−1.59–0.23)	0.15		0.16 (−0.70–1.03)	0.73	
Minimal two food types during lunch ** (% yes)	0.90 (0.24–3.35)	0.87		0.99 (0.33–2.98)	0.99	
School water consumption (0–3)	0.32 (−0.15–0.79)	0.19		−0.51 (−0.99−−0.03)	0.04	
Study years 1–4	1.31 (0.94–1.69)	<0.01	1.28	−0.38 (−0.76−0.00)	0.05	−0.37
Study years 5–8	0.99 (0.71–1.27)	<0.01	0.97	0.13 (0−0.16–0.42)	0.38	0.12
	Weight status					
Sedentary (% per day at school)	−1.62 (−5.73–2.50)	0.44		0.74 (−2.90–4.37)	0.58	
Light PA (% per day at school)	0.98 (−2.48–4.45)	0.58		−1.16 (−4.23–192)	0.46	
MVPA (% per day at school)	0.66 (−0.65–1.96)	0.32		0.44 (−0.70–1.59)	0.45	
Minimal two food types during lunch ** (% yes)	0.68 (0.12–3.99)	0.67		2.33 (0.52–10.36)	0.27	
School water consumption (0–3)	−0.14 (−0.35–0.07)	0.19		−0.02 (−0.23–0.20)	0.89	
	SES *					
Sedentary (% per day at school)		≥0.22			≥0.48	
Light PA (% per day at school)		≥0.42			≥0.54	
MVPA (% per day at school)		≥0.12			≥0.13	
Minimal two food types during lunch ** (% yes)		≥0.22			≥0.60	
School water consumption (0–3)		≥0.26			≥0.15	

Table 3. Cont.

	Full HPSF vs. Control			Partial HPSF vs. Control		
	B (95% C.I.)	p	ES	B (95% C.I.)	p	ES
	Gender					
	PA-related parental practices *					
Sedentary (% per day at school)		≥0.83			≥0.37	
Light PA (% per day at school)		≥0.88			≥0.42	
MVPA (% per day at school)		≥0.58			≥0.21	
	Nutrition-related parental practices *					
Minimal two food types during lunch ** (% yes)		≥0.24			≥0.32	
School water consumption (0–3)		≥0.37			≥0.47	

* The subgroups of SES and parenting practices are more than two (SES: low/middle/high; Parenting practices: four different clusters). To investigate the potential moderation, pairwise comparisons were conducted. The lowest p-value of the interaction terms was presented in the table (≥p-value). A complete overview of all interaction terms of each pairwise comparison is presented in Supplementary file 3. ** Binary outcome: A generalised estimating equation is used. Interaction term is Exp(B), which is the odds ratio of the first subgroup (e.g., boys) divided by the odds ratio of the second subgroup (e.g., girls), in which the odds ratio of the second group (girls) is the reference group. Analysed by linear mixed model analyses (continuous outcomes) or generalised estimating equations (binary outcomes), adjusted for baseline, gender, study year at T0, SES, ethnicity, and BMI z-score at T0. Significance level for the interaction term: $p < 0.10$. Significance level for each specific category of the subgroups with a significant interaction term (highlighted in green): $p < 0.05$. Abbreviations: HPSF: Healthy Primary School of the Future; CI: confidence interval; p: p-value; ES: effect size; PA: physical activity; MVPA: moderate-to-vigorous physical activity; na: not applicable.

3.2.3. Moderators of Intervention Effects at Home

Fewer moderators of intervention effects at home were found in the full HPSF than in the partial HPSF (3 vs. 5 significant moderators; Table 4). In both the full and partial HPSF, SES moderated the intervention effects on children's PA behaviours at home. In general, adverse effects or trends at home were found for the children in the lowest SES tertile and favourable effects or trends for the children in the highest SES tertile. In the full HPSF, a significant favourable effect on the time spent sedentary (ES = −0.34) was found for the children in the highest SES tertile. In the partial HPSF, a significant adverse effect for sedentary time (ES = 0.46) and light PA (−0.52) was found for the children in the lowest SES tertile. Supplementary file 3 presents all pairwise comparisons. The comparison between the lowest and highest SES tertile consistently shows a different effect at home compared to the effects at school. The results showed consistent differences in effect between the lowest and highest SES tertiles regarding PA behaviours at home (B > 1 in 5 out of 6 comparisons, Supplementary file 3 Table S2c), whereas no differences in effect were found at school (B < 1 in all six comparisons, Supplementary file 3 Table S2b). As an exception, this pattern was not found for children's breakfast intake. No other significant moderations were found in the full HPSF for children's PA and dietary behaviours at home. In the partial HPSF, the intervention effects at home on sedentary time, light PA, and on the consumption of at least two food types during breakfast were also moderated by weight status. Favourable trends were found at home in overweight children and adverse trends or effects were found in non-overweight children.

Table 4. Effect modifiers of HPSF on intervention effects at home.

	Full HPSF vs. Control			Partial HPSF vs. Control		
	B (95% C.I.)	p	ES	B (95% C.I.)	p	ES
Gender						
Sedentary (% per day at home)	1.22 (−1.59–4.04)	0.39		0.55 (−2.22–3.31)	0.70	
Light PA (% per day at home)	−1.32(−3.40–0.76)	0.21		−0.20 (−2.24–1.85)	0.85	
MVPA (% per day at home)	0.12 (−1.14–1.39)	0.85		−0.33 (−1.58–0.91)	0.60	
Minimal two food types during breakfast ** (% yes)	0.41 (.22–0.77)	0.15		0.38 (0.14–1.04)	0.12	
Study year						
Sedentary (% per day at home)	−2.22 (−5.16–0.73)	0.14		0.88 (−2.08–3.84)	0.56	
Light PA (% per day at home)	−1.17 (−1.03–3.36)	0.30		−0.45 (−2.65–1.76)	0.69	
MVPA (% per day at home)	1.07 (−0.24–2.38)	0.11		−0.43 (−1.74–0.88)	0.52	
Minimal two food types during breakfast ** (% yes)	1.12 (0.31–4.04)	0.86		1.23 (0.62–2.43)	0.76	
Weight status						
Sedentary (% per day at home)	2.27 (−2.01–6.55)	0.30		3.03 (−0.55–6.61)	0.10	
Non-overweight	0.00 (−1.60–1.61)	1.00	0.00	1.90 (0.33–3.47)	0.02	0.26
Overweight	−2.27 (−6.18–1.64)	0.26	−0.31	−1.13 (−4.32–2.06)	0.49	−0.15
Light PA (% per day at home)	−1.46 (−4.58–1.67)	0.36		−2.65 (−5.29−−0.01)	0.05	
Non-overweight	0.01 (−1.17–1.20)	0.99	0.00	−1.74 (−2.90−−0.58)	<0.01	−0.33
Overweight	1.47 (−1.40–4.32)	0.31	0.28	0.91 (−1.44–3.26)	0.45	0.17
MVPA (% per day at home)	−0.88 (−2.75–1.00)	0.36		−0.38 (−1.98–1.23)	0.65	
Minimal two food types during breakfast ** (% yes)	1.03 (0.20–5.21)	0.97		3.98 (0.87–18.33)	0.08	
Non-overweight	1.16 (0.59–2.29)	0.32	na	0.71 (0.35–1.40)	0.32	na
Overweight	1.20 (0.28–5.15)	0.81	na	2.81 (0.72–10.92)	0.14	na
SES *						
Sedentary (% per day at home)		≥0.05			≥0.02	
Lowest tertile	0.96 (−1.59–3.51)	0.46	0.13	3.36 (0.93–5.79)	<0.01	0.46
Middle tertile	0.26 (−2.26–2.77)	0.84	0.04	1.47 (−0.96–3.90)	0.24	0.20
Highest tertile	−2.44 (−4.80−−0.09)	0.04	−0.34	−0.50 (−2.85–1.85)	0.68	−0.07
Light PA (% per day at home)		≥0.03			≥0.03	
Lowest tertile	−1.18 (−3.06–0.70)	0.22	−0.23	−2.70 (−4.50–0.91)	<0.01	−0.52
Middle tertile	0.43 (−1.42–2.29)	0.65	0.08	−1.21 (−3.00–0.59)	0.19	−0.23
Highest tertile	1.70 (−.04–3.44)	0.06	0.32	0.11 (−1.63–1.84)	0.91	0.02
MVPA (% per day at home)		≥0.06			≥0.15	
Lowest tertile	0.20 (−0.95–1.35)	0.74	0.06	−0.68 (−1.78–0.42)	0.22	−0.20
Middle tertile	−0.66 (−1.80–0.47)	0.25	−0.19	−0.26 (−1.35–0.83)	0.64	−0.08
Highest tertile	0.79 (−.27–1.85)	0.14	0.23	0.42 (−0.63–1.48)	0.43	0.12
Minimal two food types during breakfast ** (% yes)		≥0.12			≥0.12	

Table 4. *Cont.*

	Full HPSF vs. Control			Partial HPSF vs. Control		
	B (95% C.I.)	*p*	ES	B (95% C.I.)	*p*	ES
	Gender					
	PA-related parental practices *					
Sedentary (% per day at home)		≥0.30			≥0.77	
Light PA (% per day at home)		≥0.34			≥0.47	
MVPA (% per day at home)		≥0.21			≥0.46	
	Nutrition-related parental practices *					
Minimal two food types during breakfast ** (% yes)		≥0.46			≥0.37	

* The subgroups of SES and parenting practices are more than two (SES: low/middle/high; Parenting practices: four different clusters). To investigate the potential moderation, pairwise comparisons were conducted. The lowest *p*-value of the interaction terms was presented in the table (≥p-value). A complete overview of all interaction terms of each pairwise comparison is presented in Supplementary file 3. ** Binary outcome: A generalised estimating equation is used. Interaction term is Exp(B), which is the odds ratio of the first subgroup (e.g., boys) divided by the odds ratio of the second subgroup (e.g., girls), in which the odds ratio of the second group (girls) is the reference group. Analysed by linear mixed model analyses (continuous outcomes) or generalised estimating equations (binary outcomes), adjusted for baseline, gender, study year at T0, SES, ethnicity, and BMI z-score at T0. Significance level for the interaction term: $p < 0.10$. Significance level for each specific category of the subgroups with a significant interaction term (highlighted in green): $p < 0.05$. Abbreviations: HPSF: Healthy Primary School of the Future; CI: confidence interval; p: p-value; ES: effect size; PA: physical activity; MVPA: moderate-to-vigorous physical activity; na: not applicable.

4. Discussion

The current study aimed to unravel the effects of HPSF on children's dietary and PA behaviours. It investigated the intervention effects of HPSF at school and at home. The results showed that the time children spent in MVPA at school had increased in both the full and partial HPSF. However, children of the full HPSF did not compensate at home for the improved health behaviours at school, while in the partial HPSF, the results indicated that the children did compensate by becoming less active at home. Children's dietary behaviours at school improved in the full HPSF, without compensating for these improvements at home.

The current study also investigated whether child characteristics or the home context moderated the intervention effects of HPSF. The results showed that the effects in the partial HPSF were influenced more often by moderators (in total, 13 significant moderators (18.6%)) than in the full HPSF (in total, six significant moderators (8.6%)), which indicates that the full HPSF had a more equal beneficial effect for all children. The findings indicated that the intervention effects of HPSF on children's PA and dietary behaviours were mainly moderated by SES and study year. This is in contrast to a previous study on the effects of HPSF on children BMI z-scores, in which no moderators emerged (18). An explanation for the contrasting results may be that the effect on children's BMI z-score is a result of the co-existence and interaction of the children's nutrition and PA behaviours [33]: a moderating impact on one health behaviour may therefore not automatically lead to moderation of intervention effects on children's BMI z-score.

The effects on children's PA behaviours at school were moderated by study year in both the full and partial HPSF: older children benefitted consistently more from HPSF than younger children. This may indicate that the activities in school were more appropriate for the older children. This is in line with the results and conclusions of several studies that indicated that children of different ages have different needs regarding PA activities [6,34]. Previous research has for example shown that older children's activity levels were more negatively affected by the number of peers present, while younger children were more negatively affected by the number of supervisors [35]. Therefore, it is recommended when implementing PA-related activities to ensure that either they are appropriate for all children or that age-specific PA activities are implemented.

The findings in this study showed that HPSF succeeded in creating equal effects on children's PA and dietary behaviours at school, independent of the children's backgrounds (SES, parenting practices).

However, the findings also showed that the children's socioeconomic background did influence the effects at home. The children with the lowest SES scores did not improve their PA behaviours at home; results even showed compensating behaviours of PA in these children at home. For the children from the highest SES group in the full HPSF, however, a transfer of the effects on PA was found from school to the home context. This suggests that the changes in the full HPSF schools have led to such an impact that these children also engaged in more PA after school. In contrast, these favourable effects at home did not occur in the children with the lowest SES scores. The compensation of PA at home in the lowest SES group has led to opposite effects at school and at home for these children: at school, their PA behaviours became more favourable; at home, they became less favourable. Since these opposite effects were especially found for the children with the lowest SES scores, it may contribute to an increased socioeconomic health equity gap. In addition, the partial HPSF also showed a moderating effect of SES on children's overall dietary behaviours, with less favourable, and even adverse effects for the children with lower SES scores. Children in these schools, in contrast to children in the full HPSF, brought all foods and drinks that they consumed at school from home. This means that the dietary behaviours that are included in this outcome are actually dietary behaviours that have their origin in the home context. The moderating effect of SES on this outcome in the partial HPSF seems to indicate that not only children's PA behaviours at home, but also their dietary behaviours at home are moderated by SES, with consistently less favourable effects for children with lower SES scores. It should be noted though that since all the schools are located in a low SES area, the SES tertiles used in this study are relative and not absolute scores. This means that the average SES score of children in this study sample is low compared to the average of the Netherlands [36]. Nevertheless, the differences in effect at home among children with lower and higher socioeconomic background demonstrate the interaction between two main microsystems of a child, i.e., school and home. This underlines that the school is an open system and interacts with other microsystems, such as home or the neighbourhood, to shape a child's health and well-being [6,7]. According to a study by Gubbels et al., larger consistency across microsystems leads to more favourable effects on children's health behaviours [37]. Therefore, it can be recommended for school health promotion efforts to include the home context in the HP changes, e.g., homework assignments that include parents, and/or to focus directly on health promotion in the home context [38]. In this way, the child's environment enables healthier choices both at school and at home. This creates more consistency between the different microsystems of a child, particularly for children with lower socioeconomic backgrounds [39].

No moderating effect of parenting practices was found in the current study, which indicates that the effects of HPSF were not strengthened or weakened by parenting practices at home. This is in line with the results of a previous Dutch study conducted in secondary schools, which investigated whether family environmental factors affected changes in adolescent's dietary behaviour who participated in a school health promotion program [40]. These findings indicate that it is not so much the parenting practices that explain the differences in home effects across SES groups, but that other aspects in the home context, such as the physical environment in the neighbourhood, may explain these differential intervention effects at home.

Strengths and Limitations

The quasi-experimental design can be seen as a limitation of this study, since we were unable to (cluster-) randomise schools. To deal with this limitation, we controlled for BMI z-score at T0, gender, study year at T0, SES score, and ethnicity in all analyses. However, despite the lack of randomization, the design enabled us to test the effectiveness in terms of differences in children's health behaviours between the three school groups over time, and we were able to enrol schools on the basis of motivation, which reflects the real-life situation of school health promotion. Another limitation is the multiple statistical testing in this study, which may increase the likelihood that the observed statistical differences have arisen by chance. Methodological strengths of this study include the objectively measured PA levels, all collected in the same season, and the matching of all measurements in the same week to prevent overburdening of the people in the school. Furthermore, since we had insight into the specific school hours of all included schools, we were able to separate children's PA behaviours at school and at home. Another strength of this study is that child-reported data were collected regarding both their breakfast and lunch. This created the possibility to investigate the effects of HPSF on specific dietary behaviours of children at school and at home. It should be mentioned though that by categorizing the consumption of breakfast as a dietary behaviour at home, the assumption was made that children consumed their breakfast at home. Even though this is very common in the Netherlands, we do not have the data to confirm this assumption. Moreover, to investigate as much as possible children's actual dietary behaviours during these meals, the answers of children without interference of parents were used. The specific effects of HPSF on both meals became more visible due to the use of comparable questions. In general, the assessment of children's dietary behaviours had its limitations as only questionnaires were used, which are subjective measurements and may lead to socially desirable answers [41]. To assess children's dietary behaviours more objectively, future research could include image collection methods. The parenting practices questionnaire, which also had these subjectivity limitations, was based on a validated questionnaire by Gevers et al. [23]. However, we were not able to include all practices described by Gevers et al., due to limitations in the length of the questionnaire as many other aspects were included in this questionnaire. The reduction in assessed practices was based on expert judgement; practices were only deleted when they were more or less similar to another practice. Due to this systematic approach, we were still able to conduct a cluster analysis, which led to the same four clusters [22]. The findings of this cluster analysis seem to indicate that the four patterns are also visible in another study sample, which is a next step in the validation of these patterns of parenting practices. Future research is needed to validate these findings and to investigate whether these clusters are also applicable in other study samples.

5. Conclusions

The effect of the full HPSF on children's dietary and PA behaviours was not only larger, but also more equally beneficial for all children than that of the partial HPSF. In both the full and partial HPSF, less favourable effects at school were found for younger children. At home, less favourable effects were found for children with lower SES scores. It is recommended to include the home and neighbourhood context in health promotion efforts in order to create more consistency across the different microsystems of a child. This may particularly benefit children from lower socioeconomic backgrounds.

Supplementary Materials: The following are available online at http://www.mdpi.com/2072-6643/11/9/2119/s1. Supplementary file 1: Clustering of parenting practices, Supplementary file 2: Characteristics of study sample, Supplementary file 3: Pairwise comparisons of the effect modifiers of HPSF.

Author Contributions: N.B., P.v.A., S.K., H.S., and M.J. were part of designing the intervention. N.B. collected the data for the manuscript, analysed the data and drafted and revised the manuscript. P.v.A., S.K., H.S., D.G. and M.J. critically reviewed the manuscript during the writing process. All authors have read and approved the final manuscript.

Funding: This study was funded by the Limburg provincial authorities, Project Number 200130003, by Friesland Campina, Project Number LLMV00, and by Maastricht University. None of the funding bodies had a role in the design of this study or the writing of this manuscript, nor a role in the data collection, analysis, interpretation of data, and writing of publications.

Acknowledgments: We are grateful to all the schools, the children and other collaborating partners participating in the project. We furthermore thank the PhD candidates and research assistants for their help in data collection.

Conflicts of Interest: The authors declare no conflict of interests.

References

1. Gubbels, J.S.; van Assema, P.; Kremers, S.P. Physical activity, sedentary behavior, and dietary patterns among children. *Curr. Nutr. Rep.* **2013**, *2*, 105–112. [CrossRef]
2. Sahoo, K.; Sahoo, B.; Choudhury, A.K.; Sofi, N.Y.; Kumar, R.; Bhadoria, A.S. Childhood obesity: Causes and consequences. *J. Fam. Med. Prim. Care* **2015**, *4*, 187–192.

3. Dooris, M.; Poland, B.; Kolbe, L.; De Leeuw, E.; McCall, D.S.; Wharf-Higgins, J. Healthy settings. In *Global Perspectives on Health Promotion Effectiveness*; Springer: Berlin, Germany, 2007; pp. 327–352.
4. Langford, R.; Campbell, R.; Magnus, D.; Bonell, C.P.; Murphy, S.M.; Waters, E.; Komro, K.A.; Gibbs, L.F. The WHO Health Promoting School framework for improving the health and well-being of students and their academic achievements. *Cochrane Database Syst. Rev.* **2014**, *4*. [CrossRef]
5. Verrotti, A.; Penta, L.; Zenzeri, L.; Agostinelli, S.; De Feo, P. Childhood obesity: Prevention and strategies of intervention. A systematic review of school-based interventions in primary schools. *J. Endocrinol. Investig.* **2014**, *37*, 1155–1164. [CrossRef]
6. Gubbels, J.S.; Van Kann, D.H.; de Vries, N.K.; Thijs, C.; Kremers, S.P. The next step in health behavior research: The need for ecological moderation analyses-an application to diet and physical activity at childcare. *Int. J. Behav. Nutr. Phys. Act* **2014**, *11*, 52. [CrossRef]
7. Lohrmann, D.K. A complementary ecological model of the coordinated school health program. *Public Health Rep.* **2008**, *123*, 695–703. [CrossRef]
8. Rowland, T.W. The biological basis of physical activity. *Med. Sci. Sports Exerc.* **1998**, *30*, 392–399. [CrossRef]
9. Rabia, M.; Knäuper, B.; Miquelon, P. The eternal quest for optimal balance between maximizing pleasure and minimizing harm: The compensatory health beliefs model. *Br. J. Health Psychol.* **2006**, *11*, 139–153. [CrossRef]
10. Lorenc, T.; Petticrew, M.; Welch, V.; Tugwell, P. What types of interventions generate inequalities? Evidence from systematic reviews. *J. Epidemiol. Community Health* **2013**, *67*, 190–193. [CrossRef]
11. Cook-Cottone, C.; Casey, C.M.; Feeley, T.H.; Baran, J. A meta-analytic review of obesity prevention in the schools: 1997–2008. *Psychol. Sch.* **2009**, *46*, 695–719. [CrossRef]
12. Golan, M.; Crow, S. Parents are key players in the prevention and treatment of weight-related problems. *Nutr. Rev.* **2004**, *62*, 39–50. [CrossRef]
13. Stewart-Brown, S. *What Is the Evidence on School Health Promotion in Improving Health or Preventing Disease and, Specifically, What Is the Effectiveness of the Health Promoting Schools Approach?* World Health Organization, Regional Office for Europe: Copenhagen, Denmark, 2006.
14. Bartelink, N.; van Assema, P.; Jansen, M.; Savelberg, H.; Willeboordse, M.; Kremers, S. The Healthy Primary School of the Future: A Contextual Action-Oriented Research Approach. *Int. J. Environ. Res. Public Health* **2018**, *15*, 2243. [CrossRef]
15. Willeboordse, M.; Jansen, M.; van den Heijkant, S.; Simons, A.; Winkens, B.; de Groot, R.; Bartelink, N.; Kremers, S.; van Assema, P.; Savelberg, H. The Healthy Primary School of the Future: Study protocol of a quasi-experimental study. *BMC Public Health* **2016**, *16*, 639. [CrossRef]
16. WHO. *Health Promoting Schools: A Framework for Action*; World Health Organization Western Pacific Region: Manila, Philippines, 2009.
17. Bartelink, N.H.; van Assema, P.; Kremers, S.P.; Savelberg, H.H.; Oosterhoff, M.; Willeboordse, M.; van Schayck, O.C.; Winkens, B.; Jansen, M.W. One-and Two-Year Effects of the Healthy Primary School of the Future on Children's Dietary and Physical Activity Behaviours: A Quasi-Experimental Study. *Nutrients* **2019**, *11*, 689. [CrossRef]
18. Bartelink, N.H.; van Assema, P.; Kremers, S.P.; Savelberg, H.H.; Oosterhoff, M.; Willeboordse, M.; van Schayck, C.P.; Winkens, B.; Jansen, M.W. Can the Healthy Primary School of the Future offer perspective in the on-going obesity epidemic in young children? A Dutch quasi-experimental study. *BMJ Open*. (2019 submitted).
19. Vermeer, A.J.M.; Boot, N.M.W.M.; Hesdahl, M.H.; Janssen-Goffin, M.J.H.; Linssen, E.C.A.J.; Rutten, N.; Hajema, K.J. *Lokale Rapporten Volksgezondheid Toekomst Verkenning: Een Nieuwe Kijk op Gezondheid in Heerlen, Kerkrade, Landgraaf en Brunssum*; Local Reports on Public Health Development: A New Perspective on Health in Heerlen, Kerkrade, Landgraaf and Brunssum; GGD Zuid Limburg: Geleen, The Netherlands, 2014.
20. Cole, T.J.; Bellizzi, M.C.; Flegal, K.M.; Dietz, W.H. Establishing a standard definition for child overweight and obesity worldwide: International survey. *BMJ* **2000**, *320*, 1240. [CrossRef]
21. Shavers, V.L. Measurement of socioeconomic status in health disparities research. *J. Natl. Med. Assoc.* **2007**, *99*, 1013–1023.
22. Gevers, D.W.; Kremers, S.P.; de Vries, N.K.; van Assema, P. Patterns of food parenting practices and children's intake of energy-dense snack foods. *Nutrients* **2015**, *7*, 4093–4106. [CrossRef]
23. Gevers, D.; Kremers, S.; de Vries, N.; van Assema, P. The Comprehensive Snack Parenting Questionnaire (CSPQ): Development and Test-Retest Reliability. *Int. J. Env. Res. Public Health* **2018**, *15*, 862. [CrossRef]

24. O'Connor, T.M.; Cerin, E.; Hughes, S.O.; Robles, J.; Thompson, D.I.; Mendoza, J.A.; Baranowski, T.; Lee, R.E. Psychometrics of the preschooler physical activity parenting practices instrument among a Latino sample. *Int. J. Behav. Nutr. Phys. Act.* **2014**, *11*, 3. [CrossRef]
25. Choi, L.; Liu, Z.; Matthews, C.E.; Buchowski, M.S. Validation of accelerometer wear and nonwear time classification algorithm. *Med. Sci. Sports Exerc.* **2011**, *43*, 357–364. [CrossRef]
26. Jago, R.; Sebire, S.J.; Turner, K.M.; Bentley, G.F.; Goodred, J.K.; Fox, K.R.; Stewart-Brown, S.; Lucas, P.J. Feasibility trial evaluation of a physical activity and screen-viewing course for parents of 6 to 8 year-old children: Teamplay. *Int. J. Behav. Nutr. Phys. Act.* **2013**, *10*, 31. [CrossRef]
27. Dössegger, A.; Ruch, N.; Jimmy, G.; Braun-Fahrländer, C.; Mäder, U.; Hänggi, J.; Hofmann, H.; Puder, J.J.; Kriemler, S.; Bringolf-Isler, B. Reactivity to accelerometer measurement of children and adolescents. *Med. Sci. Sports Exerc.* **2014**, *46*, 1140–1146. [CrossRef]
28. Migueles, J.H.; Cadenas-Sanchez, C.; Ekelund, U.; Nyström, C.D.; Mora-Gonzalez, J.; Löf, M.; Labayen, I.; Ruiz, J.R.; Ortega, F.B. Accelerometer data collection and processing criteria to assess physical activity and other outcomes: A systematic review and practical considerations. *Sports Med.* **2017**. [CrossRef]
29. Evenson, K.R.; Catellier, D.J.; Gill, K.; Ondrak, K.S.; McMurray, R.G. Calibration of two objective measures of physical activity for children. *J. Sports Sci.* **2008**, *26*, 1557–1565. [CrossRef]
30. Van Assema, P.; Brug, J.; Ronda, G.; Steenhuis, I. The relative validity of a short Dutch questionnaire as a means to categorize adults and adolescents to total and saturated fat intake. *J. Acad. Nutr. Diet.* **2001**, *14*, 377–390. [CrossRef]
31. Lokale en Nationale Monitor Jeugdgezondheid [Local and National Youth Health Monitor]. Standaardvraagstelling Voeding [Standard Questionnaire Nutrition]. Available online: https://www.monitorgezondheid.nl/jeugdindicatoren.aspx (accessed on 16 March 2015).
32. Brookes, S.T.; Whitely, E.; Egger, M.; Smith, G.D.; Mulheran, P.A.; Peters, T.J. Subgroup analyses in randomized trials: Risks of subgroup-specific analyses;: Power and sample size for the interaction test. *J. Clin. Epidemiol.* **2004**, *57*, 229–236. [CrossRef]
33. Hill, J.O.; Wyatt, H.R.; Melanson, E.L. Genetic and environmental contributions to obesity. *Med. Clin. N. Am.* **2000**, *84*, 333–346. [CrossRef]
34. O'Connor, J.P.; Temple, V.A. Constraints and facilitators for physical activity in family day care. *Aust. J. Early Child.* **2005**, *30*, 1–9. [CrossRef]
35. Gubbels, J.S.; Kremers, S.P.; Van Kann, D.H.; Stafleu, A.; Candel, M.J.; Dagnelie, P.C.; Thijs, C.; De Vries, N.K. Interaction between physical environment, social environment, and child characteristics in determining physical activity at child care. *Health Psychol.* **2011**, *30*, 84–90. [CrossRef]
36. Boudewijns, E.; Pepels, J.; van Kann, D.; Konings, K.; van Schayck, C.; Willeboordse, M. Non-response and external validity in a school-based quasi-experimental study 'The Healthy Primary School of the Future': A cross-sectional assessment. *Prev. Med. Rep.* **2019**, *14*, 100874. [CrossRef]
37. Gubbels, J.S.; Stessen, K.; van de Kolk, I.; de Vries, N.K.; Thijs, C.; Kremers, S.P. Energy balance-related parenting and child-care practices: The importance of meso-system consistency. *PLoS ONE* **2018**, *13*, e0203689. [CrossRef]
38. Verjans-Janssen, S.R.; van de Kolk, I.; Van Kann, D.H.; Kremers, S.P.; Gerards, S.M. Effectiveness of school-based physical activity and nutrition interventions with direct parental involvement on children's BMI and energy balance-related behaviors–A systematic review. *PLoS ONE* **2018**, *13*, e0204560. [CrossRef]
39. PHE. *Whole Systems Approach to Obesity: A Guide to Support Local Approaches to Promoting a Healthy Weight*; PHE: London, UK, 2019; Gateway number: GW-534.
40. Martens, M.; Van Assema, P.; Knibbe, R.; Engels, R.C.; Brug, J. Family environmental factors do not explain differences in the behavioral effect of a healthy diet promotion program in lower vocational schools among 12- to 14-year-old adolescents. *Am. J. Health Promot.* **2010**, *24*, 182–185. [CrossRef]
41. Nederhof, A.J. Methods of coping with social desirability bias: A review. *Eur. J. Soc. Psychol.* **1985**, *15*, 263–280. [CrossRef]

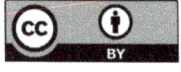

© 2019 by the authors. Licensee MDPI, Basel, Switzerland. This article is an open access article distributed under the terms and conditions of the Creative Commons Attribution (CC BY) license (http://creativecommons.org/licenses/by/4.0/).

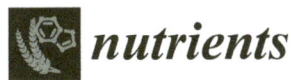

Article

The Reform of School Catering in Hungary: Anatomy of a Health-Education Attempt

Anna Kiss [1], József Popp [2], Judit Oláh [3,*] and Zoltán Lakner [1]

[1] Faculty of Food Science, Szent István University, Budapest 1118, Hungary; kiss.anna891@gmail.com (A.K.); lakner.zoltan@etk.szie.hu (Z.L.)
[2] Institute of Sectoral Economics and Methodology, Faculty of Economics and Business, University of Debrecen, Debrecen 4032, Hungary; popp.jozsef@econ.unideb.hu
[3] Institute of Applied Informatics and Logistics, Faculty of Economics and Business, University of Debrecen, Debrecen 4032, Hungary
* Correspondence: olah.judit@econ.unideb.hu; Tel.: +36-20-2869-085

Received: 14 January 2019; Accepted: 25 March 2019; Published: 27 March 2019

Abstract: School lunch nutrition standards are an important carrier of messages on healthy eating and an efficient way of changing the nutritional behaviour of new generations. Many countries in Europe have a compulsory system of school meals; the Hungarian government also wanted to take action in order to improve the nutrition requirements of the school catering service. The Hungarian Ministry of Human Resources established some limits in the school catering system. However, increasing public pressure forced the legislating organ to considerably modify this regulation. The aim of this study is to analyse the causes of this failure, based on a conceptual framework of institutional economics and a strategic modelling of different institutes by examining the results of 72 interviews (33 experts, 26 parents and 13 teachers) conducted with representatives of different stakeholders. The results highlight the lack of preparation for the introduction of the new regulatory framework, as well as the inefficient communication between the different stakeholders. In order to support children in eating healthfully, a complex nutrition education program and continuous dialogue is needed between teachers, parents, catering staff and the government.

Keywords: institutional economics; MACTOR model; nutrition policy; prevention; semi-quantitative methods; strategic analysis

1. Introduction

Parallel with increasing awareness of the adverse effects of non-communicable diseases, e.g., the effects of obesity and obesity-related diseases on the health condition and mortality of the population [1–3], the inappropriate diets and eating habits of children and adolescents is a much-debated problem all over Europe [4–6]. Growing anxiety concerning the proliferation of the unhealthy eating habits of new generations [7], as well as the increasing number of overweight and obese children [8–10], has increased attention towards different methods of influencing children's and adolescents' health behaviour [11,12]. This is an especially important problem in Hungary where the obesity rate is high. The overall prevalence of overweight and obesity among children and adolescents is 40% and 32%, respectively, and in women overweight and obesity are both at 32% [13]. This causes a considerable burden for the social security and health care system [13,14] according to the categorisation of nutritional status of people based on the body mass index (BMI) [15].

Obesity has been described by the World Health Organization (WHO) as "a global epidemic" due to its high prevalence. It is well known that there are different methods for evaluation of nutritional status of children [16]. Hungary has applied different categorization of nutritional status of children and youth, for example percentiles [17], waist circumference [18] or BMI [19]. All of the researchers have agreed that increasing of obesity is a continuous trend in Hungary. The school catering system (SCS) has a predominant place in the formation of nutrition behaviour [20–22], even if the efficiency of the SCS in the prevention of obesity has not been proven satisfactorily by rigorous, long-range studies [23,24]. School lunch nutrition standards are the basis for improving the nutritional intake of all schoolchildren. All member states of the EU have policies to help schools to provide nutritionally balanced meals. The state of school feeding is considered as a question of strategic importance all over the world [25]. All member states of the EU have policies to help schools to provide nutritionally balanced meals [26]. Based on the EU survey [26] and the cluster analysis [27], we have constructed a general synoptic table (Supplement 1, Table S1). It is obvious that there are considerably differences in the school feeding policy of various EU member states (Figure 1). The Hungarian regulation is rather similar to the Spanish and Danish systems.

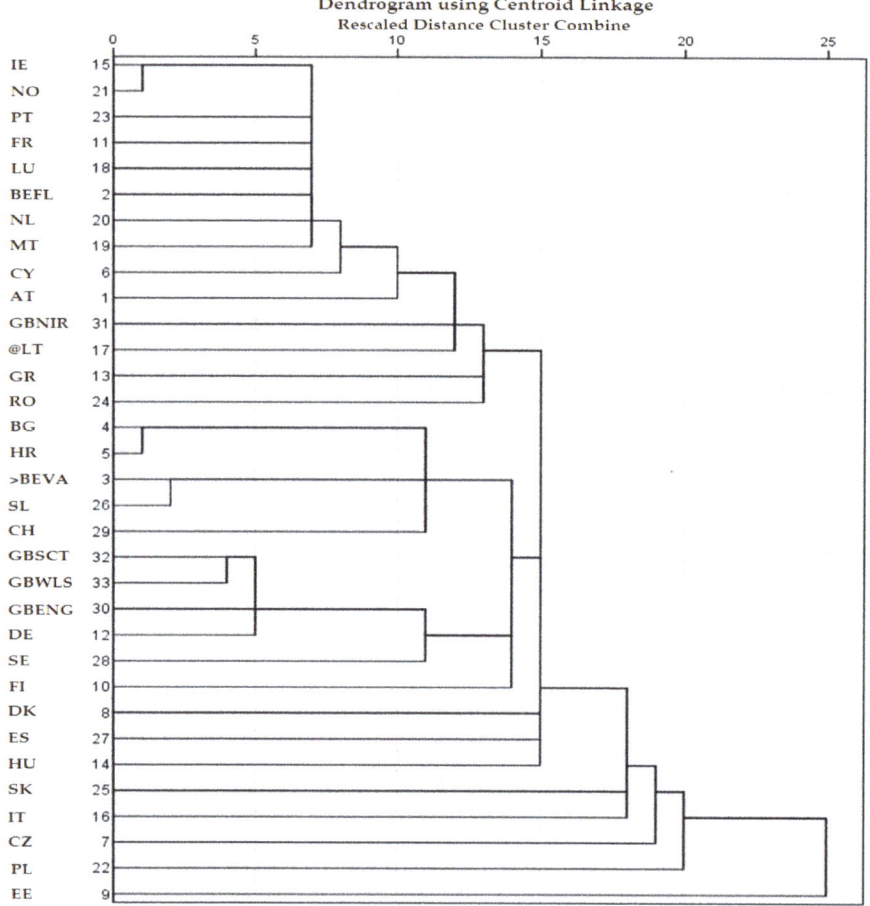

Figure 1. Results of cluster analysis of different EU member states based on their school feeding policy. Source: Authors' own construction, based on EU [28].

It can be stated that in developed countries, there is an increasing tendency to apply the SCS not just as a part of school logistics and the social system, but also as means of health and family-life education. That is why the importance of SCS has increased rapidly. The quality of the Hungarian SCS has been a highly debated issue for generations [29]. There are different business models: the majority of kitchens are owned by local authorities; however, several kitchens are run by catering service provider enterprises. Hungary's SCS is a subsidised system where meals are offered by a reduced price, and in some cases (based on social position) the school meal is free. The Hungarian National Survey of SCS (called as Canteen Panorama) is a regular report of the National Institute of Pharmacy and Nutrition (former Hungarian Office of Food and Nutrition) [30–32]. The monitoring and enforcement of the school meal standards is a mandatory regular activity of the National Food Safety Office (NFSO) with government functions. The essential results of the last three surveys are summarised in Table 1. Vending machines and snack bars are not considered as a part of SCS, but their product portfolio is strictly regulated.

Table 1. Summary of the surveys of school catering systems.

Characteristic Features/Indicators	Canteen Panorama 2008	Canteen Panorama 2013	Canteen Panorama 2017
No. of schools (educational institutions)	3099	260 representatively chosen	139 elementary schools
Elementary schools in the sample (%)	62	62	100
Secondary schools in the sample (%)	17	31	
Elementary and secondary schools (%)		7	
Schools offering warm meal at least once a day with canteen (%) *	92	17	100
School milk program (%)	15	35	72
Free fruits and vegetables (%)	14	78	95
Free drinking water outside the bathroom (%)	36	58	75
Proportion of students eating at the school canteen (in %)	85	87	88
Primary (7–10 years)			
Lower secondary (%) (10–14 years)	47	63	61
Secondary school (%) (14–18 years)	20	27	
Survey of children's satisfaction conducted by the schools (%)	29		
Qualified food catering manager (%)	76.5	83	no data
Food planning with involvement of a dietitian (%)	10	29	38
Energy and nutrients content calculation (%) **	22	57	no data
Net food budget calculated for raw material ***	0.72 EURO	1.2 EURO	1.15 EURO
School snack bar in institutions (%)	45	50	44
Vending machines (%)	30	34	no data

* In each elementary school, and proportion of secondary schools without boarding; ** Energy and nutrient content calculation is based on official nutrient and energy content information, the age-specific menu is calculated based on this information and in some cases even a specific menu planning sotftware is applied. *** Hungarian currency converted to EURO on yearly average conversion rate. Source: Authors' own construction, based on Martos [30], Bakacs et al. [32] and Bakacs et al. [31].

The Hungarian SCS is an evolving system, which is characterised by considerable backwardness and delayed development, compared to Western-European school boarding solutions. The national averages hide important regional differences. According to the Canteen Panoramas [30–32], the school snack bars and vending machines are significant competitors for the SCS, and have an improving product portfolio. At the same time, the SCS is not capable of meeting changing demands. A good indicator of this is the rapidly decreasing take up rate as children's age increases. Another indicator of problems is the fact that according to the school canteen survey Bakacs et al. [32], 85% of parents prepared some kind of prepacked food for their children in 2013. Prepacked food was mainly sandwiches, with vegetables (41%) or without vegetables (37%), and refreshing soft drinks (50%).

Generally speaking, the Hungarian SCS faces substantial long-standing, unsolved problems, which can be attributed to the lack of monetary resources and the lack of attention from responsible organs. This motivated the government to take action to update the nutrition requirements of the public catering service, including school meals, in 2011. In 2011, the Office of the Hungarian Chief Medical Officer issued the 'Recommendation for Public Caterers' with nutritional standards [33]. This recommendation provided a checklist enabling to monitor the adherence to the recommendations. This document was the basis of the 37/2014 decree of Ministry of Human Capacities (MHC) on public catering [34].

The aim of the school meal provision was to reduce the prevalence of obesity and non-communicable diseases (NCDs) among Hungarian children and adolescents, as well as promote healthier environments, especially in schools. The most important elements of the decree are summarised in Table 2. This rather ambitious regulation has tried to increase the fruit, vegetable, cereals and milk consumption and decrease the consumption of fat, sugar and salt. When comparing the content of the Decree with dietary guidelines of other member states of the EU, our nation's dietary guidelines seem to be in line with the nutrition policy of most EU member states. However, the public acceptance of this new regulation has been mixed, and mainly negative. Overall take up rates were generally low, according to the comments of school children. Pupils refused the dishes that conformed to the requirements and both children and their parents rebelled against the rules. In 2015, the Hungarian Association of Dietitians carried out a survey among dietitian food-service managers about the practical feasibility of Hungarian Regulation No. 37/2014 on nutrition requirements in the provision of public food services. Of the 56 food-service managers interviewed, 19 represented child nutrition institutions. Since the introduction of the regulation in 36 of 56 institutions interviewed, satisfaction with nutrition care had decreased. In 13 cases, the rate of dissatisfaction was 30% or more, and the amount of daily food waste increased significantly. The majority of catering service providers (62%) requested some alterations to the regulations because the prescribed composition of the food was not in line with children's demands. The greatest cause of dissatisfaction among parents and children derived from the control of salt content, and the attempt to provide the prescribed quantity of dairy products and added sugars [35]. To date, there are no representative, academically well-founded empirical studies on pupils' consumption of the new school meals [36]. That is why, in 2016, the regulatory framework was changed [37]. The new decree significantly modified the prescriptions. The most important features of the original and the modified decree and the energy limits of school feeding are summarised in Tables 2 and 3.

Table 2. The energy limits of school feeding *.

	1–3 years	4–6 years	7–10 years	11–14 years	15–18 years
Boarding school	4600–5450	5643–6900	7100–8600	8360–10000	8360–10,900
Nursery	3340–4000				
Three meals/day		3800–4600	4600–5500	5500–6500	5400–7100
One meal/day		1880–2500	2500–3200	3000–3500	3000–3800

* Original values in kcal, converted to KJ and rounded. Source: EMMI [38].

Table 3. The most important changes in the public catering decrees.

	2014 * Food-Based Standards	2016 ** Food-Based Standards
Specific foods and food groups have to be provided daily for all age groups (for one person)		
5 meals/day (in a boarding institution the public caterer is obliged to offer main meals three times and two snacks two times)	4 portions of fruits or vegetables per day, at least one of which should be raw *** 3 portions of cereals, at least one which should be whole grain 0.5 l milk or a diary product with an adequate amount of calcium	4 portions of fruits or vegetables per day, at least one of which should be raw 3 portions of cereals, at least one which should be whole grain Removed
Nursery (1 to <3 years) (75% of the daily energy requirement should be covered by two main meals and two snacks)	3 portions of fruits or vegetables per day, at least one of which should be raw 2 portions of cereals, at least one of which should be whole grain 0.4 l milk or a diary product with an adequate amount of calcium	3 portions of fruits or vegetables per day, at least one of which should be raw 2 portions of cereals, at least one of which should be whole grain Removed
3 meals/day (by offering boarding 65% of daily energy requirement should be covered by one main meal and two snacks)	2 portions of fruits or vegetables per day, at least one of which should be raw 2 portions of cereals, at least one of which should be whole grain 0.3 l milk or a diary product with an adequate amount of calcium	2 portions of fruits or vegetables per day, at least one of which should be raw 2 portions of cereals, at least one of which should be whole grain Removed
1 meal/day (offering one main meal (dinner), 35% of daily energy content) Supplementation	1 portion of fruits or vegetables per day, at least three of which should be raw over a 10-day catering period	1 portion of fruits or vegetables per day, at least three of which should be raw over a 10-day catering period If pre-primary, 5 or 3 meals are provided a day, milk or a diary product with an adequate amount of calcium should be served every day
Regulations, limitations and prohibitions of using certain foods and products		
Fat content of milk	2.8% or 3.6% milk fat milks should be served for age group 1–3 years; 1.5% or <1.5% milk fat milks should be served above 3 years old	2.8% or 3.6% milk fat milks should be served for age group 1–3 years; 2.8% or <2.8% milk fat milks should be served above 3 years old
Water	Constant access to fresh water (outside of bathrooms)	Constant access to fresh water (outside of bathrooms)
Added sugar	Free sugar should not exceed 8% of total energy in a 10-day catering period	Free sugar should not exceed 10% of total energy in a 10-day catering period
Salt and free sugar	Salt and sugar should not be placed on dining table	Salt or sugar containers should be labelled: "Excessive salt intake could cause cardiovascular diseases, obesity and diabetes!"
Salt content	Daily salt intake should be reduced to 5 g/day up to 1st of September 2021 At the age bracket 7–10 years salt intake should be reduced to 3.5 g/day up to 1st of September 2021. If the institute offers one meal/day the salt content of the main meal should be reduced up to 2 g/day at age bracket 7–10 years up to 1st of September 2021	

* Public Catering Decree EMMI (Ministry of Human Capacities), Decree 37/2014 (came into force in September 2015). ** Decree on modification of EMMI (Ministry of Human Capacities), Decree 37/2014 (came into force in December 2016). *** The ration of the raw fruit/vegetable requirement is not included in the legislation but it is assumed that this can be explained by higher vitamin content of these goods [39]. Source: MHC [34] and MHC [37].

The Hungarian SCS is a highly complex, dynamic system. The last Decree on Public Catering has yielded important results: the quality of meals has been increasing in the last few years [40]; however, numerous unresolved problems have remained. The new regulatory framework of the SCS is more liberal, although in numerous points it represents a step back from the goals of the former Decree. The aim of this study is to uncover the causes of this phenomenon. In a wider context, our goal is to understand the justification of the low acceptance of the SCS towards a regulatory attempt to manage a long-standing, generally accepted problem, namely childhood obesity. What is the main reason that the regulation could not be put into practice? How can we explain that the take up rate of the SCS has not increased considerably since the introduction of the new decree? To achieve this goal, the authors have applied an innovative, semi-quantitative method for the analysis of social bargaining.

2. Materials and Methods

2.1. The Methodological Framework of the Research

The fundamental theoretical paradigms of the analysis were institutional economic theory [41,42], principle-agent theory [43] and the concept of strategic planning [44]. According to the basic theory of the so-called "French school of strategy", the different social systems can be considered as a playground in which different groups of participants (the actors) take part with the purpose of making their specific interests prevail. In the opinion of [45], if one can adequately simplify the actors and the most characteristic features of their systems of interests and strategies, then it is possible to analyse the chances of different actors realizing their goals. The method of the systematic analysis of social bargaining can be described by using the MACTOR model. One of the key concepts of the model is that actors may influence other actors in terms of their potential to put pressure on other actors directly or indirectly in order to affect their behaviour. The influence of one actor (A) on another actor (C) is the sum of the direct and indirect influences of actor A on actor C.

Based on unstructured interviews, the key actors of the catering system were determined. In the next phase the intensity of mutual direct influences was characterized using a rectangular matrix offering a good overview of the MACTOR method. The cells of the matrix, by definition, reflect the intensity of the influence of any actor in a row on any actor in a column. The intensity of the direct influence by one actor on another was measured on a 0–4 scale ranging from no influence to absolute influence.

The importance of different goals from the point of view of each actor was expressed by the Matrix of Actor-Objective. This was the so-called 1MAO matrix. Each cell of the matrix contained the attitude of a given actor towards a given goal in the form of a positive, 0 or negative sign. In the second phase the 2MAO matrix is determined, which contains the intensity of these attitudes determined from the point of view of different actors and quantified on a −4 ... +4 scale, where −4 denotes the high importance and total negation of the given goal, and +4 denotes the high importance and total support.

The mathematical methodology of the MACTOR method is presented in the literature [46].

2.2. Setting Up the Input Data System

The data collection for the analysis was a multiphase process (Figure 2).

In the present study we applied a self-designed interview method. Besides analysis of publicly available papers, press releases, newspaper articles and the blogosphere, face-to-face expert estimations were made with 24 stakeholders related to the field of Hungarian catering. This series of preliminary interviews were conducted with the purpose of determining the set of relevant actors and interests. The interviews were carried out in 2015 and 2016. The aim of this preliminary phase of interviews was to outline the most important stakeholder groups and the set of the potential objectives of the stakeholders identified in the Supplementary Information (Table S2). As a result of these preliminary investigations, a robust and relatively well-manageable set of actors and goals could be identified. In setting up a pool of experts a specific procedure was followed. In this phase we pursued the following logic. We considered experts to be people (1) who have a direct "field" experiences in catering functions as parents or teachers; (2) people whose job directly involves a catering business with relatively long experience in the practice of SC and whose existence directly depends on this enterprise S; (3) independent experts, preferably those who have been especially active in professional social debates concerning the catering regulations in the printed and electronic media; (4) experts who have been actively involved in the preparation and enforcement of the new regulatory framework of the SCS. The attitude of experts towards school catering has not been taken into consideration, neither in the choice of experts, nor in the interview phase.

The second phase of research was a semi-quantitative interview. The list of potential participants was collected on the basis of intensive research into publications (including professional conferences, various formal and informal meetings of professional communities, the blogosphere and the grey literature), membership of professional organizations and the personal recommendations of other experts.

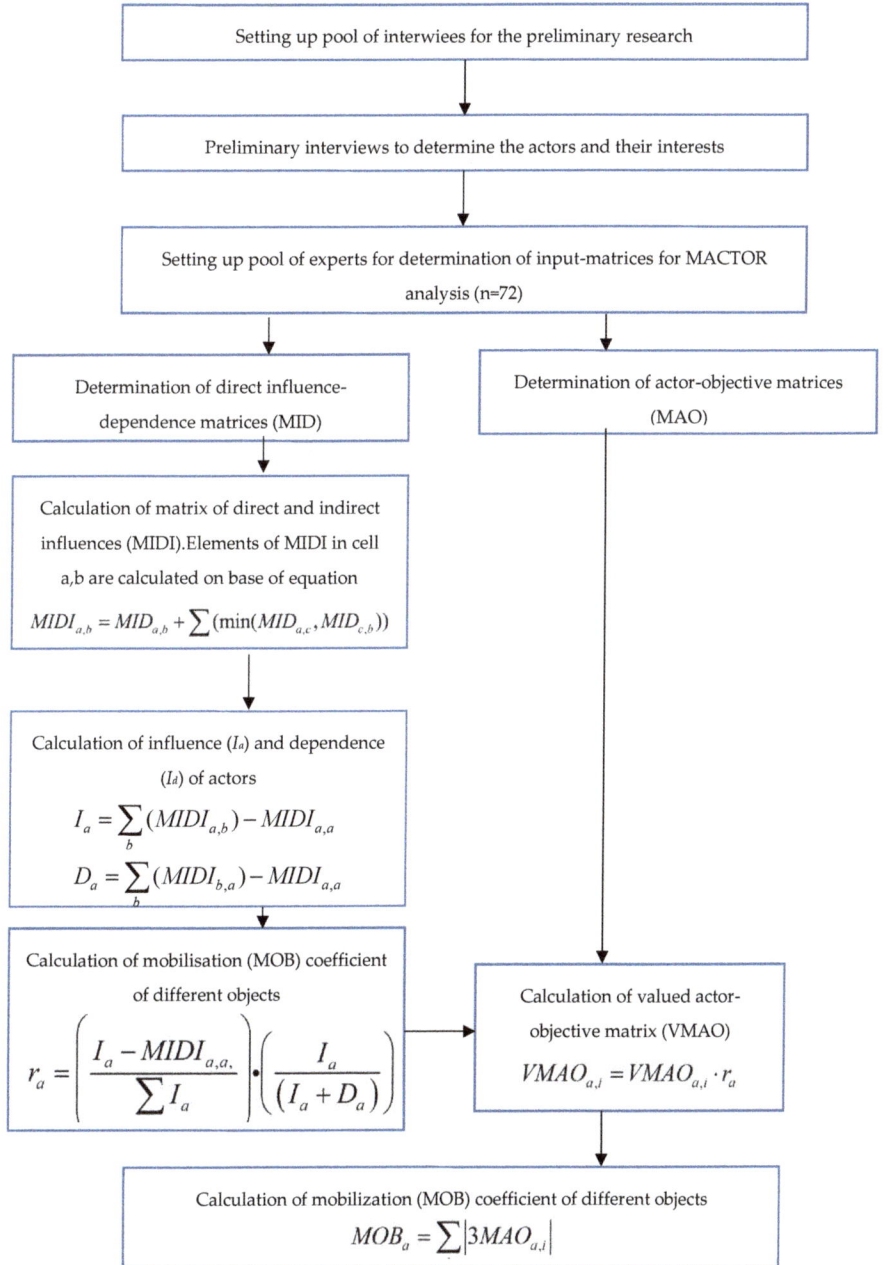

Figure 2. Flowchart of investigations.

In summary, the names of 321 experts were collected (not including parents and teachers). Out of these experts, we tried to make contact with specialists who supposedly, in the opinion of at least two members of the community of authors, have a more 'holistic' approach to the SCS universe without taking into consideration their attitude to the SCS question. In the process of our study, all relevant stakeholders were taken into consideration. In this way, 78 experts were selected. We contacted 61 of them; 45 respondents expressed their willingness to participate in the research. Due to time and financial constraints, 33 expert-interviews were carried out, all of them face-to-face. Additionally, we interviewed 26 parents and 13 teachers. Specific attention was paid to choose parents and teachers from relatively well-off and less developed regions of Hungary: cities like Budapest and Szeged, a small town (Hajós) and a village (Báta). Personal acquaintance played an important role in the choice of teachers and parents. The characteristic features of interviewees are summarised in the Supplementary Information (Table S3).

The quantification of the intensity of actor–actor influences, as well as the actor–objective relations has been developed in a step-by-step manner. As we have experienced with our previous research [47], filling out the input matrices in the form of MS Excel worksheets for research was a very time-consuming (and in some cases a rather boring) process often leading to internal contradictions because it was very difficult to achieve a general common interpretation of different scales. That is why a semi-structured interview was used [48]. The conversion of the verbal estimations was carried out in the personal interview phase with the help of the researchers. The only task of the researchers was to help interpret the different scales. This method proved to be an efficient method for achieving internal consistency in the input data for analysis [49].

In the framework of the interviews, we asked the respondents to evaluate the bargaining power of each actor in comparison with another actor (e.g., Government vs. Teachers, Government vs. Catering service managers etc ...) on a 0–4 scale. The interpretation of this scale was the following:

0—no direct influence.
1—actor A can eliminate the tactical steps of actor B.
2—actor A can jeopardize/eliminate the projects of actor B.
3—actor A can jeopardize/eliminate the strategic goals of actor B.
4—actor A can substantially influence/dominate actor B.

In the second phase of interviews, we asked the interviewees to evaluate the attitudes of actors (stakeholders) towards different elements of goal set on a −4 ... 0 ... +4 scale. The interpretation of the scale was as follows:

−4 the objective is against the vital interest/jeopardizes the existence of the actor
−3 the objective jeopardizes the strategic mission of actors
−2 the objective jeopardizes the tactical goals of the actors
−1 the objective jeopardizes the operative goals of the actor
0 the actors' attitude towards the goal is neutral
+1 the objective falls in line with the operative goals of the actor
+2 the objective falls in line with the tactical goals of the actors
+3 the objective considerably supports the strategic goals of the actor
+4 the objective is a vital interest of the actor

The participants received the cumulated input-matrices and their interpretation by e-mail, and had the opportunity to suggest some modifications. The results of the MACTOR analysis were discussed in detail with a representative pool of respondents in a group discussion and in face-to-face interviews. This phase of the research was an explorative one since our ambition was not to create a representative sample but rather to collect a relatively wide range of opinions.

The research topics were considered very important and interesting questions by all participants, which is why the willingness to participate in the interviews was very high. People evaluated their participation in the research very positively and they were cooperative. Participants were willing to share their experiences and views with others on different problems related to the school catering system development.

2.3. Ethics

The Inter-Faculty Research Ethics Committee of the faculty of Budapest Corvinus University approved both the concept and procedure of the research (Ref. No.15/12/2014). All of the participants signed an informed consent, which described the procedure of the research in detail.

3. Results

3.1. Identification of Key Actors

The framework of individual comprehensive interviews with 24 experts offered a favourable opportunity for understanding the views of different expert actors and their key goals. It was very interesting to see the convergence in the opinions of the respondents concerning the estimation of the goal structures of different actors.

3.1.1. Governments

All respondents agreed that the role of government was essential in the SCS, and that neither the national nor local governmental organs consider the development of the SCS as a priority because it is much less spectacular (i.e., it offers much less possibility to increase the number of votes) than the delivery of a new sports complex or Christmas gift for older voters. This rather curious behaviour is an integrated part of the paternalistic political culture of Hungary [50]. This phenomenon can serve as an explanation of the fact that up to 2010 no significant efforts were made to change the rather negative trends of obesity among children and adolescents.

At the same time, the efforts of the government to change the traditional SCS in Hungary were weakened by the differences of approaches of various ministries and public administration institutions. The attention of governmental organs was divided among different goals and dispersed projects aiming at changing the SCS in Hungary. A possible explanation for this is the scattered structure of the Hungarian public administration and governmental system: the SCS, as a catering service, is supervised by the state secretariat of Health Care at the Ministry of Human Capacities; as a service operated in schools, it is subordinated to the state secretariat of Public Education of the same ministry; as a part of the food chain, it is controlled by the Ministry of Agriculture. Under these conditions a wide range of actions were taken by different actors and lobbies. In the opinion of our interview partners, the SCS is regarded as an important market for local products by the Hungarian Ministry of Agriculture. It is not a coincidence that that the ministry intensively supported the Canteen-Pattern (in Hungarian: Minta Menza®) project, which aims to sell local products in the SCS, often involving specific ingredients (e.g., game-meat, locally grown mushrooms, quail eggs). The project mainly focused on increasing the diversity of dishes and marketing [51]. Children were considered in this framework as consumers, and not as real partners in development. Another state-supported program was the Canteen Reform (in Hungarian: Mensareform®) project developed by some Hungarian celebrity chefs. The goal of this project was the diversification of dish portfolios in the SCS, streamlining the traditional dishes by the introduction of such dish names as "bang-bang crazy chicken" as well upgrading the knowledge of local chefs by a sophisticated qualification system. Both of these programs lost their impetus in the absence of government support [52].

The question arises of what the reason was for launching different programs in parallel. In the opinion of our interview partners, the reason is not just the activity of different lobbies and governmental organs: each public servant tries to highlight his/her importance with the management of one or more programs. For that reason, numerous small-scale projects were initiated, often without any real chance of accomplishment (e.g., "Start with breakfast!", or "Happy week" to increase tap water consumption).

Under these conditions the initiative of the Healthcare secretariat was not able to mobilize the agricultural lobby, nor the catering system providers.

3.1.2. Local Authorities

Local authorities have played an important role in the development of the SCS because the operative running of schools is their responsibility. All of the respondents agreed that (1) the decisions, taken by local authorities concerning the SCS are considerably influenced by policy, namely by the central government and local lobbies, (2) local authorities have a relatively high level of influence on business enterprises, because they can allocate additional financial resources to increase the per-capita financial subsidy for school catering by agreements with SCS firms, (3) the SCM plays an important role in the welfare system as under these conditions the relative availability of food and school services can be considered a political question par excellence.

3.1.3. The Catering Service Providers

There is an increasing number of municipalities that buy the catering service for schools from specific enterprises, which run the kitchen at schools or run the finishing kitchens, where they heat and serve the meals prepared in the central kitchens of the enterprises. The catering service provision has been considered a flourishing business.

3.1.4. Catering Service Managers

The catering service managers are the bosses of kitchens or finishing kitchens. In general, their work consists of the procuration of raw materials, food preparation and management of serving process.

All respondents agreed that local managers are extremely important in the SCS but their scope of decision is rather limited due to budget limits and the difficult systems of regulations. A surprising phenomenon has occurred, namely the burnout the catering managers.

A catering manager said: "I am sick and tired of hearing from early morning to late night each day the snivelling spoiled children. They encourage each other to refuse to eat our food, and they complain about the bad meals we prepare."

The catering managers are frontline solders of the system; however, they felt abandoned. They complained in the following way: "From these limited material resources (i.e., a lack of money) we are not able to buy the raw materials for the kind of food which could satisfy the requirements of Decree ... I do not know enough recipes to prepare a diverse menu to satisfy the requirements—we did not receive any help to do this."

3.1.5. The Parents

Our interviews highlighted that in numerous cases parents do not have enough time to cook, and often even go to fast-food restaurants. This phenomenon decreases families' influence on the healthy nutrition of children and adolescents. All of the respondents agreed that due to the considerable differences within the socio-economic structure in Hungary, it is hard to speak about parents as a homogenous group, because (1) there are parents who simply do not have energy/time to care about the food consumption of their children. There are those (2) who worry about the low quality/quantity of food served to their children in school canteens, which is why they pack them sandwiches or give them money to buy additional food, while (3) in the case of poor families the school canteen plays an important role in relieving families (and their budgets) from the burden of daily food provision. It was a very frequent reflection that: "There is so much talking about school feeding but this is the first time that my opinion is important for someone". Or, as one parent formulated: "This is a very long-lasting problem and a crucial issue but lack of money and attention is an obstacle to improve the situation, so there is not too much to expect". One school canteen manager said: "The most important days for us are Mondays and Fridays: on Monday we have to prepare to energy-rich food, because the children wants nutrient rich food after the unsatisfactory food consumption in the weekend, and on Friday we have to "fill up" the children with copious food".

3.1.6. The Children

Our interviews highlighted that the current world of the SCS is quite distant from the demands of children. There is old, adolescent-sized furniture and sometimes rude and un-motivated kitchen staff (mainly older, often burnt-out female employees), who acquired their experiences in years of relative food shortage and are not able to communicate in an appropriate way with children. Catering reform will only be successful if pupils like and choose to eat these meals, but this aspect has been neglected in Hungary.

The majority of specialists agreed that time has passed the old-style catering infrastructure by, and it has not been renovated for decades. This contrasts noticeably with the vivid colours and modern interiors of the majority of fast-food restaurants which target the younger generation. Under these conditions there is just a relatively low chance of attracting young consumers, who often consider traditional food as old-style.

Children were not included in our evaluation/interview because we focussed on the socio-economic arena of SCS. The primary aim of our investigation was the determination of optimal (qualitative and quantitative) parameters of school meals.

3.1.7. Teachers

Our interview partners agreed that, theoretically, teachers play a very important role in the formation of the eating behaviours and eating habits of children. The teachers eat mainly the same food as the children, if they are eating in the same canteen.

Under these conditions, there is an increasing tendency towards overburdened, burnt-out teachers. As one teachers formulated it: "I have a lot of problems in school and in my private life, I am simply too tired to deal with such problems as the nutrition of the children". As another formulated it: "I am fed up with the fact that society tries to push all its problems onto the schools and teachers. I do not feel it to be my responsibility to care about what children eat under such conditions, when I have to teach them the most elementary rules of social behaviour, just because their parents are playing with their smartphones or lingering on social websites."

3.2. Analysis of Actors' Positions and Strategies Using the MACTOR Method

By using the results of extensive interviews, we determined the set of key actors, and the set of strategic goals, which were determined for one or more actors.

The matrix of the direct influences of actors is shown in Table 4. Based on the actor–goal matrix, we have depicted the position of different actors by the analysis of correspondence [53]. This method is widely applied for the visualization of the relative position of different actors to each other.

The goals in this table are based on preliminary interviews. This is a rectangular matrix. The main diagonal of the matrix (the influence of a given actor on itself) is by definition zero. The actor considered as the influencer is placed in the row, and the influenced party is situated in the column. The values in the cells of matrix are the simple averages of responses obtained as a result of discussion. To be on the safe side we have calculated the averages by group of actors (e.g., teachers, parents, catering managers etc.), but we have not been able to prove significant differences between the two methods. The in-depth analysis of standard deviations according to interviewees could go beyond the limits of the current research.

Some remarks about the results of the matrix of direct influences based on in-depth interviews are indicated as follows:

—The matrix highlights the considerable influence of the government on the behaviour of catering service providers and on the SCS in general, because the government has a considerable influence on the monetary resources for school catering.

—Local authorities can exercise an important influence on catering service providers because they have the possibility to select the SCS provider for different schools in the framework of the public procurement procedure.

—In the opinion of interview partners, a basically positive tendency has occurred over the last years: the increasing influence of parents' organizations on the life of schools. At the same time, due to the lack of democratic roots and traditions it is quite difficult to achieve a situation in which parents' influence is based on an absolute majority of the parents and not just on a relative majority of a small group with active and noisy members. Due to the lack of democratic roots and traditions, it is quite difficult to achieve parents' influence based on an absolute majority of the parents and not just on a small group with active and noisy members. The interest relation of the different actors is summarized in Table 5. This is a not a rectangular matrix. The actors are placed in rows and the different goals are located in columns. The values in the cells of matrix are the simple averages of responses obtained as a result of discussion.

Table 4. The matrix of direct influences on actors measured on a 0–4 scale (0—no direct influence, 4—very strong influence).

	GOV	MUNICIP	PARENTS	CHILDREN	MANAGERS	BUSINESS	TEACHERS
Government GOV	0	3	1	0	1	4	2
Local authorities MUNICIP	1	0	1	0	1	4	0
PARENTS	1	3	0	3	0	0	2
CHILDREN	0	0	2	0	0	0	1
Catering service managers MANAGERS	0	0	0	2	0	0	1
Catering service providers BUSINESS	1	1	0	0	3	0	0
TEACHERS	1	2	2	3	1	1	0

Table 5. The actors' interest relations measured on a −4 ... +4 scale.

	Good Taste of the Meal (TASTE)	Healthiness of the Food (HEALTH)	Healthy Children (HEALTHYCHI)	Vote maximisation (VOTE)	Feeling of Being sated (SATED)	Minimisation of Expenditure on Health Promotion (CPOSTMIN)	Simplicity of Food Preparation (SIMPLE)
GOV	1	3	4	4	3	3	0
MUNIICIP	2	1	4	4	3	4	0
PARENT	4	3	4	0	2	3	0
CHILD	4	1	4	0	2	0	0
CATERING	3	0	0	0	2	4	4
BUSINESS	3	0	0	0	2	2	4
TEACHERS	3	1	3	0	3	1	0

Interpretation: −4 the objective is against the vital interest/jeopardizes the existence of the actor, +4 the objective is a vital interest of the actor.

The health of children is a generally accepted goal for all participants, but this goal is relatively more distant in time, which means it is difficult to translate into operative actions. Local authorities are in direct connection with the population, so the taste of food is especially important for them. The children's acceptance of food is important for the parents, too, because in this way they can reduce their household expenditure on feeding their children. A well-fed child can be managed easily so the taste and acceptance of food is important for teachers, as well. It should be highlighted that cost minimization is quite an important question for the majority of actors.

According to our findings, school feeding was important for parents. It can be assessed as a positive point, that, at least on the verbal level, the healthiness of school feeding was evaluated as a question of great importance. This can be considered as a favourable tendency. The bargaining position of different actors has been depicted on a two-dimensional coordinate system. On one ordinate of the system, we have indicated the level of influence of the given actor. This value has been calculated based on Table 4 by the summation and normalization of direct influences for each given actor in relation to another actor [47]. The dependence of actors has been calculated in a similar manner.

Analysing the map of influences and dependences between actors (Figure 3), it is obvious that the government has a relatively favourable bargaining position because it has a relatively high level of influence and a low level of dependence. The direct socio-economic environment of children's food consumption is the following: the triangle of teachers, local authorities and parents have roughly the same position, namely a relatively high level of influence and a low level of dependence. The owners of the SCS firms have approximately the same level of dependence as the former three actors, with a much lower influence. The two key actors of the SCS system, the children and the catering service managers, have an extremely low level of influence, which—especially in the case of the children—is accompanied by high dependence. In other words, the two critical actors of the systems, namely the actual service providers and the children, have the least possibility to influence the operation of the system.

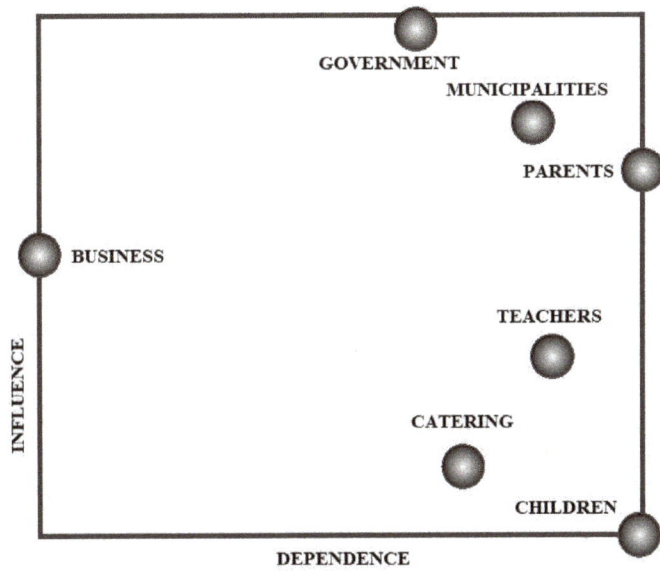

Figure 3. The influence–dependence relations of actors.

The analysis of influence dependence matrix offers information on estimated power relationships between actors and also on the way of thinking of respondents. It can be considered as a rather negative tencency that interviewees evaluated the catering system as a set of different, relativevly separated actors instead of a coherent system with numerous relations. This fact is experessed in a high number of zeroes indicating no infuence.

The indicator "mobilizing force" of different goals has been calculated based on the acceptance of differing goals weighted by bargaining power (influence) on actors.

Analysing the mobilizing force of the different interests, good taste and children's health have the highest value (Table 6). Notwithstanding, it is important to stress that the mobilizing force of the cost minimization of health expenditure promotion and simplicity is much higher than the healthiness of food criteria.

Table 6. Mobilising force of different goals.

Goal	Mobilising Force
good taste of the meal	12.8
healthy food	17.1
healthy children	17.8
vote maximisation	8.6
feeling of being sated	10.2
minimisation of expenditure on health promotion	17.4
simplicity of food preparation	2.4

4. Discussion and Conclusions

The results of this survey highlight that government support has been rather weak so far because the majority of parents accept the importance of healthy eating, but they avoid the conflicts with their children. The overburdened teachers have done little to change the eating habits of the students. The caterers and the catering service managers support the best solution for themselves. At the same time the direct influence of catering managers is relatively low; however, their behaviour and attitude are of great interest in any reform. It is a contradiction that they have not been prepared to make use of these reforms. Neither the government nor the local municipalities have been determined enough to mobilize additional financial and intellectual sources to change the situation and consequently follow the policy. In general, it can be stated that the MACTOR method has been an efficient tool to uncover the direct and indirect force relations and motivations of different actors.

Our results are consistent with conclusions drown by another actors. For example, in the opinion of Gaál et al. [54], the central government of Hungary has almost exclusive power to formulate and realize strategic decisions and shape the regulatory framework of the health care system, as well as make public-health-related interventions. The majority of schools (with the exception of schools owned by foundations and churches) are in state ownership.

Due to a wide agreement on the long-term instability of the Hungarian health-care system [55–58], preventive measures should be given priority.

It is a contradiction that while all Hungarian governmental programs [59–62] have highlighted the importance of prevention in the health-care system, obesity among the young population groups has been increasing in the last few decades [63,64].

It should be highlighted that neither schools, teachers, nor parents can be considered homogenous groups [65]. There are significant differences in parents' attitudes and behaviour in relation to the school catering system. The results of van Zenten [66] and Raveaud and van Zanten [67] highlight that upper- or middle-class parents have a much higher level of aspiration to participate in the decision-making process in the framework of the school than working-class parents, who are more 'loyal' to local schools [68].

The importance of school feeding for parents was a surprising result. It can be regarded as positive that the healthiness of school feeding has been evaluated as a question of great interest. This can be considered a favourable tendency.

The results of investigations have demonstrated clearly that children are key players in the Hungarian SCS but have little influence on the system. In Hungary, there does not exist any mechanism to survey the opinion and test the preference system of children. The most reliable indicators are the cleaners, who can furnish some information on the quantity of food and the amount leftover. There are neither experiences nor resources or mechanisms to uncover the drivers behind children's behaviour [69].

The average uptake level is low, varying from 40% to 95%; the highest take up rate in Europe is in Finland (over 90%), probably because school lunch plays a central role in education [70].

Based on our analyses, the failure of the new regulation of the SCS was predictable because children have not accepted dishes with low salt content and milk with low fat content. The uptake level of the reform was extremely low as children were not involved in the new and rapidly introduced changes. The reluctance of children induced a chain reaction: neither the parents nor the teachers were motivated, nor did they have any background knowledge to argue for the positive aspects of the reform. The catering service providers and the local managers experienced a high level of food waste. These negative views were reinforced by the media, which over-emphasized the negative aspects of the new regulations. Under these conditions, it was relatively easy to forge a coalition between parents, catering service providers and managers, teachers and local authorities to choose the easier option: i.e., to force the government to substantially modify the original legislation. The fate of this regulation, based on sound professional arguments, lends itself to an analysis of the failures leading to the collapse of the regulation. The most important failures can be summarized as follows:

1. There was no general, well-designed study and testing of the effects of the regulation in the framework of a pilot study.
2. There was no multilateral communication between the government and the stakeholders, mainly with catering service providers and catering managers.
3. The teachers did not have the necessary background to discuss the issue with children due to their total illiteracy in the field of nutrition.
4. Children do not have to learn practically any nutrition or food skills during their studies in the primary and secondary school, so they did not have the capacity to understand the reason for the changes.
5. The energy and resources of different governmental organs were scattered among different, partially competing, goals.

The school lunch provides an excellent opportunity to learn healthy eating habits, promote nutrient-rich foods, involve children in foodservice planning and improve the nutritional intake of school children. There is an urgent need to improve the situation, taking into account the WHO tool for the development of school nutrition programmes in the European Region [71]. The policy paper emphasizes that healthy food and nutrition should be given a high priority on every school agenda and school meals are an indispensable part of a whole school approach to health promotion. To ensure effective implementation, stakeholders should review the available information on nutritional status and eating patterns before developing school lunch standards and issuing any regulation on nutrition requirements in public food-services.

As a conclusion of this study, it can be determined that the position and the system of interests of different actors must be taken into consideration before setting up SCS-related regulations. Children play a central role because they will be able indirectly influence parents and teachers. From this it follows that considerable resources should be mobilized to understand the driving forces of children's behaviour and their taste. On the other hand, from a retrospective perspective it is obvious that the government wanted to improve the SCS "by force", following top-down logic, with minimal mobilization of material and human resources on education and widening the possibilities of raw material procuration.

Cooperation among all the different stakeholders is crucial when working out a school food and nutrition policy [72]. Moreover, one can even state that cooperation between different players, including coopetition, is a fundamental issue in today's world [73,74].

Representatives of teachers, parents, pupils, caterers and representatives from a school's governing body should develop an action plan and introduce a comprehensive education program. The study of policy itself can be an educational tool. Teaching about food and nutrition policies in schools would make students active participants throughout the policy process [75]. The SCS should be better integrated into the general education program. For example, the participation of children in food preparation and servicing could promote family-life education and a more harmonious division of work between the genders, too. In order to establish a successful and effective strategy, a continuous dialogue is needed between parents, health promotion experts, teachers and their organizations. It should be emphasized that there is no universal solution: the specific needs of children should be taken into consideration because a good school meal is an investment in the future.

Supplementary Materials: The following are available online at http://www.mdpi.com/2072-6643/11/4/716/s1, Table S1: Synoptic table of school-feeding policy and regulation based on (EU, 2018). Legend: 1 - there is a recommendation/legislation, Table S2: Structure of participants in preliminary phase of research, Table S3: The socio-economic characteristic features of participants (n = 72).

Author Contributions: Conceptualization, A.K. and Z.L.; methodology, Z.L.; software, Z.L.; validation, J.P. and J.O.; formal analysis, J.P.; investigation, A.K.; resources, J.O.; data curation, J.P.; writing—original draft preparation, A.K.; writing—review and editing, J.P.; visualization, J.O.; supervision, J.P.; project administration, A.K.; funding acquisition, A.K.

Funding: This research was supported by the ÚNKP-18-4 New National Excellence Program of the Ministry of Human Capacities and by the János Bolyai Research Scholarship of the Hungarian Academy of Sciences and Food Science Doctoral School of Szent István University and the research fond: EFOP-3.6.3-VEKOP-16-2017-00005.

Conflicts of Interest: The authors declare no conflict of interest.

References

1. Malik, V.S.; Willett, W.C.; Hu, F.B. Global obesity: Trends, risk factors and policy implications. *Nat. Rev. Endocrinol.* **2013**, *9*, 13–27. [CrossRef]
2. McPherson, K. Reducing the global prevalence of overweight and obesity. *Lancet* **2014**, *384*, 728–730. [CrossRef]
3. Nurwanti, E.; Uddin, M.; Chang, J.-S.; Hadi, H.; Syed-Abdul, S.; Su, E.; Nursetyo, A.; Masud, J.; Bai, C.-H. Roles of sedentary behaviors and unhealthy foods in increasing the obesity risk in adult men and women: A cross-sectional national study. *Nutrients* **2018**, *10*, 704. [CrossRef]
4. van Dijk, S.J.; Molloy, P.L.; Varinli, H.; Morrison, J.L.; Muhlhausler, B.S.; Buckley, M.; Clark, S.J.; McMillen, I.C.; Noakes, M.; Samaras, K. Epigenetics and human obesity. *Int. J. Obes.* **2015**, *39*, 85–97. [CrossRef] [PubMed]
5. Koletzko, B. Childhood obesity: Current situation and future opportunities. *J. Pediatr. Gastroenterol. Nutr.* **2016**, *63*, 18–21. [CrossRef]
6. Grasgruber, P.; Cacek, J.; Hrazdíra, E.; Hřebíčková, S.; Sebera, M. Global Correlates of Cardiovascular Risk: A Comparison of 158 Countries. *Nutrients* **2018**, *10*, 411. [CrossRef] [PubMed]
7. Lobstein, T.; Jackson-Leach, R.; Moodie, M.L.; Hall, K.D.; Gortmaker, S.L.; Swinburn, B.A.; James, W.P.T.; Wang, Y.; McPherson, K. Child and adolescent obesity: Part of a bigger picture. *Lancet* **2015**, *385*, 2510–2520. [CrossRef]
8. Dietz, W.H. Critical periods in childhood for the development of obesity. *Am. J. Clin. Nutr.* **1994**, *59*, 955–959. [CrossRef] [PubMed]
9. Elmadfa, I.; Freisling, H. Nutritional status in Europe: Methods and results. *Nutr. Rev.* **2009**, *67*, 130–134. [CrossRef] [PubMed]
10. Karnik, S.; Kanekar, A. Childhood obesity: A global public health crisis. *Int. J. Prev. Med.* **2012**, *3*, 1–7.
11. Waddingham, S.; Stevens, S.; Macintyre, K.; Shaw, K. Most of them are junk food but we did put fruit on there and we have water. What children can tell us about the food choices they make. *Health Educ.* **2015**, *115*, 126–140. [CrossRef]

12. Swinburn, B.; Kraak, V.; Rutter, H.; Vandevijvere, S.; Lobstein, T.; Sacks, G.; Gomes, F.; Marsh, T.; Magnusson, R. Strengthening of accountability systems to create healthy food environments and reduce global obesity. *Lancet* **2015**, *385*, 2534–2545. [CrossRef]
13. Rurik, I.; Torzsa, P.; Móczár, C.; Ungvári, T.; Iski, G.; Sándor, J.N. Prevalence and economic burden of obesity in Hungary. *Ann. Nutr. Metabol.* **2015**, *67*, 331–332.
14. Iski, G.; Rurik, I. The estimated economic burden of overweight and obesity in Hungary. *Orvosi Hetilap* **2014**, *155*, 1406–1412. [CrossRef]
15. Jaqueline, D.S.F.; Paula, D.D.M.; Elza, D.M. Subjective global assessment of nutritional status—A systematic review of the literature. *Clin. Nutr.* **2015**, *34*, 785–792.
16. Cole, T.J.; Faith, M.S.; Pietrobelli, A.; Heo, M. What is the best measure of adiposity change in growing children: BMI, BMI%, BMI z-score or BMI centile? *Eur. J. Clin. Nutr.* **2005**, *59*, 419. [CrossRef] [PubMed]
17. Bodzsar, E.B.; Zsakai, A. Recent trends in childhood obesity and overweight in the transition countries of Eastern and Central Europe. *Ann. Hum. Biol.* **2014**, *41*, 263–270. [CrossRef]
18. Kovacs, V.A.; Gabor, A.; Fajcsak, Z.; Martos, E. Role of waist circumference in predicting the risk of high blood pressure in children. *Int. J. Pediatr. Obes.* **2010**, *5*, 143–150. [CrossRef] [PubMed]
19. Ahrens, W.; Pigeot, I.; Pohlabeln, H.; De Henauw, S.; Lissner, L.; Molnár, D.; Moreno, L.; Tornaritis, M.; Veidebaum, T.; Siani, A. Prevalence of overweight and obesity in European children below the age of 10. *Int. J. Obes.* **2014**, *38*, 99–107. [CrossRef]
20. Briggs, M. Position of the American dietetic association, school nutrition association, and society for nutrition education: Comprehensive school nutrition services. *J. Am. Diet. Assoc.* **2010**, *110*, 1738–1749. [CrossRef]
21. Ganann, R.; Fitzpatrick-Lewis, D.; Ciliska, D.; Peirson, L.J.; Warren, R.L.; Fieldhouse, P.; Delgado-Noguera, M.F.; Tort, S.; Hams, S.P.; Martinez-Zapata, M.J. Enhancing nutritional environments through access to fruit and vegetables in schools and homes among children and youth: A systematic review. *BMC Res. Notes* **2014**, *7*, 422. [CrossRef] [PubMed]
22. Meiklejohn, S.; Ryan, L.; Palermo, C. A Systematic Review of the Impact of Multi-Strategy Nutrition Education Programs on Health and Nutrition of Adolescents. *J. Nutr. Educ. Behav.* **2016**, *48*, 631.e631–646.e631. [CrossRef]
23. Brown, T.; Summerbell, C. Systematic review of school-based interventions that focus on changing dietary intake and physical activity levels to prevent childhood obesity: An update to the obesity guidance produced by the National Institute for Health and Clinical Excellence. *Obes. Rev.* **2009**, *10*, 110–141. [CrossRef] [PubMed]
24. Jaime, P.C.; Lock, K. Do school based food and nutrition policies improve diet and reduce obesity? *Prev. Med.* **2009**, *48*, 45–53. [CrossRef]
25. World Food Programme (WFO). School Feedign Policy (Revised). 2013; Available online: https://documents.wfp.org/stellent/groups/public/documents/communications/wfp263529.pdf?_ga=2.233517214.1895239352.1553180739-536407624.1553180739 (accessed on 3 March 2019).
26. Storcksdieck, S.; Kardakis, T.; Wollgast, J.; Nelson, M.; Caldeira, S. *Mapping of National School Food Policies across the EU28 Plus Norway and Switzerland*; 2014; Available online: http://publications.jrc.ec.europa.eu/repository/bitstream/JRC90452/lbna26651enn.pdf (accessed on 3 March 2019).
27. Norušis, M.J. *IBM SPSS Statistics 19 Statistical Procedures Companion*; Prentice Hall: Upper Saddle River, NJ, USA, 2012.
28. EU. School Food Policy Country Factsheets. 2018; Available online: https://ec.europa.eu/jrc/en/publication/school-food-policy-country-factsheets (accessed on 3 March 2019).
29. Tarján, R. Evaluation of school feeding programmes in some European countries. In *Nutrition and Technology of Foods for Growing Humans*; Karger Publishers: Rüschlikon-Zürich, Switzerland, 1973; pp. 280–288.
30. Martos, E. *Országos Iskolai Menza Körkép. Iskolai Táplálkozás-Egészségügyi Környezetfelmérés. Gyosrjelentés*; Országos Élelmezés-és Táplákozástudományi Intézet: Budapest, Hungary, 2008. Available online: https://www.ogyei.gov.hu/dynamic/oeti_forms/menza2008.pdf (accessed on 3 March 2019).
31. Bakacs, M.; Cs, K.; Nagy, B.; Varga, A.; Zentai, A. *Menza Parorama 2017*; Országos Gyógyszerészeti és Élelmezés-Egészségügyi Intézet (OGYÉI): Budapest, Hungary, 2018. Available online: https://www.ogyei.gov.hu/dynamic/Orszagos%20iskolai%20MENZA%20k%C3%B6rkep%202017%20webre.pdf (accessed on 3 March 2019).
32. Bakacs, M.; Martos, E.; Schrebiberne-Monlár, E.; Zentai, A. *Menza Panorama, 2013*; Országos Gyógyszerészeti és Élelmezés-egészségügyi Intézet (OGYÉI): Budapest, Hungary, 2013; Available online: https://www.researchgate.net/publication/291986522_Orszagos_Iskolai_MENZA_Korkep_2013 (accessed on 3 March 2019).

33. HCMFO. A Rendszeres Étkezést Biztosító, Szervezett Élelmezési Ellátásra Vonatkozó Táplálkozás-Egészségügyi Ajánlás Közétkeztetők Számára No.1/2011 [Nutritional Recommendations for Organizations, Offering Regular, Organized Catering Service], Hungarian Chief Medical Officer's Office. 2011; Available online: https://www.antsz.hu/data/cms30236/szervezett_elelmezesi_ellatasra_vonatkozo_taplalkozas_egeszsegugyi_ajanlas_kozetkeztetoknek_20110805.pdf (accessed on 2 February 2019).
34. MHC. Rendelet a Közétkeztetésre Vonatkozó Táplálkozás-Egészségügyi Előírásokról, No. 37/2014 [Decree on Nutirional Regulations in Public Catering, in Hungarian]. 2014; Available online: https://net.jogtar.hu/jogszabaly?docid=A1400037.EMM (accessed on 2 February 2019).
35. Erdélyi-Sipos, A. Survey among dietetian-foodservice managers on the application of the 37/2014 Hungarian Regulation on nutrition requirements for the public foodservices. *ÚJ Diéta* **2016**, *2–3*, 18–23.
36. Kliestik, T.; Misankova, M.; Valaskova, K.; Svabova, L. Bankruptcy Prevention: New Effort to Reflect on Legal and Social Changes. *Sci. Eng. Ethics* **2018**, *24*, 1–13. [CrossRef]
37. MHC. Rendelet a Közétkeztetésre Vonatkozó Táplálkozás-Egészségügyi Előírásokról Szóló 37/2014 EMMI Rendelet Módosításáról No.36/2016 [Decree on Change of 37/2014 Decree on Nutirional Regulations in Public Catering, in Hungarian]. 2016; Available online: https://net.jogtar.hu/jogszabaly?docid=A1600036.EMM&timeshift=ffffff4&txtreferer=00000001.TX (accessed on 2 February 2019).
38. EMMI. 36/2016. (XII. 8.) EMMI rendelet a közétkeztetésre vonatkozó táplálkozás-egészségügyi előírásokról szóló 37/2014. (IV. 30.) EMMI rendelet módosításáról. Available online: https://net.jogtar.hu/jogszabaly?docid=A1600036.EMM&timeshift=ffffff4&txtreferer=00000001.TXT (accessed on 2 February 2019).
39. Chemat, F.; Rombaut, N.; Meullemiestre, A.; Turk, M.; Perino, S.; Fabiano-Tixier, A.-S.; Abert-Vian, M. Review of green food processing techniques. Preservation, transformation, and extraction. *Innov. Food Sci. Emerg. Technol.* **2017**, *41*, 357–377. [CrossRef]
40. Varga, A.; Bakacs, M.; Zentai, A.; Nagy, B.; Nagy-Lőrincz, Z.; Erdei, G.; Illés, É.; Varga-Nagy, V.; Sarkadi Nagy, E.; Cserháti, Z. Assessment of the public catering act in primary schools in Hungary: Anita Varga. *Eur. J. Public Health* **2018**, *28*, cky213 681. [CrossRef]
41. Hannan, M.T.; Freeman, J.H. Structural inertia and organisational change. *Am. Sociol. Rev.* **1984**, *49*, 149–164. [CrossRef]
42. Dacin, M.T.; Goodstein, J.; Scott, W.R. Institutional theory and institutional change: Introduction to the special research forum. *Acad. Mang. J.* **2002**, *45*, 45–47. [CrossRef]
43. Eisenhardt, K. Agency Theory: An Assessment and Review Acad. *Manag. Rev.* **1989**, *14*, 57–74. [CrossRef]
44. Mintzberg, H. The fall and rise of strategic planning. *Harv. Bus. Rev.* **1994**, *72*, 107–114. Available online: https://hbr.org/1994/01/the-fall-and-rise-of-strategic-planning..
45. Godet, M. Actors' moves and strategies: The mactor method: An air transport case study. *Futures* **2003**, *23*, 605–622. [CrossRef]
46. Bendahan, S.; Camponovo, G.; Pigneur, Y. Multi-issue actor analysis: Tools and models for assessing technology environments. *J. Decis. Syst.* **2004**, *13*, 223–253. [CrossRef]
47. Popp, J.; Oláh, J.; Fári, M.; Balogh, P.; Lakner, Z. The GM-regulation game-the case of Hungary. *Int. Food Agribus. Manag. Rev.* **2018**, *27*, 945–968. [CrossRef]
48. Lindlof, T.R.; Taylor, B.C. *Qualitative Communication Research Methods*; SAGE Publications: Thousand Oaks, CA, USA, 2010; p. 377. ISBN 978-1412974738.
49. Kliestik, T.; Kovacova, M.; Podhorska, I.; Kliestikova, J. Searching for key sources of goodwill creation as new global managerial challenge. *Pol. J. Manag. Stud.* **2018**, *17*, 144–154. [CrossRef]
50. Enyedi, Z. Paternalist populism and illiberal elitism in Central Europe. *J. Political Ideol.* **2016**, *21*, 9–25. [CrossRef]
51. Takács, S. Környezet-ember; gondolatok az új tudományos megállapításokról (Environment-humans; thoughts about the new scientific observations). *Egészségtudomány* **2012**, *LVII*, 61–67.
52. Báti, A. Paradicsomlevestől a fürjtojásig: A gyermekétkeztetés néprajzi vizsgálata budapesti példa nyomán. *Ethno-Lore Magy. Tud. Akad. Népr. Kutatóint. Kv.* **2014**, *31*, 201–259. Available online: http://real.mtak.hu/20816/1/Bati_Aniko_u_173810.586803.pdf (accessed on 3 March 2019).
53. Greenacre, M. *Correspondence Analysis in Practice*; Chapman and Hall/CRC: New York, NY, USA, 2017.
54. Gaál, P.; Szigeti, S.; Csere, M.; Gaskins, M.; Panteli, D. Hungary health system review. *Health Syst. Trans.* **2010**, *13*, 1–266.
55. Docteur, E.; Oxley, H. Health care: A quest for better value. *Observer* **2003**, *238*, 1–18.

56. Boncz, I.; Nagy, J.; Sebestyén, A.; Kőrösi, L. Financing of health care services in Hungary. *Eur. J. Health Econ. Form.* **2004**, *5*, 252–258. [CrossRef] [PubMed]
57. Gaal, P.; Evetovits, T.; McKee, M. Informal payment for health care: Evidence from Hungary. *Health Policy* **2006**, *77*, 86–102. [CrossRef] [PubMed]
58. Tchouaket, É.N.; Lamarche, P.A.; Goulet, L.; Contandriopoulos, A.P. Health care system performance of 27 OECD countries. *Int. J. Health Plan. Manag.* **2012**, *27*, 104–129. [CrossRef] [PubMed]
59. Romsics, I. *Magyar Kormányprogramok (Programs of Hungarian Governments) II*; Magyar Hivatalos Közlönykiadó: Budapest, Hungary, 2004; Volumn 2.
60. Gyurcsány, F. *New Hungary—Freedom and Solidarity (Governmental Program for Successful, Modern and Fair Hungary)*; Hungarian Government: Budapest, Hungary, 2006.
61. Bajnai, G. *Válságkezelés és Bizalomerősítés (Crysis Management and Enhancement of Confidence)*; Hungarian Governmnent: Budapest, Hungary, 2009.
62. Orbán, V. *Program of National Cooperation*; Hungarian Parliament: Budapest, Hungary, 2010.
63. Tóth, G.A.; Molnár, P.; Suskovics, C. Trends in Body Mass Index in School-age children in Central-Europe. *Hum. Biol. Rev.* **2014**, *3*, 167–174.
64. Kopia, J.; Kompalla, A.; Buchmüller, M.; Heinemann, B. Performance measurement of management system standards using the balanced scorecard. *Amfiteatru Econ.* **2017**, *19*, 981–1002.
65. van Zanten, A. Competitive arenas and schools' logics of action: A European comparison. *Comp. A J. Comp. Int. Educ.* **2009**, *39*, 85–98. [CrossRef]
66. van Zenten, A. Middle-class parents and social mix in French urban schools: Reproducion and transfromation of class relations in education. *Int. Stud. Sociol. Educ.* **2003**, *13*, 107–124. [CrossRef]
67. Raveaud, M.; van Zanten, A. Choosing the local school: Middle class paenets' values and social and ethnic mix in London and in Paris. *J. Educ. Policy* **2006**, *22*, 107–124. [CrossRef]
68. Hirschman, A. *Exit, Voice and Loyalty. Responses to Decline in Firms, Organisations and States*; Harvard University Press: Cambridge, UK, 1970; ISBN 0-674-27660-4.
69. DeCosta, P.; Møller, P.; Frøst, M.B.; Olsen, A. Changing children's eating behaviour-A review of experimental research. *Appetite* **2017**, *113*, 327–357. [CrossRef]
70. Harper, C.; Wood, L.; Mitchell, C. *The Provision of School Food in 18 Countries*; School Food Trust: London, UK, 2008.
71. World Health Organization. *Food and Nutrition Policy for Schools: A Tool for the Development of School Nutrition Programmes in the European Region*; WHO Regional Office for Europe: Copenhagen, Denmark, 2006; Available online: https://apps.who.int/iris/handle/10665/107797 (accessed on 3 March 2019).
72. Djokic, N.; Grubor, A.; Milicevic, N.; Petrov, V. New Market Segmentation Knowledge in the Function of Bioeconomy Development in Serbia. *Amfiteatru Econ.* **2018**, *20*, 700–716. [CrossRef]
73. Cygler, J.; Sroka, W. Coopetition disadvantages: The case of the high tech companies. *Inz. Ekon.-Eng. Econ.* **2017**, *28*, 494–504. [CrossRef]
74. Cygler, J.; Sroka, W.; Solesvik, M.; Dębkowska, K. Benefits and drawbacks of coopetition: The roles of scope and durability in coopetitive relationships. *Sustainability* **2018**, *10*, 2688. [CrossRef]
75. McKenna, M.; Brodovsky, S. School food and nutrition policies as tools for learning. In *Learning, Food, and Sustainability*; Sumner, J., Ed.; Palgrave Macmillan: New York, NY, USA, 2016; pp. 201–220.

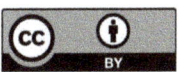

© 2019 by the authors. Licensee MDPI, Basel, Switzerland. This article is an open access article distributed under the terms and conditions of the Creative Commons Attribution (CC BY) license (http://creativecommons.org/licenses/by/4.0/).

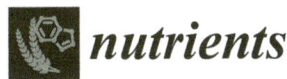

Article

Food Consumed by High School Students during the School Day

Almudena Garrido-Fernández [1], Francisca María García-Padilla [1,*,†], José Luis Sánchez-Ramos [1], Juan Gómez-Salgado [2,3,*,†], Gabriel H. Travé-González [4] and Elena Sosa-Cordobés [5]

1. Department of Nursing, University of Huelva, 21007 Huelva, Spain; almudena.garrido@denf.uhu.es (A.G.-F.); jsanchez@denf.uhu.es (J.L.S.-R.)
2. Department of Sociology, Social Work and Public Health, University of Huelva, 21007 Huelva, Spain
3. Safety and Health Postgraduate Programme, Universidad Espíritu Santo, 092301 Guayaquil, Ecuador
4. Department of Pedagogy, University of Huelva, 21007 Huelva, Spain; gabriel.trave@dedu.uhu.es
5. Doctoral Programme, University of Huelva, 21007 Huelva, Spain; elenasosacordobes@gmail.com
* Correspondence: fmgarcia@denf.uhu.es (F.M.G.-P.); salgado@uhu.es (J.G.-S.); Tel.: +34-9-5921-8321 (F.M.G.-P.); +34-6-9999-9568 (J.G.-S.)
† These authors are corresponding authors.

Received: 21 December 2019; Accepted: 10 February 2020; Published: 14 February 2020

Abstract: The development of healthy eating habits in adolescence is perceived as an effective strategy to avoid health problems in adulthood. The involvement of educational centres' governing boards, as well as the Educational State and Regional Administrations', may be necessary to create healthy food environments during the school day. The objective of this study is to identify the relationship between students' eating habits during the school day and sociodemographic, family and physical activity variables, as well as the existence of a school cafeteria. For this, a cross-sectional study in a stratified random sample of 8068 students of Public Secondary Education High Schools of Andalusia (Spain) has been carried out. The results show that students who are 14 years old or older are more likely to skip breakfast at home (odds ratio (OR): 1.81, 95% confidence interval (CI): 1.55–2.12) than those under this age. Students whose mothers do not have a university education are more likely to consume incomplete breakfasts (OR: 1.83, 95% CI: 1.26–2.65). Snacks with sweets (OR: 1.93, 95% CI: 1.67–2.23), candy in general (OR: 2.75, 95% CI: 2.38–3.19), and bagged crisps (OR: 3.06, 95% CI: 2.65–3.54) were more likely to be consumed in schools with a cafeteria. The factors that significantly influence the eating habits of secondary students in Andalusia include age, sex, parental level of education, physical activity and the existence of a cafeteria.

Keywords: nutrition; adolescent; breakfast; school

1. Introduction

The regular practice of physical activity and adequate nutrition are fundamental habits for improving quality of life [1] and reducing some public health problems that affect the population worldwide, such as being overweight and obesity; these problems are closely related to low-quality diets and sedentary lifestyles [2–6]. With regard to eating, diverse studies suggest that the progressive loss of a varied and balanced traditional diet can lead to an overweight condition and obesity. In the Spanish adolescent population, the consumed food deviates from the Mediterranean diet by exceeding the caloric intake because of an excessive consumption of meat, fat and sweets and a shortage of fruits, cereals, legumes, and fish [2–6].

Several studies have been performed in Spain that confirm the significant impact these unhealthy habits have on the population [2,7,8]. Currently, there is also significant awareness regarding healthy eating habits [9–12]. School age is an important time to develop healthy eating and physical activity habits, which improve the feeling of well-being by more successfully developing school activities and reducing the risk of chronic diseases in adulthood [13,14]. An increasing number of studies correlate poor physical and intellectual performance with inadequate caloric intake, low nutritional quality in their diet and the omission of breakfast [7,15]. Previous studies have shown that when young people eliminate breakfast or consume an incomplete breakfast, they may compensate by consuming unhealthy products, many of which are purchased in the school cafeteria itself [16].

These findings suggest that institutions must ensure an affordable food supply of acceptable nutritional quality in the educational environment and encourage educational interventions aimed at achieving this objective. The training and involvement of different educational and community agents in the promotion of a healthy diet in secondary education high schools (SEHS) is a high priority [17].

Healthy-eating education seems to occupy an insignificant place in the secondary school curriculum. In addition, fundamentally prescriptive approaches and ineffective recommendations are used with respect to substantial changes in student habits [18]. Finally, in a more recent study in which the role of the family was analysed, parents were reported to emphasize the importance of education in the acquisition of healthy habits and in the responsibility and control on the part of the family, although they identify certain difficulties such as lack of time, convenience and the negative influence of the market [19]. These results are relevant for the present study as they show family-related variables such as type of family, parents' level of education and employment situation, which have been used here as independent variables.

This study is integrated into the ANDALIES project and is dedicated to the promotion of healthy eating in the school environment. A summary of the research has been distributed in secondary education centres in Andalusia [20].

Objectives

In the context of the SEHS of Andalusia (Spain), the objective of this study was to explore the relationships between students' eating habits during the school day, sociodemographic and family characteristics, the existence of a cafeteria in the educational centre, and the practice of physical activity. The time frequency comprises the time lapse between 8 am and 3 pm.

2. Materials and Methods

2.1. Design and Sample

This was a cross-sectional exploratory study based on a multistage sample stratified by clusters. The study population was randomly selected and stratified by province and size of town of residence of the 95 SEHS. The students were chosen by the systematic sampling of classrooms. The sample comprised 8068 students, assuming a sampling error of ±2% for a confidence level of 95.5% in the estimate of the prevalence of dietary habits during the school day. After the data collection, an SEHS has been eliminated as the students' characteristics greatly differed from the rest of the sample. This is a centre which is located in the South of Andalusia, in the province of Cadiz, where a high proportion of immigrants from Northern Africa arrive. These have dietary habits and sociodemographic characteristics that greatly differ from the rest of the Andalusian population. Thus, of the 95 initially selected centres, only 94 remained under study.

Information on the sizes of each aggregate and stage was obtained from the database of the Council of Education of the Andalusia Council and the Confederation of Parent Associations for Public Education (*Confederación de Asociaciones de Padres y Madres por la Enseñanza Pública CODAPA*).

Reserve samples were selected to replace the secondary schools that refused to participate, by the same primary selection procedure. Only 6 centres have been replaced: 3 for refusing to participate in the study, 2 due to errors in the databases (non-existent centres), and 1 due to methodological criteria (the sampling was stratified by province and, in one of the provinces, many centres were found without a school cafeteria. The methodological criteria followed was to substitute one of these centres by one from our reserve sample that had a school cafeteria).

2.2. Variables and Data Collection

The following information on eating habits during the school day was collected: breakfast at home and type of breakfast; intake at school and characteristics of the school snack; and the consumption of candy, bagged crisps, and pastries (sugary products and products high in salt and saturated fats, which are not recommended for a healthy diet). In addition, information was obtained on sociodemographic and family characteristics (age, sex, province, parents educational level, type of family, parents' employment situation), the existence of a cafeteria in the school, physical activity performed, and self-assessment of the students' physical activity levels. In case there is no school cafeteria available in the centre, students bring their own snack or buy it in nearby shops.

The questionnaire was self-administered and was previously submitted for review by expert judges and applied to a sample of 30 students from different populations, sexes, ages and social statuses. The existence of a cafeteria in the SEHS was verified by observation. To inform and request access to the school, the Provincial Delegations of Education were contacted. Subsequently, visits to the SEHS were arranged with a school official from the centre's management team by telephone or email.

The questionnaire was composed of 13 questions, where three of them were open-ended and the remaining 10 were closed-ended, with several possible answers. These questions surveyed information on the students' sociodemographic and family characteristics (8 questions), and on their dietary habits for breakfast and during their school day (5 questions). The questions surveyed about "generally" or "typically" during the school day and asked for a typical meal (see Supplementary Files 3.1 and 3.2). Given the variability of the types of breakfast and afternoon snack, these data were assessed through direct responses to open questions. Three researchers categorised the types of breakfast and afternoon snack independently. As for breakfast, a consensus of 8 types of breakfast was reached by assessing the nutritional composition of the different foods declared (Table 1). In descriptive terms, these 8 types of breakfast were grouped into three categories (Table 1), and in analytical terms, they were classified as dichotomous. The dichotomisation was made by considering the variables "full breakfast" (types 1 and 2) and "incomplete breakfast" (types 3–8). The reference category was full breakfast.

Table 1. Type of breakfast.

Category	Type	Designation	Ingredients
Full breakfast (B1)	1	Full breakfast with bread or breakfast cereals	Milk drink, bread (toast or sandwich) and a piece of fruit or natural fruit juice
	2	Full breakfast with pastries	Milk drink, biscuits or breakfast cereals and a piece of fruit or natural fruit juice
Incomplete breakfast (B2)	3	Incomplete breakfast with bread and/or breakfast cereals	Drink (milk or juice …) and a toast or sandwich
	4	Incomplete breakfast with pastries	Drink and any pastry (muffins, sponge cake or biscuits)
	5	Incomplete breakfast with pastries or bread	Drink (milk or juice …), bread and/or breakfast cereals and pastries (including processed baked goods)
	6	Solid incomplete breakfast	Solid food, may include a toast, sandwich or piece of fruit
	7	Liquid incomplete breakfast	Liquid food, may be milk products like milk, milk with cocoa powder, liquid yogurt, or juice
Low nutritional quality breakfast (B3)	8	Low nutritional quality breakfast	Fizzy drink and/or crisps and/or processed baked goods, or any other product which is not recommended in a healthy diet

As for the type of afternoon snack, 8 typologies were identified according to their ingredients, grouping them into four categories (Table 2) regarding descriptive terms. In analytical terms, these were dichotomised in an afternoon snack without sweets (types 1–3), and an afternoon snack including sweets (types 4–8). The reference category was snack without sweets.

The variables sweets and processed baked goods consumption, bagged crisps consumption, and candy consumption were independently measured through a specific question in the questionnaire (question 11 on the attached questionnaire).

Table 2. Type of afternoon snack.

Category	Type	Designation	Ingredients
Afternoon snack without sweets (S1)	1	Solid and liquid food	A combination of high nutritional quality food and food which could be improved, plus a liquid product
	2	Solid and liquid food, plus fruit	A combination of the previous group, plus a piece of fruit
	3	Food from three groups	A combination of food from three groups: cereals + fruit + diary product
Afternoon snack including sweets (S2)	4	Solid food plus non-recommended products	A combination of solid food (sandwich) and processed baked goods, pastries, crisps and/or candy
	5	Solid and liquid food plus non-recommended products	A combination of the previous group plus a liquid product
	6	Liquid food plus non-recommended products	A combination of liquid food plus processed baked goods, pastries, crisps and/or candy
Liquid varied afternoon snack (S3)	7	Liquid food	Only liquid food: milk drink, juice …
Only sweets (S4)	8	Only non-healthy food	Only candy, crisps, both, or processed baked goods

2.3. Data Analysis

The data were analysed using the statistical package SPSS version 19. The percentages of each eating habit were obtained for the descriptive analysis. For the relationships between variables, through the descriptive data in Tables 3 and 4, a univariate logistic regression was used for each of the seven dietary habits previously dichotomised, assessing the predictive role of the sociodemographic variables, physical activity, existence of school cafeteria, and relatives.

To estimate the unbiased influence of each of the factors on eating habits, seven multiple logistic regression analysis were performed, using as predictive variables those which showed more relevance in the initial analysis and a significance level of relationship of $p < 0.1$. Odds ratio (OR) associated to each factor, with 95% confidence interval for each habit, were estimated.

2.4. Ethical Considerations

The approval of the Research Ethics Committee of the Public Health System of Andalusia in Huelva was obtained, as well as the approval of the Bioethics Committee of the University of Huelva. Participation in the study was voluntary and free. An informed consent form was delivered to the participants to be signed by their legal guardians, ensuring the confidentiality of the data and their exclusive use for this study. (See Supplementary Files 1.1, 1.2, 2.1 and 2.2)

3. Results

Of the total sample, 50.9% were boys and 49.1% were girls. The average age of the surveyed students was 15.71 years (standard deviation (SD) = 3.65). A total of 65.4% of the students attended compulsory secondary education, 20.9% were baccalaureate students, and 13.6% were in another type of educational programme. The most common type of family was a first-generation nuclear family (71.8%). In terms of physical activity, 5891 students (73%) reported to perform physical activity outside school.

The descriptive data related to the study variables can be seen in Tables 3 and 4. It is worth highlighting that a total of 78.2% of the students had breakfast at home, although it was incomplete for 74.1% due to low caloric intake. Recess school snacks included sandwiches (90.8%), packaged juices (63.3%) and a large variety of bagged crisps, industrial pastries and sweets (75%). Table 5 shows the results of the crude analysis of the different factors associated with dietary habits during the school day. From these results obtained from the tables, the predictive variables included in the multiple regression analysis in Table 6 are identified.

3.1. Skipping Breakfast at Home

In the multiple regression analysis (Table 6), students aged 14 years and older had a higher probability of not having breakfast before going to school than students aged 12 and 13 years old, with an OR of 1.81 (95% CI: 1.55–2.12). Moreover, girls (OR: 1.43, 95% CI: 1.25–1.62) and students who belonged to families other than those considered first-generation or extended (OR: 1.44, 95% CI: 1.23–1.69) had the highest probability of not having breakfast. The presence of a cafeteria, although to a lesser degree, increases the probability of not having breakfast at home before going to school (OR: 1.23, 95% CI: 1.03–1.46). Those who did not perform physical activity had a higher probability of not having breakfast (OR: 1.46, 95% CI: 1.27–1.68).

3.2. Incomplete Breakfast

The probability of consuming an incomplete breakfast was 41% lower in students aged 14 and older (OR: 0.59, 95% CI: 0.40–0.85). The students whose mothers did not have a university education had a higher probability of having an incomplete breakfast (OR: 1.83, 95% CI: 1.26–2.65), as did students whose both parents did not have a university education (OR: 1.48, 95% CI: 1.01–2.17). There was a greater probability of consuming an incomplete breakfast if the student did not perform physical activity (OR: 1.74, 95% CI: 1.09–2.76) (Table 6).

3.3. No Snacks at School

The probability of not having a snack in school was somewhat higher for students aged 14 or older (OR: 1.19, 95% CI: 1.05–1.36) and whose families were other than first-generation or extended (OR: 1. 32, 95% CI: 1.15–1.52). The presence of a cafeteria also increased this probability (OR: 1.28, 95% CI: 1.10–1.50). There was a weaker association with parents' employment situations. The students whose parents were unemployed had a higher probability of not snacking at school (OR: 1.16, 95% CI: 1.01–1.34) (Table 6).

3.4. Type of Snack

The existence of a cafeteria increased the probability of consumption of unhealthy school meals (OR: 1.93, 95% CI: 1.67–2.23). Students aged 14 and older had a somewhat higher probability of consuming this type of snack (OR: 1.16, 95% CI: 1.04–1.30), as did students who did not perform physical activity outside the school (OR: 1.14, 95% CI: 1.01–1.28). Belonging to the provinces of eastern Andalusia decreased this probability by 15% (OR: 0.85, 95% CI: 0.77–0.93) (Table 6).

3.5. Consumption of Bagged Crisps

The existence of a cafeteria in the school was strongly related to the consumption of bagged crisps, with an OR of 3.06 (95% CI: 2.65–3.54). Girls were more likely to consume bagged crisps during the school day (OR: 1.36, 95% CI: 1.23–1.50) (Table 6).

3.6. Consumption of Candy

The existence of a cafeteria was once again related to a greater likelihood of consuming candy at school (OR: 2.75, 95% CI: 2.38–3.19). Students aged 14 years and older had an 18% lower probability of consuming candy than those under 14 years of age (OR: 0.82, 95% CI: 0.73–0.93). This probability was also 35% lower in those who belonged to the provinces of eastern Andalusia (OR: 0.65, 95% CI: 0.58–0.71). Meanwhile, girls were more likely to consume candy than boys (OR: 1.48; 95% CI: 1.33–1.64), as were students whose mothers and fathers did not have a university education (OR: 1.25, 95% CI: 1.08–1.45 and OR: 1.20, 95% CI: 1.02–1.38, respectively) (Table 6).

Table 3. Eating habits according to sociodemographic characteristics, the existence of a cafeteria and physical activity.

		Breakfast at Home n %		Type of Breakfast (B1, B2, B3) n %				Snack in the SEHS n %		Type of Snack (S1, S2, S3, S4) n %						Candy Consumption n %		Bagged Crisps Consumption n %		Sweets and Pastries Consumption n %	
Age	12–13	1743	86.2	1654	97.1	42	2.5	1575	78.2	1198	64.6	559	30.1	77	4.2	21	1.1	1094	56.3	963	50.6	614	32.4
	14–16	2775	78	2583	96.4	88	3.3	2679	75.3	1943	60.9	1036	32.5	161	5	49	1.5	1912	56.2	1677	50.1	1223	36.2
	>16	1766	71.8	1604	94.9	80	4.7	1792	72.8	1294	59.6	662	30.5	184	8.5	30	1.4	1048	44.7	1117	47.7	902	38.3
Sex	Male	3340	82	3072	95.4	132	4.1	3094	76.1	2334	62.6	1146	30.7	202	5.4	48	1.3	1875	48.3	1775	45.9	1340	34.6
	Female	2915	74.2	2742	97	77	2.7	2920	74.3	2081	60.3	1099	31.8	219	6.3	52	1.5	2166	57.3	1971	53.3	1391	37.3
Province	Huelva	783	83.7	736	97.1	19	2.5	638	68.3	383	47.8	282	35.2	92	11.55	44	5.5	496	56.7	456	52.6	168	19.8
	Almería	700	79.9	624	95.4	30	4.6	632	72.4	444	58.6	213	28.1	90	11.9	11	1.5	232	27.9	251	30.8	239	28.3
	Cádiz	733	74.9	672	95.9	26	3.7	774	79	606	65.8	269	29.2	37	4	9	1	597	62.6	553	58.2	271	28.5
	Córdoba	569	78.1	546	97	17	3	568	78.1	434	62.3	235	33.7	21	3	7	1	376	53.2	361	52	199	28.5
	Sevilla	1373	77.2	1284	96.3	39	2.9	1353	76.2	996	62.6	520	32.7	59	3.7	15	0.9	917	54.9	974	58.6	652	39.5
	Málaga	970	75.1	906	96	35	3.7	1012	78.1	904	73.3	291	23.6	37	3	2	0.2	649	52.2	589	47.8	538	43.2
	Granada	659	79.7	607	95.6	26	4.1	615	74.3	414	59.7	233	33.6	43	6.2	4	0.6	408	51.2	344	44.3	385	48.7
	Jaén	497	79.9	466	96.3	18	3.7	454	72.8	254	48.9	214	41.2	43	8.3	8	1.5	379	62.2	229	38.4	287	47.6

Table 3. Cont.

		Breakfast at Home n %		Type of Breakfast (B1, B2, B3) n %				Snack in the SEHS n %		Type of Snack (S1, S2, S3, S4) n %					Candy Consumption n %		Bagged Crisps Consumption n %		Sweets and Pastries Consumption n %	
Cafeteria	Yes	5254	77.6	169	3.3	4887	96.3	18	0.4	5039	74.5	3604	59.3	2007	33	374	6.1	97	1.6	3647	56	3437	53.4	2279	35.3
	No	1030	81	41	4.1	654	95.5	4	0.4	1007	79.3	831	73.4	250	22.1	48	4.2	3	0.3	407	34.7	320	27.7	460	39.1
Outside physical activity	Yes	4765	80.8	180	3.9	4401	95.7	19	0.45	4462	75.7	3328	62.5	1634	30.7	290	5.5	69	1.3	2943	51.9	2735	48.8	1974	35.1
	No	1418	70.3	28	3.9	1347	95.7	3	0.2	1495	74	1047	58.6	587	32.8	124	6.9	29	1.6	1061	55	973	51.4	724	37.7
Physical activity self-evaluation	Sedentary	713	72.5	16	2.3	670	97.5	1	0.1	743	75.8	519	60.1	269	31.2	63	7.3	12	1.4	464	49.6	471	50.6	348	36.9
	Moderate	1681	78.6	74	4.5	1547	95.1	6	0.4	1614	75.4	1178	61.5	587	30.7	123	6.4	26	1.4	1068	52	1015	49.7	733	35.7
	Active	1771	79.6	54	3.1	1661	96.6	4	0.2	1681	75.6	1248	62.2	641	32	94	4.7	22	1.1	1108	51.8	1010	48.2	739	35
	Very active	1109	81.2	51	4.8	1013	94.5	8	0.7	1048	76.8	799	63.6	371	29.5	64	5.1	22	1.8	697	53.6	643	50.3	471	36.7
	Don't know	837	75.9	11	1.4	787	96.3	3	0.4	797	72	572	58.2	329	33.5	64	6.5	17	1.7	619	58.5	530	50.6	374	35.9

B1: Complete breakfast; B2: Incomplete breakfast; B3: Breakfast of low nutritional quality. S1: Combined snack without sweets (healthy snack); S2: Combined snack with sweets; S3: Varied liquid snack; S4: Exclusive ingestion of sweets. SEHS: Secondary Education High Schools. Missing values: Breakfast at home (31) Type of breakfast (1810) Snack in the SEHS (31) Type of snack (854) Candy consumption (378) Bagged crisps consumption (471) Sweets and pastries consumption (437).

Table 4. Eating habits according to family characteristics.

		Breakfast at Home n %		Type of Breakfast (B1, B2, B3) n %		Snack in the SEHS n %		Type of Snack (S1, S2, S3, S4) n %								Candy Consumption n %		Bagged Crisps Consumption n %		Sweets and Pastries Consumption n %	
Mother's education	Does not know how to read/write	39	72.2	35	96.4	34	63	18	50	16	44.4	1	2.8	1	2.8	33	62.3	33	63.5	27	51.9
	No education	259	73.8	247	97.6	257	72	198	60.6	104	31.8	19	5.8	6	1.8	199	59.2	172	52.1	134	40.6
	Incomplete primary education	547	74.4	515	97.5	534	72.8	412	62.2	199	30.1	39	5.9	12	1.8	397	56.5	342	49.1	248	35.4
	Primary education	1568	77.3	1482	97.4	1530	75.5	1140	62.8	544	30	10.	5.6	31	1.7	1094	56.2	973	50.5	672	34.9
	Secondary education	2429	78.6	2259	96	2365	76.8	1704	61.2	879	31.6	168	6	34	1.2	1556	52.7	1465	50.4	1071	36.6
	University education	1106	82.5	994	93.5	1010	75.4	713	59.9	409	34.4	56	4.7	12	1	590	45.9	597	46.7	437	34.1
Father's education	Does not know how to read/write	22	61.1	20	100	25	69.4	16	53.3	12	40	2	6.7	0	0	24	64.9	18	52.9	16	44.4
	No education	268	73.2	253	96.9	268	72.2	198	59.1	111	33.1	20	6	6	1.8	206	59.2	172	49.6	144	42
	Incomplete primary education	640	76.4	601	97.1	635	75.7	463	61.6	227	30.2	46	6.1	16	2.1	463	57.7	399	50	291	36.2
	Primary education	1483	76.7	1398	97.2	1474	76.2	1061	61.3	533	30.8	102	5.9	34	2	1066	57.2	943	51.3	672	36.4
	Secondary education	2284	79.4	2138	96.3	2181	75.9	1622	62.2	811	31.1	144	5.5	29	1.1	1416	51.7	1355	50.2	961	35.3
	University education	1043	83	934	93.7	960	76.6	674	61.5	372	33.5	56	5	8	0.7	564	46.6	579	48.2	391	32.8

Table 4. Cont.

		Breakfast at Home n %		Type of Breakfast (B1, B2, B3) n %			Snack in the SEHS n %		Type of Snack (S1, S2, S3, S4) n %						Candy Consumption n %		Bagged Crisps Consumption n %		Sweets and Pastries Consumption n %	
Family type	1st gen. nuclear fam	4602	78.3	4315	96.4	148 3.3	14 0.3	4403	76.6	3213	61.7	1645	31.6	280	5.4	73	1.4	2952	53.4	2691	49.4	1846	33.8
	Extended family	397	78.3	369	96.6	12 3.1	1 0.3	386	76.1	269	61.7	137	31.4	26	6	4	0.9	249	53	226	47.9	193	40.3
	Single parent	532	72.5	479	94.9	21 4.2	5 1	506	68.9	384	60.5	204	32.1	40	6.3	7	1.1	355	50.4	351	50.75	310	44.9
	2nd gen. nuclear family	211	72.8	196	98	3 1.5	1 0.5	187	64.7	148	58.7	85	33.7	15	6	4	1.6	142	51.8	142	53	117	43
	Only grandparents	151	75.5	140	97.2	4 2.8	0 0	161	80.5	116	61.7	61	32.4	5	2.7	6	3.2	120	62.5	108	56.2	61	32.3
	Other	375	70.4	327	93.7	21 6	1 0.3	382	71.8	296	63.1	115	24.5	53	11.3	5	1.1	226	44.8	232	46.2	211	41.3
Mother's employment	Working	3336	79.2	3110	96.1	113 3.5	12 0.4	3187	75.8	2301	61	1203	31.9	211	5.6	55	1.5	2109	52.5	1986	50	1448	36.3
	Unemployed	630	74.9	583	95.3	25 4.1	4 0.7	601	71.5	469	62.4	234	31.1	43	5.7	6	0.8	446	55.4	383	48.3	310	38.7
	Domestic chores	2114	78.6	1973	96.7	62 3	6 0.3	2047	76.1	1503	61.9	752	30.9	137	5.6	38	1.6	1390	53.6	1260	49.4	862	33.7
	Retired	24	72.7	22	95.7	1 4.3	0 0	24	72.7	21	67.7	7	22.6	3	9.7	0	0	12	36.4	14	42.4	12	36.4
	Student	4	80	3	75	1 25	0 0	5	100	3	75	1	25	0	0	0	0	4	80	2	40	2	40

Table 4. Cont.

		Breakfast at Home n %		Type of Breakfast (B1, B2, B3) n %				Snack in the SEHS n %		Type of Snack (S1, S2, S3, S4) n %								Candy Consumption n %		Bagged Crisps Consumption n %		Sweets and Pastries Consumption n %	
Father's employment	Working	4760	79.5	153	3.3	4461	96.3	16	0.3	4572	76.3	3303	61.1	1717	31.8	300	5.6	85	1.6	3032	52.8	2843	50	1974	34.7
	Unemployed	898	75.3	31	3.6	826	96.2	2	0.2	868	73	669	63.4	316	30	63	6	7	0.7	643	56.9	562	50.6	440	39
	Domestic chores	79	76.7	2	2.8	70	97.2	0	0	77	74	48	53.3	34	37.8	6	6.7	2	2.2	54	55.1	47	49.5	37	38.1
	Retired	119	77.3	5	4.3	110	95.7	0	0	122	79.7	92	67.6	37	27.2	7	5.1	0	0	72	48.3	63	43.8	55	37.2
	Student	2	100	0	0	2	100	0	0	2	100	0	0	2	100	0	0	0	0	1	50	1	50	1	50

B1: Complete breakfast; B2: Incomplete breakfast; B3: Breakfast of low nutritional quality. S1: Combined snack without sweets (healthy snack); SEHS: Secondary Education High Schools; S2: Combined snack with sweets; S3: Varied liquid snack; S4: Exclusive ingestion of sweets. Missing values: Breakfast at home (31) Type of breakfast (1810) Snack in the SEHS (31) Type of snack (854) Candy consumption (378) Bagged crisps consumption (471) Sweets and pastries consumption (437).

Table 5. Factors associated with eating habits during the school day (crude).

	No Breakfast at Home OR 95% CI (OR)	Incomplete Breakfast OR 95% CI (OR)	No Snack at SEHS OR 95% CI (OR)	Unhealthy Snack OR 95% CI (OR)	Candy Consumption OR 95% CI (OR)	Bagged Crisps Consumption OR 95% CI (OR)	Sweets and Pastries Consumption OR 95% CI (OR)
Age (>14 y)	**2.031** **1.76–2.33**	0.633 0.44–0.89	1.170 1.05–1.29	**1.150** **1.04–1.26**	0.823 0.74–0.91	0.942 0.85–1.04	**1.228** **1.10–1.37**
Sex (Girl)	**1.585** **1.42–1.76**	**1.530** **1.15–2.03**	1.102 0.96–1.22	1.10 1.00–1.21	**1.435** **1.31–1.57**	**1.342** **1.22–1.46**	1.123 1.02–1.23
Province (Eastern)	1.004 0.90–1.11	0.745 0.56–0.98	1.028 0.92–1.13	0.897 0.81–0.98	0.702 0.64–0.76	0.549 0.50–0.60	**1.580** **1.43–1.73**
Father no university degree	**1.411** **1.20–1.65**	**2.182** **1.59–2.98**	1.052 0.91–1.21	0.963 0.84–1.09	**1.391** **1.22–1.57**	1.095 0.96–1.24	**1.166** **1.02–1.33**
Mother no university degree	**1.381** **1.18–1.61**	**2.334** **1.72–3.15**	0.994 0.86–1.14	0.927 0.81–1.05	**1.425** **1.26–1.60**	**1.165** **1.03–1.31**	1.097 0.96–1.24
Other than 1st gen and extended family	**1.527** **1.35–1.72**	0.796 0.57–1.10	**1.370** **1.21–1.54**	1.022 0.91–1.14	**1.131** **1.01–1.26**	1.045 0.93–1.16	**1.392** **1.24–1.55**
Mother unemployed	1.095 0.98–1.22	1.054 0.79–1.39	1.040 0.93–1.15	0.958 0.87–1.05	0.962 0.87–1.05	1.057 0.96–1.15	0.203 0.85–1.03
Father unemployed	**1.273** **1.01–1.47**	0.914 0.61–1.35	**1.192** **1.03–1.37**	0.907 0.79–1.03	**1.179** **1.03–1.34**	1.025 0.90–1.16	**1.207** **1.05–1.37**
SEHS cafeteria existence	**1.232** **1.05–1.43**	1.243 0.87–1.76	**1.313** **1.13–1.52**	**1.898** **1.64–2.18**	**2.396** **2.10–2.72**	**2.982** **2.59–3.42**	0.848 0.74–0.96
No physical activity outside SEHS	**1.772** **1.57–1.98**	**1.968** **1.31–2.94**	1.097 0.97–1.23	**1.180** **1.05–1.31**	1.134 1.02–1.25	**1.113** **1.00–1.23**	1.115 1.00–1.24
Sedentary	**1.431** **1.23–1.66**	1.589 0.94–2.66	0.968 0.82–1.13	1.066 0.92–1.23	0.862 0.75–0.98	1.047 0.91–1.20	1.054 0.91–1.21

SEHS: Secondary Education High Schools; CI = Confidence Interval; OR = Odds ratio. Bolden values = significance $p < 0.005$.

Table 6. Multivariate regression analysis. Factors associated with unhealthy eating habits during the school day.

	B	P	OR	Lower limit CI (OR)	Upper limit CI (OR)
NO BREAKFAST AT HOME					
14 and over	0.596	<0.001	1.816	1.552	2.124
Girl	0.358	<0.001	1.43	1.259	1.625
Mother no university degree	0.17	0.078	1.185	0.981	1.431
Father no university degree	0.126	0.194	1.134	0.938	1.371
Family other than 1st gen. or extended	0.369	<0.001	1.446	1.236	1.691
Unemployed father	0.131	0.105	1.14	0.973	1.335
Cafeteria existence	0.207	0.02	1.23	1.033	1.466
No physical activity	0.384	<0.001	1.468	1.276	1.688
Sedentary	0.139	0.121	1.149	0.964	1.369
INCOMPLETE BREAKFAST					
14 and over	−0.53	0.005	0.589	0.407	0.851
Girl	0.225	0.165	1.252	0.912	1.72
Western Andalusia	−0.187	0.219	0.83	0.616	1.117
Mother no university studies	0.604	<0.001	1.83	1.263	2.651
Father no university studies	0.396	0.042	1.485	1.015	2.174
No physical activity	0.555	0.018	1.741	1.098	2.761
Sedentary	0.574	0.061	1.775	0.974	3.233
NO SNACK IN SEHS					
14 and over	0.181	0.005	1.198	1.056	1.36
Girl	0.057	0.304	1.059	0.95	1.18
Family other than 1st gen. or extended	0.283	<0.001	1.327	1.153	1.528
Father unemployed	0.156	0.032	1.169	1.014	1.347
Cafeteria existence	0.25	0.002	1.284	1.099	1.499
SNACK WITH SWEETS					
14 and over	0.152	0.009	1.165	1.04	1.304
Girl	0.06	0.247	1.062	0.959	1.176
Eastern Andalusia	−0.164	<0.001	0.849	0.77	0.937
Cafeteria existence	0.659	<0.001	1.934	1.674	2.234
No physical activity	0.136	0.022	1.146	1.019	1.288
CANDY CONSUMPTION					
14 and over	−0.189	0.002	0.828	0.737	0.931
Girl	0.395	<0.001	1.485	1.338	1.648
Eastern Andalusia	−0.432	<0.001	0.649	0.587	0.719
Mother no university degree	0.228	0.002	1.256	1.084	1.456
Father no university degree	0.177	0.019	1.194	1.029	1.384
Family other than 1st gen. or extended	0.05	0.465	1.051	0.92	1.201
Cafeteria existence	1.015	<0.001	2.759	2.386	3.19
No physical activity	0.041	0.509	1.042	0.922	1.179
Sedentary	−0.128	0.104	0.88	0.755	1.027
BAGGED CRISPS CONSUMPTION					
Girl	0.311	<0.001	1.365	1.235	1.508
Eastern Andalusia	−0.009	0.417	0.991	0.969	1.013
Mother no university degree	0.069	0.282	1.071	0.945	1.214
Cafeteria existence	1.12	<0.001	3.065	2.653	3.54
No physical activity	0.022	0.706	1.023	0.911	1.148

Table 6. Cont.

	B	p	OR	Lower limit CI (OR)	Upper limit CI (OR)
CONSUMPTION OF SWEETS AND PASTRIES					
14 and over	0.115	0.062	1.122	0.994	1.267
Girl	0.081	0.144	1.084	0.973	1.209
Eastern Andalusia	0.448	<0.001	1.565	**1.41**	**1.738**
Father no university degree	0.152	**0.035**	1.164	**1.011**	**1.339**
Family other than 1st gen. or extended	0.324	**<0.001**	**1.383**	**1.206**	**1.585**
Unemployed father	0.14	**0.046**	**1.151**	**1.003**	**1.321**
Cafeteria existence	−0.243	**<0.001**	**0.784**	**0.68**	**0.903**
No physical activity	0.076	0.238	1.079	0.951	1.223

Family other than 1st gen. or extended: Family other than first-generation or extended; SEHS: Secondary Education High Schools. The coefficients and OR of each factor are adjusted by the covariables present in each model. CI = Confidence Interval; OR = Odds ratio; p = significance level; B = regression coefficient. Bolden values = significance $p < 0.005$.

3.7. Consumption of Sweets and Pastries

Students belonging to the provinces of eastern Andalusia had a higher probability of consuming sweets and pastries (OR: 1.56, 95% CI: 1.41–1.73), as did students belonging to families other than first-generation or extended (OR: 1.38, 95% CI: 1.20–1.58). In schools with a cafeteria, there was a 20% lower probability of consuming sweets and pastries than in schools that lacked a cafeteria (OR: 0.80; 95% CI: 0.68–0.90). There was a weaker relationship between the level of education and the employment situation of the parents. Students whose parents did not have a university education (OR: 1.16, 95% CI: 1.01–1.33) and students whose parents were unemployed (OR: 1.15, 95% CI: 1.00–1.32) were more likely to consume sweets and pastries (Table 6).

4. Discussion

The data in this study show that age influenced the different studied eating habits, particularly regarding eating breakfast at home and consuming candy. This factor was also associated with the type of breakfast the students consumed. Students over 14 years were more likely to skip breakfast and not snack in the SEHS, although students younger than 14 consumed incomplete breakfasts and candy the most. Performing regular physical activity outside the school resulted in the acquisition of other healthy habits, such as healthy eating habits. Thus, students who performed physical activity ate breakfast at home more frequently than those who did not and were more likely to consume a complete breakfast.

The existence of a cafeteria in the school had a strong association with the type of snack that students consumed, particularly regarding the intake of candy and bagged crisps. Likewise, there was an inverse association between the existence of a cafeteria and the consumption of sweets and pastries, with schools having a cafeteria seeing a lower consumption of sweets and pastries. This observation can be attributed to greater sensitivity to recommendations by public administrations, media and/or schools to reduce the consumption of industrial baked goods. These entities have decreased the supply of such products in school cafeterias to lower consumption [21] but have not been as sensitive regarding other non-recommended products (candy or bagged crisps). Therefore, we urge that the recommendations be followed and that the provisions of the Spanish Food Safety and Nutrition Act be met to reduce consumption of the remaining non-recommended products. In one of the reviewed articles, where selling healthy products at school is proposed, we find satisfaction among the students, creating a positive effect on healthy food accessibility [22].

Finally, we emphasise that the educational level of the mother and father is closely related to the type of breakfast consumed before going to school, as well as the consumption of candy. Students whose mothers and fathers did not have a university education were more likely to have incomplete breakfasts at home and to consume sweets at school.

The data obtained in this study are self-declared, so they share the usual limitation of data quality regarding self-declared food intake, in this case. A possible weakness of this study is the lack of questionnaire responses regarding the parents' professions due to ignorance or confusion about their real professions. Additionally, the participants reported the contents of a "typical" breakfast, and so within-person variability in food consumption was not examined. Certain discrepancies between the answers to "Snack in SEHS" and "Type of snack" are possible, as they were obtained from two different questions of the questionnaire. Because this is a cross-sectional study, the relationships found cannot be considered causal. Among the strengths of the study we can highlight the sample size, as well as its representative capacity for the whole Andalusian region. As far as we are concerned, this is the first study specifically aimed at knowing the dietary habits of secondary education students during the school day.

Most of the studies reviewed were based on the evaluation of breakfast [13,23–30], on the analysis of adolescents' daily consumption or on overall eating habits [31–38] and on the relationship of diet with physical activity [39–42] or with school performance [15,43–45]. We also found some educational interventions [42,46–52] and studies that focused on adherence to the Mediterranean diet [53,54]. Of special interest are those relating emotional state [55] or social support [56,57] with breakfast among adolescents. The scarcity of research on adolescent eating habits during the school day [16–20,56] justifies the relevance of this line of research and supports the need for policies that favour the creation of healthy environments.

As mentioned above, we have not identified previous studies that focus on the eating habits of young people during the school day. Therefore, we consider this study to provide novel data that can be a reference for promoting healthy eating habits in the school environment.

Our results agree with those of other studies that high school students eat some breakfast at home [27,29,39,40] and that a large portion of them eat a poor breakfast [15,30,33,39]. Moreover, as in our study, age and sex are predictive factors of omitting breakfast or having breakfast at home before going to the SEHS. Several studies show that girls tend to skip breakfast more frequently than boys, as well as older students as compared to younger ones [15,23,29]. This last fact is also widespread among those students whose parents have a higher educational level [55] and among those who do not perform physical activity [55].

Most reviewed studies conclude that having a full and healthy breakfast is vital for the mental and physical health status of secondary education students. Also, performing interventions aimed at these practices are both necessary and effective, although there is little research on the importance of school snacks, the consumption of non-recommended products during the school day, or the real need for school cafeterias, thus stating breakfast as the key and only responsible element composing dietary health regarding the school day.

Knowing about dietary habits during adolescence, related social determinants, regulations and resources of the school will be very useful in the design of plans and strategies towards health promotion. Performing interventions that consolidate good lifestyle habits, that create health-promoting environments and decrease the risks associated with unhealthy eating in adulthood is a commitment for the future in the context of community health. Moreover, the creation and continuity of future research must continue to focus on adolescent eating habits during the school day and take into account the other agents involved, including family, teachers, administration, parents' associations and community health teams.

5. Conclusions

The factors that significantly influence the eating habits of secondary students in Andalusia include age, sex, parental level of education, physical activity and the existence of a cafeteria.

More concretely, among the dietary habits of students during the school day, the following associations can be highlighted:

Skips breakfast at home: students over 14 years old, girls, students who do not perform physical activity outside the school and those who belong to a family other than first-generation or extended tend to more frequently skip breakfast at home before going to school. In schools with a cafeteria, students eat less at home.

Consumes incomplete breakfast: students under 14 years of age who do not perform physical activity or whose parents do not have a university education consume an incomplete breakfast more frequently.

Does not snack at the SEHS: there is a greater probability of not snacking at school for students aged 14 or older, those with an unemployed father and those who belong to families other than the extended or first-generation families. Curiously, there is less snacking in schools with a cafeteria than in schools without a cafeteria.

Type of snack: unhealthy snacks are consumed more frequently among students whose schools have a cafeteria and among those in western Andalusia. Students who are 14 years or older and those who do not perform physical activity have the highest probability of consuming unhealthy snacks.

Consumption of bagged crisps: the consumption of bagged crisps is higher in schools with a school cafeteria and in girls.

Consumption of candy: having a cafeteria in the SEHS also increases the consumption of candy. The study sample presents a greater consumption of candy in girls, students under 14 years of age, those whose parents do not have a university education and those from western Andalusia.

Consumption of sweets and pastries: the probability of consuming sweets and pastries during the school day is greater in the provinces of eastern Andalusia, in students belonging to families other than first-generation or extended families and in students whose fathers do not have a university education or are unemployed. Consumption is lower in schools with a cafeteria.

Supplementary Materials: The following are available online at http://www.mdpi.com/2072-6643/12/2/485/s1: Supplementary File 1.1. Ethics Committee Report Spanish; Supplementary File 1.2. Ethics Committee Report English; Supplementary File 2.1 University Ethics Committee Report Spanish; Supplementary File 2.2. University Ethics Committee Report English; Supplementary File 3.1. Data collection questionnaire in Spanish; Supplementary File 3.2. Data collection questionnaire in English.

Author Contributions: Conceptualization, A.G.-F. and F.M.G.-P.; Data curation, A.G.-F., F.M.G.-P. and G.H.T.-G.; Formal analysis, A.G.-F., F.M.G.-P., J.L.S.-R., E.S.-C. and G.H.T.-G.; Funding acquisition, F.M.G.-P. and G.H.T.-G.; Investigation, A.G.-F.; Methodology, A.G.-F., F.M.G.-P., J.L.S.-R., J.G.-S. and G.H.T.-G.; Project administration, A.G.-F.; Resources, J.L.S.-R., E.S.-C. and J.G.-S.; Software, E.S.-C.; Supervision, F.M.G.-P. and J.G.-S.; Validation, J.L.S.-R., E.S.-C. and G.H.T.-G.; Visualization, A.G.-F., F.M.G.-P., J.L.S.-R., J.G.-S. and G.H.T.-G.; Writing—original draft, A.G.-F., F.M.G.-P. and J.L.S.-R.; Writing—review and editing, E.S.-C., J.G.-S. and G.H.T.-G. All authors have read and agreed to the published version of the manuscript.

Funding: This research received no external funding.

Acknowledgments: We thank all students who completed the questionnaires. Special thanks to the School Head teachers and teachers who actively participated in the implementation of the initiative. We are grateful to the Andalusian Community Nursing Association, the Confederation of Associations of Fathers and Mothers for Public Education in Andalusia and the Nursing Department of the University of Huelva.

Conflicts of Interest: The authors declare no conflict of interest.

References

1. Pérez López, I.; Tercedor Sánchez, P.; Delgado Fernández, M. Effects of school programmes on the promotion of physical activity and nutrition in Spanish adolescents: Systematic review. *Nutr. Hosp.* **2015**, *32*, 534–544.
2. Study ALADINO. Monitoring study of growth, nutrition, physical activity, child development and obesity in Spain 2015. In *Spanish Agency of Consumer Affairs, Food Safety and Nutrition*; Ministry of Health, Social Services and Equality: Madrid, Spain, 2016.
3. Ayechu, A.; Durá, T. Quality of eating habits (adherence to the Mediterranean diet) in students of compulsory secondary education. *Sist. Sanit. Navar.* **2010**, *33*, 35–42.

4. Palenzuela Paniagua, S.M.; Pérez Milena, A.; Pérula de Torres, L.A.; Fernández García, J.A.; Maldonado Alconada, J. Food consumption patterns among adolescents. *Sist. Sanit. Navar.* **2014**, *37*, 47–58. [CrossRef]
5. Gómez Candela, C.; Lourenzo Nogueira, Y.; Loria Kohen, V.; Marín Caro, M.; Martínez Álvarez, J.R.; Pérez Rodrigo, C.; Polanco, I. Analysis of eating habits surveys carried out in the student population during the 4th National Nutrition Day (NND) 2005. *Nutr. Clín. Diet Hosp.* **2007**, *27*, 32–40.
6. Moreno, C.; Ramos, P.; Rivera, F.; Sánchez Queija, I.; Jiménez Iglesias, A.; García Moya, I.; Moreno Maldonado, C.; Paniagua, C.; Villafuente Díaz, A.M.; Morgan, A. Behaviours Related to the Health and Development of Andalusian Adolescents. Summary of the Health Behaviour in School-Aged Children study in Andalusia (HBSC-2011). University of Seville. Available online: http://www.juntadeandalucia.es/salud/export/sites/csalud/galerias/documentos/c_3_c_1_vida_sana/adolescencia/hbsc_estudio_andalucia_def.pdf (accessed on 5 October 2019).
7. Serra Majem, L.; Ribas Barba, L.; Aranceta Bartrina, J.; Pérez Rodrigo, C.; Saavedra Santana, P.; Peña Quintana, L. Childhood and adolescent obesity in Spain. Results of the Kid Study (1998–2000). *Med. Clin. (Barc.)* **2003**, *121*, 725–732. [CrossRef]
8. White Paper on Nutrition in Spain. Spanish Nutrition Foundation. Ministry of Health, Social Services and Equality. Available online: http://www.seedo.es/images/site/documentacionConsenso/Libro_Blanco_Nutricion_Esp-2013.pdf (accessed on 5 October 2019).
9. World Health Organization. *European Food and Nutrition Action Plan 2015–2020*; World Health Organization: Copenhagen, Denmark, 2014.
10. Naos Strategy. Strategy for Nutrition, Physical Activity and Prevention of Obesity. Spanish Food Safety Agency. Ministry of Health and Consumer Affairs, 2005. Available online: http://www.aesan.msssi.gob.es/AESAN/docs/docs/publicaciones_estudios/nutricion/maqueta_NAOS1.pdf (accessed on 5 October 2019).
11. White Paper. *European Strategy on Health Problems Related to Food, Overweight and Obesity*; European Commission: Brussels, Belgium, 2007.
12. Guideline. *Sugars Intake for Adults and Children*; World Health Organization: Geneva, Switzerland, 2015.
13. Galiano Segovia, M.; Moreno Villares, J. Breakfast in childhood: More than a good habit. *Madr. Acta Pediatr. Esp.* **2010**, *68*, 403–408.
14. Aguilar Jurado, M.A.; Gil Madrona, P.; Ortega Dato, J.F.; Rodríguez Blanco, O.F. Mejora de la condición física y la salud en estudiantes tras un programa de descansos activos. *Rev. Esp. Salud. Pública* **2018**, *92*, e201809068.
15. Fernández Morales, I.; Aguilar Vilas, M.V.; Mateos Vega, C.J.; Martínez Para, M.C. Relationship between the quality of breakfast and academic performance in adolescents in Guadalajara (Castilla-La Mancha). *Nutr. Hosp.* **2008**, *23*, 383–387.
16. García Padilla, F.M.; González Rodríguez, A.; Martos Cerezuela, I.; González Delgado, A. Food profile of secondary school students in Andalusia during the school day. *Nutr. Clín. Diet Hosp.* **2013**, *33*, 129.
17. García Padilla, F.M.; González Rodríguez, A.; González de Haro, M.D.; Frigolet Maceras, J. Encouraging healthy eating in secondary education: Consensus on assessment indicators. *Rev. Esp. Nutr. Comunitaria* **2012**, *18*, 143–148.
18. González Rodríguez, A.; García Padilla, F.M.; Silvano Arranz, A.; Fernández Lao, I. Do Andalusian secondary schools promote the Mediterranean diet? *Ann. Nutr. Metab.* **2013**, *62*, 55.
19. González Rodríguez, A.; García Padilla, F.M.; Garrido Fernández, A. The role of the family in feeding secondary education students during the school day. II Ibero-American Congress on Epidemiology and Public Health: Santiago de Compostela, Spain. *Gac. Sanit.* **2015**, *29*, 246.
20. González Rodríguez, A.; García Padilla, F.M.; Martos Cerezuela, I.; Silvano Arranz, A.; Fernández Lao, I. Project ANDALIES: Consumption, supply and promotion of healthy eating in the secondary education centres of Andalusia. *Nutr. Hosp.* **2015**, *31*, 1853–1862. [PubMed]
21. García Padilla, F.M.; González Rodríguez, A. Cafeteria services and promoting health in the school environment. *Aten Primaria.* **2017**, *49*, 271–277.
22. Kim, K.; Hong, S.A.; Yun, S.H.; Ryou, H.J.; Lee, S.S.; Kim, M.K. The effect of a healthy school tuck shop program on the access of students to healthy foods. *Nutr. Res. Pract.* **2012**, *6*, 138–145. [CrossRef]
23. Díez-Navarro, A.; Martín-Camargo, A.; Solé-Llussà, A.; González Montero de Espinosa, M.; Marrodán Serrano, M.D. Influence of breakfast on excess weight in the population of children and adolescents in Madrid. *Nutr. Clin. Diet Hosp.* **2014**, *34*, 9–17.

24. Quintero Gutiérrez, A.G.; González Rosendo, G.; Rodríguez Murguía, N.A.; Reyes Navarrete, G.E.; Puga Díaz, R.; Villanueva Sánchez, J. Skipping breakfast, nutritional status and eating habits of children and adolescents of public schools in Morelos, Mexico. *CyTA J. Food.* **2014**, *12*, 256–262.
25. Herrero Lozano, R.; Fillat Ballesteros, J.C. Breakfast in a group of adolescents. *Nutr. Clin. Diet Hosp.* **2010**, *30*, 26–32.
26. Díaz, T.; Ficapal-Cusí, P.; Aguilar Martínez, A. Breakfast habits in primary and secondary students: Possibilities for school-based nutritional education. *Nutr. Hosp.* **2016**, *33*, 909–914.
27. Infantozzi, F.G.; Giordano, C. Characteristics associated with skipping breakfast in Montevidean adolescents attending private schools. *Enfermería Cuid. Humaniz.* **2017**, *6*, 4–19.
28. Nanney, M.S.; Shanafelt, A.; Wang, Q.; Leduc, R.; Dodds, E.; Hearst, M.; Kubik, M.Y.; Grannon, K.; Harnack, L. Project BreakFAST: Rationale, design, and recruitment and enrollment methods of a randomized controlled trial to evaluate an intervention to improve school breakfast program participation in rural high Schools. *Contemp. Clin. Trials Commun.* **2016**, *3*, 12–22. [CrossRef] [PubMed]
29. Ukegbu, P.; Okoli, C.; Uwaegbute, A. Nutrition knowledge and breakfast habits of a group of adolescents in public secondary schools in anambra state, nigeria. *Ann. Nutr. Metab.* **2017**, *71*, 647.
30. Sygit, K.M.; Sygit, M.; Wojtyła-Buciora, P.; Lyubinets, O.; Stelmach, W.; Krakowiak, J. Environmental variations of nutritional mistakes among Polish school-age adolescents from urban and rural áreas. *Ann. Agric. Environ. Med.* **2019**, *26*, 483–488. [CrossRef] [PubMed]
31. Martí, A.; Martínez, J.A. Adolescent nutrition: The need to act now. *Sist. Sanit. Navar.* **2014**, *37*, 1–8.
32. Campos, K.B.A.C.; Silva, A.R.V.; Nadabe e Silva, A.; Da Silva, G.R.F.; De Freitas, R.W.J.; De Almeida, P.C. Food habits of school teens. *J. Nurs. UFPE* **2012**, *6*, 2161–2166.
33. González Jiménez, E.; Río Valle, J.S.; García López, P.A.; García García, C.J. Analysis of food intake and nutritional habits in a population of adolescents in the city of Granada. *Nutr. Hosp.* **2013**, *28*, 779–786.
34. Espejo Almazán, T.; Cros Otero, S.J.; Torti Calvo, J.; Bolivar Ruano, M.; Moreno García, M.M. Eating habits in compulsory secondary school students of Villa de Puerto Real (Cadiz). *Rev. Paraninfo Digit.* **2013**, *18*. Available online: http://www.index-f.com/para/n18/022d.php (accessed on 20 December 2019). (In Spanish).
35. Kolahdooz, F.; Nader, F.; Daemi, M.; Jang, S.L.; Johnston, N.; Sharma, S. Adherence to Canada's Food Guide recommendations among Alberta's multi-ethnic youths is a major concern: Findings from de WHY ACT NOW project. *J. Hum. Nutr. Diet* **2018**, *31*, 658–669. [CrossRef]
36. De Cock, N.; Van Camp, J.; Kolsteren, P.; Lachat, C.; Huybregts, L.; Maes, L.; Deforche, B.; Verstraeten, R.; Vangeel, J.; Beullens, K.; et al. Development and validation of a quantitative snack and beverage food frecuency questionnaire for adolescents. *J. Hum. Nutr. Diet* **2016**, *30*, 141–150. [CrossRef]
37. Sygit, K.M.; Sygit, M.; Wojtyła-Buciora, P.; Lyubinets, O.; Stelmach, W.; Krakowiak, J. Effects of dietary lifestyle education program for adolescents in middle schools: Study design of a cluster randomized controlled trial. *Ann. Nutr. Metab.* **2013**, *63*, 726–727.
38. Anton-Paduraru, D.T.; Mocanu, V.; Popescu, V.; Boiculese, L.V.; Gotca, I.; Iliescu, M.L. Evaluation of eating habits of adolescents from highschools from north-eastern part of romania. *Clin. Nutr.* **2019**, *38*, 59–296. [CrossRef]
39. Alfaro González, M.; Vázquez Fernández, M.E.; Fierro Urturi, A.; Rodríguez Molinero, L.; Muñoz Moreno, M.F.; Herrero Bregón, B. Eating habits and physical exercise in adolescents. *Rev. Pediatr. Aten. Primaria* **2016**, *18*, 221–229.
40. Lima-Serrano, M.; Guerra Martín, M.D.; Lima-Rodríguez, J.S. Lifestyles and factors associated with diet and physical activity in adolescents. *Nutr. Hosp.* **2015**, *32*, 2838–2847. [PubMed]
41. Cuervo Tuero, C.; Cachón Zagalaz, J.; Zagalaz Sánchez, M.L.; González de Mesa, C. Knowledge and interests regarding healthy eating habits and practising physical activity. A study with an adolescent population. *Aula Abierta* **2018**, *47*, 211–220. [CrossRef]
42. Llauradó, E.; Aceves-Martins, M.; Tarro, L.; Papell-Garcia, I.; Puiggròs, F.; Arola, L.; Prades-Tena, J.; Montagut, M.; Moragas-Fernández, C.M.; Solà, R.; et al. A youth-led social marketing intervention to encourage healthy lifestyles, the EYTO (European Youth Tackling Obesity) project: A cluster randomised controlled0 trial in Catalonia, Spain. *BM Public Health* **2015**, *15*, 607. [CrossRef] [PubMed]
43. Herrero Lozano, R.; Fillat Ballesteros, J.C. Study of breakfast and academic performance in a group of teenagers. *Nutr. Hosp.* **2006**, *21*, 346–352.

44. Asigbee, F.M.; Whitney, S.D.; Peterson, C.E. The link between nutrition and physical activity in increasing academic achievement. *J. Sch. Health* **2018**, *88*, 407–415. [CrossRef]
45. Burrows, T.; Goldman, S.; Pursey, K.; Lim, R. Is there an association between dietary intake and academic achievement: A systematic review. *J. Hum. Nutr. Diet.* **2016**, *30*, 117–140. [CrossRef]
46. González-Jiménez, E.; Cañadas, G.R.; Lastra-Caro, A.; Cañadas de la Fuente, G. Effectiveness of an educational intervention on nutrition and physical activity in a population of adolescents. Prevention of endocrine-metabolic and cardiovascular risk factors. *Rev. Aquichan.* **2014**, *14*, 549–559. [CrossRef]
47. Martínez, M.I.; Hernández, M.D.; Ojeda, M.; Mena, R.; Alegre, A.; Alfonso, J.L. Development of a nutritional education programme and assessment of the change in healthy eating habits in a population of compulsory secondary school students. *Nutr. Hosp.* **2009**, *24*, 504–510.
48. Pedersen, S.; Grønhøj, A.; Thøgersen, J. Texting your way to healthier eating? Effects of participating in a feedback intervention using text messaging on adolescents' fruit and vegetable intake. *Health Educ. Res.* **2016**, *31*, 171–184. [CrossRef] [PubMed]
49. Van Lippevelde, W.; Van Stralen, M.; Verloigne, M.; Bourdeaudhuij, I.; Deforche, B.; Brug, J.; Maes, L.; Haerens, L. Mediating effects of home-related factors on fat intake from snacks in a school-based nutrition intervention among adolescents. *Health Educ. Res.* **2011**, *27*, 36–45. [CrossRef] [PubMed]
50. Godin, K.M.; Patte, K.A.; Leatherdale, S.T. Examining predictors of Breakfast Skipping and Breakfast Program Use Among Secondary School Students in the COMPASS. Study. *J. Sch. Health* **2018**, *88*, 150–158. [CrossRef] [PubMed]
51. Hearst, M.O.; Shanafelt, A.; Wang, Q.; Leduc, R.; Nanney, M.S. Altering the School Breakfast Environment Reduces Barriers to School Breakfast Participation Among Diverse Rural Youth. *J. Sch. Health* **2017**, *88*, 3–8. [CrossRef] [PubMed]
52. Caspi, C.E.; Wang, Q.; Shanafelt, A.; Larson, N.; Wei, S.; Hearst, M.O.; Nanney, M.S. School Breakfast Program Participation and Rural Adolescents' Purchasing Behaviors in Food Stores and Restaurants. *J Sch. Health* **2017**, *87*, 723–731. [CrossRef]
53. Grao-Cruces, A.; Nuviala, A.; Fernández-Martínez, A.; Porcel Gálvez, A.M.; Moral García, J.E.; Martínez López, E.J. Adherence to the Mediterranean diet among rural and urban adolescents in southern Spain, satisfaction with life, anthropometry, and physical and sedentary activities. *Nutr. Hosp.* **2013**, *28*, 1129–1135.
54. Doménech Asensi, G.; Sánchez Martínez, A.; Ros Berruezo, G. Cross-sectional study to evaluate the associated factors with differences between city and districts secondary school students of the southeast of Spain (Murcia) for their adherence to the Mediterranean diet. *Nutr. Hosp.* **2015**, *31*, 1359–1365.
55. Hae Jeong Lee, H.J.; Kim, C.H.; Han, I.; Kim, S.H. Emotional State According to Breakfast Consumption in 62276 South Korean Adolescents. *Iran J. Pediatr.* **2019**, *29*, e92193. [CrossRef]
56. Mumm, J.; Hearst, M.O.; Shanafelt, A.; Wang, Q.; Leduc, R.; Nanney, M.S. Increasing Social Support for Breakfast: Project BreakFAST. *Health Promot. Pract.* **2017**, *18*, 862–868. [CrossRef]
57. Garcia-Silva, J.; Navarrete Navarrete, N.; Silva-Silva, D.; Caparros-Gonzalez, R.A.; Peralta-Ramírez, M.I.; Caballo, V.E. Escalas de apoyo social para los hábitos alimentarios y para el ejercicio: Propiedades psicométricas. *Rev. Esp. Salud Pública* **2019**, *93*, 1–13.

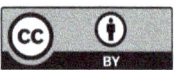

© 2020 by the authors. Licensee MDPI, Basel, Switzerland. This article is an open access article distributed under the terms and conditions of the Creative Commons Attribution (CC BY) license (http://creativecommons.org/licenses/by/4.0/).

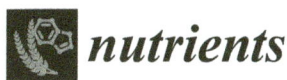

Article

Adolescents' Food Purchasing Patterns in the School Food Environment: Examining the Role of Perceived Relationship Support and Maternal Monitoring

Roel C.J. Hermans [1,2,*], Koen Smit [3,4], Nina van den Broek [3], Irma J. Evenhuis [1] and Lydian Veldhuis [1]

1. The Netherlands Nutrition Centre, 2594 AC The Hague, The Netherlands; evenhuis@voedingscentrum.nl (I.J.E.); veldhuis@voedingscentrum.nl (L.V.)
2. Department of Health Promotion, NUTRIM School of Nutrition and Translational Research in Metabolism, Maastricht University, 6299 AH Maastricht, The Netherlands
3. Behavioural Science Institute, Radboud University, 6500 HE Nijmegen, The Netherlands; k.smit@bsi.ru.nl (K.S.); n.vandenbroek@bsi.ru.nl (N.v.d.B.)
4. Trimbos Institute, Netherlands Institute of Mental Health and Addiction, 3500 AS Utrecht, The Netherlands
* Correspondence: r.hermans@maastrichtuniversity.nl; Tel.: +31-43-388-2415

Received: 31 January 2020; Accepted: 9 March 2020; Published: 11 March 2020

Abstract: The school food environment plays a role in adolescents' dietary behaviors. In this study, adolescents' food purchasing patterns in and around school and its potential relationship with perceived maternal relationship support and maternal monitoring were examined. Data were collected in The Netherlands in 2017. A total of 726 adolescents (45.8% boys; M_{age} = 13.78 ± 0.49) and 713 mothers (M_{age} = 45.05 ± 4.45) participated. Adolescents' frequency of bringing and purchasing foods was assessed via a Food Frequency Questionnaire (FFQ). Relationship support and monitoring were measured via self-report questionnaires. Structural Equation Modelling (SEM) was conducted to examine associations between adolescents' food purchasing patterns, relationship support, and monitoring. Results indicated that adolescents brought food and drinks mostly from home, and infrequently purchased these products in and around school. Yet, differences exist between subgroups of adolescents. Relationship support was positively associated with bringing fruit, vegetables and salad and negatively associated with purchasing sweet snacks. No associations were found for monitoring. These findings indicate that family-home determinants of healthy and unhealthy eating are important factors to consider when examining the impact of the school food environment on adolescents' food purchasing patterns. This has implications for policy makers who aim to develop and implement measures to improve adolescents' eating in and around school.

Keywords: school food environment; dietary behavior; food purchasing; adolescents; maternal monitoring; perceived relationship support

1. Introduction

The prevalence of overweight (including obesity) in children and adolescents in the WHO European region is alarming and considered to be one of the most serious public health challenges of the 21st century [1]. Globally, one in five children and adolescents aged 5–19 years have overweight, with levels increasing rapidly in many countries and regions in recent years [1]. The Netherlands is no exception in this case, with almost 12% of the children aged 4 to 17 years considered to have overweight in 2018 [2]. Healthy eating throughout the life-course helps prevent malnutrition in all its forms, as well as the development of a range of non-communicable diseases such as diabetes and heart disease. Furthermore, it is crucial for ensuring optimal physical and cognitive development during childhood and adolescence [3]. Yet, many children and adolescents do not meet dietary intake guidelines: they consume high levels of added sugar and/or fat, and have low intakes of fruits, vegetables, and whole grains [4–6]. Excessive consumption of energy-dense, nutrient-poor foods and drinks are a key cause of weight gain and contribute substantially to the development of overweight and obesity among youth [7]. Understanding the drivers of these unhealthy eating patterns is therefore essential to inform targeted approaches for overweight prevention in youth.

The current food environment, in particular, has been proposed to contribute importantly to the sharp increase in obesity rates worldwide [8–10]. As a consequence, there is also increasing attention to the role of the school food environment on young people's dietary behaviors (e.g., [11–13]). Adolescents are offered a variety of eating options and opportunities within their schools, varying from national lunch programs to food retailing in canteens and vending machines. In recent years, efforts have been made to create healthier school food environments [14–17]. These preventive school-based programs often focus on improving the nutritional quality of existing lunch meal programs or the food and beverage assortment in canteens and vending machines, thereby increasing the availability of healthy foods and limiting the supply of unhealthy foods. Furthermore, nudging and social marketing strategies are employed to steer adolescents towards better food choices by modifying the direct school food environment (e.g., by providing ready access to potable water or displaying fruits and salads in attractive bowls or stands). There is also a growing body of literature that recognizes the role of the local retail food environment around schools. There are studies that demonstrate, for instance, that a high fast-food outlet density in school neighborhoods is associated with increased fast-food purchasing by adolescents [18] or decreased odds of daily fruit and vegetable intake [19]. Furthermore, given that studies show that unhealthy food options (e.g., fried snacks and sugar-sweetened beverages) are more often for sale, in-store promoted or advertised in comparison with healthy options (e.g., fruit or bottled water [20]), these outlets in school neighborhoods are a key competitor of (healthy) school canteens, particularly since adolescents feel that they can get lower prices, more variety and more value for money in these outlets [21,22].

As research exploring the associations between school environments and adolescents' food purchasing behavior in European countries is sparse, the first aim of this study was to acquire more insight into the frequency at which Dutch adolescents purchase food and drinks in their school food environment. Previous work conducted in The Netherlands demonstrated that adolescents mostly bring food and drinks from home as lunch, whereas the school canteen is primarily visited to buy something extra [21,22]. Adolescents also buy their food and drinks at nearby food retailers, whenever the school permits them to leave school grounds. Demographic factors, such as adolescents' sex, age and educational level, play a role in their food purchasing behaviors. Older adolescents, for instance, may be more likely to make food purchases in and around school. Considering the potential role of these factors in adolescents' food purchasing behaviors, we also examined how these factors (i.e., adolescents' sex, age, educational level, and Body Mass Index (BMI)) are associated with adolescents' frequency of food purchasing in the school food environment. Specifically, we examined food purchasing behavior in four different food/beverage categories; fresh fruit, vegetables and salad (FVS); sugar-sweetened beverages (SSB), sweet snacks (SWS) and savory snacks (SAS), as these are associated with health promotion and disease prevention [3]. In particular, positive associations have been found between consumption of ultra-processed food and body fat during childhood and adolescence [23].

The school food environment is not the only factor that has an influence on adolescents' food purchasing patterns in and around school. Parents also play an important role in adolescents' food attitudes and behaviors. This can occur through various processes such as their own dietary intake patterns and their food-related parenting practices [24]. A recent systemic review, for instance, demonstrated that the availability of healthy foods and non-availability of unhealthy foods are associated with decreased unhealthy eating in adolescents [25]. Likewise, the effects of parental modeling on adolescents' dietary behavior have been found to be consistent and significant across studies; the frequency at which parents eat healthily and demonstrate the benefits and pleasure of eating healthily are associated with adolescents' healthy eating patterns [26]. Other food parenting practices, such as setting restrictions regarding food consumption or food monitoring, have not been found to be consistently related to adolescents' dietary behavior [26]. Inconsistent findings in this domain are often explained by the influence of general parenting [27], which is defined as the emotional climate in which specific parenting practices are expressed [28]. For example, it has been demonstrated that the use of parenting practices such as encouragement and covert control led to an increase in healthy intake and decrease in unhealthy food intake only in those children who were reared in a positive parenting context (characterized by parental warmth and guidance) [29]. As such, authoritative parenting is often found to be associated with better weight-related outcomes compared to other parenting styles such as permissive or coercive forms of parenting [27,30]. As research on the role of parental factors in explaining adolescents' food purchasing in the school food environment is scarce, a second aim of the present work was to acquire more insight into the frequency at which adolescents bring food and drinks from home. Again, we also examined how demographic factors are associated with this behavior. Finally, the present research examined for the first time whether two specific parenting factors (i.e., perceived relationship support and monitoring) were associated with adolescents' frequency of bringing and purchasing food and drinks in the school food environment. Data on the extent to which adolescents received relationship support from their mother and mothers' knowledge about their child's daily activities (i.e., maternal monitoring) were collected in a previous wave of a longitudinal lifestyle cohort study [31,32]. This final research aim, therefore, is explorative in its ambition, without having derived causal hypotheses.

2. Materials and Methods

2.1. Procedure and Materials

Data for the current study were drawn from a multi-informant, seven-wave longitudinal lifestyle cohort study (2015–2018). We aimed to recruit a nationwide representative sample of 10-to-13-year-olds and their mothers. Therefore, random sampling methods were used to recruit participants from five randomly selected regions and provinces in the Netherlands [31,32]. The regions were based on the four cardinal points (i.e., North, East, South, West). The center of The Netherlands was added as an extra region, resulting in a total of five regions. After distributing the twelve Dutch provinces across these regions, we randomly selected one province in each of the five regions using the website www.random.org. We then retrieved a list of all primary schools in these provinces via the website of Dutch Ministry of Education (n = 913). Management boards of these schools were then contacted by telephone. Of the 913 schools, 123 school boards agreed to participate (13.5%). After providing consent, schools were asked to distribute invitation letters to children in the 6th grade of primary education. Children and mothers from 104 of the 123 participating schools opted into the study. To register for the study, mothers (at baseline, n = 755) and their children (n = 755) had to provide informed consent through the research project's website. All participants were informed that their participation was voluntary, and that they could withdraw from the study at any time. The current study was conducted in accordance with the Declaration of Helsinki, and the study procedures were approved by the ethics committee of the Faculty of Social Sciences of Radboud University, Nijmegen, The Netherlands (ECSW2014-2411-272).

At baseline, paper and pencil questionnaires were administered to students in the classroom. In the same week, mothers were requested to complete the online questionnaire by e-mail. In the following three years, online questionnaires were sent to the adolescents every six months. Their mothers received their questionnaire via e-mail every twelve months. Yearly monetary incentives (€10) were provided to both adolescents and their mothers. If the mother was not available for any reason, the father could complete the questionnaires. However, these cases were excluded in the present study. The questionnaire used in this study is available in Dutch from the corresponding author upon request.

2.2. Participants

The current study used fifth wave data (2017), including 726 adolescents (46% boys, M_{age} = 13.78) and 713 mothers. Self-reported information about length (in centimeters) and weight (in kilograms) was provided by 72.8% of the adolescents, and by 91.4% of the mothers. Adolescents lived together with two parents (79%) or within a divorced household (21%). Adolescents were almost equally distributed over the three educational levels (i.e., low-medium-high) in The Netherlands (see Table 1).

Table 1. Sample characteristics.

		Adolescents	Mothers
Age; Mean (SD)		13.78 (0.49)	45.05 (4.45)
Sex	Boys	46%	-
	Girls	54%	
Educational level	Low	39.1%	11.1%
	Medium	27.4%	46.3%
	High	33.5%	42.6%
BMI; Mean (SD)		zBMI-for -age -0.33 (1.02)	24.62 (4.17)
Relationship support (0–4)		3.32 (0.45)	-
Monitoring (0–4)		3.83 (0.44)	-

Note. zBMI-for-age is the measure that can be used from age 2 to 20 years to screen for obesity, overweight, or underweight. Body Mass Index (BMI).

2.3. Measures

All of the measures relevant to the present research are outlined in detail below. Measures related to adolescents' food purchasing behavior were specifically added to the fifth wave of the longitudinal lifestyle cohort study. All the other measures were already part of the existing cohort study and also measured at the fifth wave, unless otherwise specified.

Demographic information adolescent. Adolescents' sex and birth date were assessed at baseline, their weight and height and their educational level at wave five. Adolescents' age was obtained from their reported date of birth and the date of measurement. Adolescents reported on their height in centimeters and their weight in kilograms. To calculate adolescents' zBMI-for-age, first adolescents' BMI was computed by dividing their weight in kilograms by their squared height in meters. Subsequently, adolescents' zBMI-for-age was computed by considering the age- and gender-specific growth curves for BMI, based on a Dutch representative sample of 0-to-21-year-olds [33]. Adolescents' educational level was measured with one item ('what is your level of education?'), and response categories ranged from the lowest to the highest educational level in The Netherlands. All responses were grouped in one of the three categories: low (practical and pre-vocational education), medium (higher general secondary education) to high education (pre-university education), using the standard classification of education in The Netherlands [34].

Adolescents' frequency of purchasing food and drinks in the school food environment and bringing these products from home. To assess the frequency at which adolescents purchased food and drinks in and around their school, adolescents completed a short Food Frequency Questionnaire (FFQ). This FFQ was specifically developed for the aim of the present study. In this FFQ, adolescents were asked to report how frequently they purchased items within (1) FVS (e.g., fresh fruit and vegetables), (2) SSB (e.g., soft drinks and fruit juice), (3) SWS (e.g., cookies, candies, and ice cream), and (4) SAS (e.g., sausage roll, French fries, and pizza slice) at an average school week. This was asked on a 6-point scale, ranging from "never to almost never"(0 days per week) to "all schooldays" (5 days per week). For each of these categories, adolescents were asked to separately report the frequency at which they purchased items within this category from (1) their school canteen, (2) vending machines in school, or

(3) at food retailers outside the school. The same FFQ was administered to assess the frequency at which adolescents brought food and drinks within these categories from home.

Demographic information mother. Mothers' age was obtained at baseline from the reported date of birth and the date of measurement, together with their educational level. Mothers also reported on their height in centimeters and weight in kilograms. Mothers' BMI was calculated by dividing their weight in kilograms by their squared height in meters. Mothers' educational level was measured with one item ('what is your highest level of education?'), and response categories ranged from the lowest to the highest educational level in The Netherlands. All responses were grouped in one of the three categories: low (primary, lower secondary, lower vocational education), medium (higher secondary, vocational education) and high education (university of applied sciences, university), using the standard classification of education in The Netherlands [34].

Adolescents' perceived maternal relationship support. The extent to which adolescents received relationship support from their mother was assessed by administering the short 12-item version of the Relationship Support Inventory (RSI; [35]). Adolescents indicated the degree to which they received emotional and instrumental support from their mother (e.g., "My mother supports what I do") on a 5-point scale, ranging from 0 (absolutely not true) to 4 (absolutely true). The scores on the 12 items were summed and averaged to create a total score. Cronbach's α in the present study was 0.85, indicating high internal consistency.

Maternal monitoring. Monitoring was assessed by asking mothers about their knowledge of their offspring's daily activities [36]. Mothers indicated to what degree they were up to date on their offspring's whereabouts (e.g., "Does your child need approval to leave the house at night")? The three items existed of a 5-point scale, ranging from 0 ("never") to 4 ("always"). The scores were summed and averaged to create a total score. Cronbach's α in the present study was 0.77, indicating sufficient internal consistency.

2.4. Statistical Analyses

First, descriptive analyses were conducted to provide information about the sample and the frequency at which adolescents purchased food and drinks in their school food environment or brought these products from home. The second set of analyses existed of statistical tests to assess whether demographic factors relevant to the adolescent (i.e., sex, age, zBMI-for-age, and educational level) were associated with the frequency at which adolescents purchased and brought food and drinks. We conducted *t*-tests to assess sex differences, and ANOVAs with Games-Howell post-hoc comparisons were conducted to test differences between educational levels. Moreover, bivariate correlations for age and zBMI-for-age were conducted to assess whether these factors predicted any differences in the frequency to which adolescents purchased or brought food and drinks. These analyses were performed with SPSS version 24.0 (IBM Corp., Armonk, NY, USA). Finally, Structural Equation Modelling (SEM) in Mplus 8.0 was conducted [37] to assess whether maternal monitoring and relationship support were associated with the frequency of purchasing or bringing food and drinks. The latter existed of a latent variable constructed from the three contexts in which adolescents could purchase their food and drinks (i.e., school canteen, vending machines in school, or at food retailers outside the school). The model was estimated for all food categories simultaneously, i.e., FVS, SSB, SWS, and SAS. In a second model, we controlled for adolescents' age, sex, zBMI-for-age and educational level. The model fit was assessed using the comparative fit index (CFI) and the Root Mean Square Error of Approximation (RMSEA). The CFI relates to the total variance accounted for by the model, where values close to 1, i.e., higher than 0.95, are considered adequate [38]. The RMSEA is based on the non-centrality parameter, where fit values of <0.06 are considered adequate. Full information maximum likelihood (FIML) procedures were used to account for missing data (e.g., in zBMI-for-age). We also report the Standardized Root Mean Square Residual (SRMR). Alpha was set at $p < 0.05$. See Figure 1 for the conceptual model of these analyses. The data that support the findings of this study are available from the corresponding author, upon reasonable request.

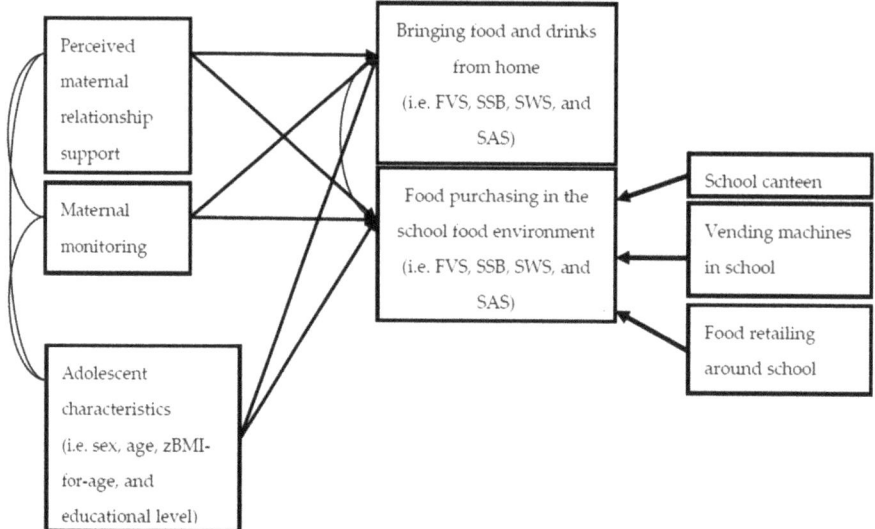

Figure 1. Conceptual model testing the associations between perceived relationship support, maternal monitoring and the frequency of bringing or purchasing food and drinks in the school food environment. Note. FVS = fresh fruit, vegetables and salad; SSB = sugar sweetened beverages; SWS = sweet snacks; SAS = savory snacks.

3. Results

3.1. Descriptive Analyses

Table 2 describes the frequency (days per week) to which adolescents (12–15 years) brought food and drinks within one of the four categories from home and how often they purchased items in these categories in their school food environment.

Table 2. Means and standard deviations (between brackets) of bringing and purchasing food and drinks in the school food environment, in days per school week ($n = 716$).

	FVS	SSB	SWS	SAS
Bringing from home	2.04 (2.08)	1.83 (2.11)	2.59 (2.06)	0.28 (0.77)
Purchasing at school canteen	0.17 (0.73)	0.28 (0.86)	0.46 (0.97)	0.36 (0.80)
Purchasing at vending machines in school	0.07 (0.50)	0.24 (0.73)	0.46 (0.83)	0.15 (0.53)
Purchasing at food retailing around school	0.10 (0.51)	0.33 (0.81)	0.51 (0.89)	0.38 (0.76)

Note. FVS = fresh fruit, vegetables and salad; SSB = sugar sweetened beverages; SWS = sweet snacks; SAS = savory snacks.

Overall, adolescents most frequently brought their food and drinks from home. Items within FVS, SSB and SWS were brought from home each about two days per week, on average. The frequency at which items within the categories were purchased in and around school was relatively low (each less than one day per week, on average).

3.2. Demographic Factors

We tested whether demographic factors (adolescents' sex, age, zBMI-for-age and educational level) predicted any differences in frequency of bringing and buying food and drinks. The results of these analyses are displayed in Tables 3 and 4.

Table 3. Differences in sex and educational level in the extent to which adolescents bring and purchase food and drinks the school food environment.

	Bringing from Home		School Canteen		Vending Machine in School		Food Retailing around School	
Sex [a]		p		p		p		p
FVS	1 < 2	<0.001	NS	0.139	NS	0.934	NS	0.519
SSB	1 > 2	<0.001	NS	0.104	NS	0.586	1 > 2	0.009
SWS	NS	0.346	1 < 2	0.036	NS	0.099	NS	0.501
SAS	NS	0.572	NS	0.711	NS	0.414	1 > 2	0.024
Educational level [b]								
FVS	NS	0.843	NS	0.177	1>2	0.018	1 > 3	0.013
SSB	1,2 > 3	<0.001	1 > 2,3	<0.001	1>2,3	<0.001	1 > 2,3	<0.001
SWS	NS	0.177	1 > 2,3	<0.001	1>3	0.012	1 > 2,3	<0.001
SAS	1,2 > 3	<0.001	1,2 > 3	0.001	1>3	0.002	1 > 3	<0.001

Note. [a] Significant differences are reported by indicating differences between boys (1) and girls (2). [b] Significant differences are reported by indicating differences between low (1), medium (2) and high (3) levels of education. Alpha is set at $p < 0.05$. NS is non-significant.

Table 4. Bivariate associations between adolescents' age and zBMI-for-age with bringing and purchasing food and drinks in the school food environment.

	Bringing from Home		Purchasing in School Canteen		Purchasing at Vending Machine in School		Purchasing at Food Retailing around School	
Age	r	p	r	p	r	p	r	p
FVS	−0.05	0.215	0.05	0.153	0.09	0.023	0.04	0.239
SSB	0.11	0.002	0.08	0.034	0.02	0.653	0.09	0.014
SWS	0.05	0.156	0.11	0.004	0.05	0.151	0.08	0.036
SAS	0.14	<0.001	0.09	0.017	0.04	0.289	0.09	0.012
zBMI-for-age	r	p	r	p	r	p	r	p
FVS	0.04	0.382	0.03	0.435	0.06	0.160	0.10	0.026
SSB	−0.02	0.725	0.01	0.850	0.09	0.029	0.09	0.028
SWS	−0.09	0.032	−0.01	0.816	0.01	0.789	0.04	0.327
SAS	−0.03	0.559	−0.03	0.557	0.06	0.197	0.05	0.240

Note: Alpha is set at <0.05.

It was found that girls more frequently brought items within FVS from home compared to boys. Boys more frequently brought items within SSB from home and purchased these items more often from food retailers around school. Moreover, it was found that girls more frequently purchased items within SWS in their school canteen, whereas boys purchased items within SAS more often from food retailers around the school. Regarding educational level, it was found that boys and girls from lower educational levels reported a higher frequency of bringing and purchasing food and drinks. Specifically, they reported to purchase items within FVS more often from vending machines and food retailers around school. They also reported to bring and purchase items within SSBs and SAS more often than adolescents from medium or high educational levels. For more specific details, see Supplementary Tables S1 and S2.

Age was found to be positively associated with bringing and purchasing different types of food, indicating that older adolescents reported to bring and buy food and drinks more often than younger adolescents. zBMI-for-age was positively associated with purchasing items within FVS and SSB at food retailers around school, indicating that those with a higher zBMI-for-age purchased these food products more often around school. Adolescents with a lower zBMI-for-age reported to bring items within SWS less frequently from home

The associations between perceived maternal relationship support, maternal monitoring and frequency of bringing and purchasing food and drinks were assessed in Structural Equation Models. The total model showed an adequate fit ($\chi^2_{(df=78)}$ = 115.03; CFI = 0.982; TLI = 0.966; RMSEA = 0.025; SRMR = 0.026).

3.3. The Role of Perceived Relationship Support

Relationship support was positively associated with bringing items within FVS from home, and negatively associated with purchasing items within SWS (see Table 5), indicating that more support from mothers was associated with bringing FVS more frequently and purchasing SWS less frequently.

Table 5. Between perceived relationship support, maternal monitoring and the frequency of bringing and purchasing food and drinks.

	Total Model				Total Model with Covariates			
	Bringing		Purchasing [a]		Bringing		Purchasing [a]	
FVS	B(SE)	p	B(SE)	p	B(SE)	p	B(SE)	p
Relationship Support	0.081 (0.037)	0.028	−0.018 (0.044)	0.686	0.059 (0.038)	0.119	−0.009 (0.050)	0.861
Monitoring	0.003 (0.038)	0.941	0.020 (0.036)	0.568	−0.004 (0.036)	0.914	0.017 (0.034)	0.623
Sex	−		−		0.168 (0.037)	<0.001	0.033 (0.048)	0.489
Age	−		−		−0.027 (0.038)	0.480	0.074 (0.045)	0.102
Educational level	−		−		0.014 (0.037)	0.705	−0.117 (0.035)	0.001
zBMI-for-age	−		−		0.035 (0.040)	0.388	0.084 (0.063)	0.186
SSB								
Relationship Support	−0.032 (0.036)	0.374	−0.087 (0.057)	0.131	0.004 (0.035)	0.901	−0.062 (0.058)	0.288
Monitoring	−0.060 (0.043)	0.159	0.010 (0.045)	0.823	−0.050 (0.039)	0.200	−0.007 (0.042)	0.861
Sex	−		−		−0.181 (0.037)	<0.001	−0.078 (0.045)	0.085
Age	−		−		0.077 (0.038)	0.042	0.032 (0.047)	0.497
Educational level	−		−		−0.130 (0.036)	<0.001	−0.232 (0.036)	<0.001
zBMI-for-age	−		−		−0.017 (0.042)	0.691	0.090 (0.063)	0.151
SWS								
Relationship Support	0.003 (0.038)	0.929	−0.135 (0.058)	0.021	0.005 (0.039)	0.903	−0.129 (0.059)	0.028
Monitoring	−0.003 (0.037)	0.953	−0.038 (0.045)	0.462	0.001 (0.035)	0.979	−0.034 (0.046)	0.464
Sex	−		−		0.040 (0.038)	0.292	0.109 (0.049)	0.027
Age	−		−		0.054 (0.038)	0.158	0.067 (0.045)	0.130
Educational level	−		−		−0.009 (0.038)	0.806	−0.234 (0.039)	<0.001
zBMI-for-age	−		−		−0.093 (0.043)	0.033	−0.010 (0.058)	0.858
SAS								
Relationship Support	−0.078 (0.043)	0.072	−0.061 (0.045)	0.168	−0.058 (0.043)	0.183	−0.045 (0.047)	0.343
Monitoring	0.021 (0.029)	0.473	−0.048 (0.049)	0.324	0.024 (0.028)	0.384	−0.045 (0.046)	0.329
Sex	−		−		−0.008 (0.037)	0.829	−0.004 (0.047)	0.934
Age	−		−		0.101 (0.044)	0.021	0.061 (0.049)	0.212
Educational level	−		−		−0.151 (0.030)	<0.001	−0.198 (0.039)	<0.001
zBMI-for-age	−		−		−0.031 (0.036)	0.391	0.055 (0.058)	0.342

Note. Effects are standardized Beta's (standard errors in brackets); Except for monitoring, all variables were reported by the adolescents; [a] latent variable constructed from three items (i.e., purchasing in the school canteen, vending machine, or at food retailing around school. Alpha is set at <0.05.

In a next model, we added adolescents' sex, age, zBMI-for-age, and educational level as covariates, again showing an adequate fit ($\chi^2_{(df=118)}$ = 204.97; CFI = 0.966; TLI = 0.937; RMSEA = 0.032; SRMR = 031). Although the association between perceived relationship support and purchasing SWS remained significant after adding these covariates, B = −0.129, SE = 0.059, p = 0.028, it became non-significant for bringing FVS from home, B = 0.059, SE = 0.038, p = 0.119, see Table 5.

3.4. The Role of Maternal Monitoring

Monitoring neither predicted frequency of bringing any food from home nor purchasing any food in or around school. Moreover, when adding covariates to the model, no significant associations were found (see Table 5).

4. Discussion

The present study aimed to get more insight into the frequency at which adolescents bring and purchase food and drinks in the school food environment. Specifically, we explored the potential associations between adolescents' demographic information (i.e., sex, age, educational level, and zBMI-for-age) and their food purchasing behaviors. Furthermore, we investigated the associations between two specific parental factors (i.e., perceived relationship support from the mother and maternal monitoring) and adolescents' food purchasing in and around their school.

One of the main findings of the present study is the observation that adolescents infrequently purchase food and drinks in and around their school. This is in line with previous work showing that self-purchasing of food and drinks in the school canteen or at vending machines in school is not very prevalent among Dutch adolescents [21,22]. Adolescents, however, also reported to infrequently visit food vendors near school. This finding is in contrast to previous studies which have suggested that adolescents more frequently spend money on food and drinks at food retailers around their school [21,22]. It should be noted, however, that the adolescents participating in this study were younger than those in previous work. An increase in food purchases in the school food environment with age may be due to an increased level of personal autonomy, greater access to own money and greater freedom to make choices about what to purchase and consume [39,40]. Indeed, Dutch adolescents aged 12–14 years receive 15–20 euros (which equals an amount of 16.5–22 US dollars) per month from their parents, and their budget increases with age as they may also generate income by means of a holiday or secondary job [41]. In future research, it would be worthwhile to further explore how adolescents' food purchasing behavior in the school food environment may increase with age, linking current data with future waves of the longitudinal lifestyle cohort study [31,32]. This also holds for potential differences between boys and girls, and those with a lower versus higher educational background, as these were also found to be associated with adolescents' food purchases in the school food environment.

Secondly, it was found that adolescents brought food and drinks mostly from home. This suggests that the availability of specific food and drinks in the home context plays a role in adolescents' consumption behavior for the simple reason that these products are (freely) available to them. This is consistent with recent reviews that have summarized the importance of the availability and accessibility of healthy (i.e., fruit and vegetables) and unhealthy foods (i.e., SSB and energy-dense snack food) in the home context as a consistent predictor of desirable and undesirable food consumption in children and adolescents [25,42].

Thirdly, we found that the degree of relationship support adolescents perceived from their mother predicted the frequency of bringing and purchasing food and drinks. Specifically, it was found that those who perceived more support from their mother indicated to bring more FVS from home to school, and to purchase SWS less frequently in and around school. Although this is the first study to investigate this specific relationship, results are in line with suggestions that the quality of the parent-adolescent relationship can have an impact on the development of adolescent health risk behaviors [43]. Such research, for instance, has demonstrated that parental warmth, involvement, and emotional support are positively associated with higher fruit and vegetable consumption and lower intakes of high fat and/or sugar food and beverage intake [44,45]. We propose that higher levels of perceived relationship support may be the result of an authorative parenting style, and in this way play a protective role in adolescents' food purchasing patterns in the school food environment. However, this is a posthoc suggestion and is speculative, so it will need to be empirically tested. Furthermore, although directions were in accordance with theory [27,29], the strengths of these associations were small. This may be explained by the notion that perceived support, as an indicator of general parenting style may be modeled at a more distal level of influence rather than at a more direct level of influence [46]. Finally, it should be noted that the relationship between perceived support and bringing FVS became non-significant when we controlled for demographic factors. This once again underscores the importance of these factors in this research area and further work is needed to gain more insight in their working mechanism.

Finally, this study found no evidence for a relationship between maternal monitoring and adolescents' food purchasing patterns. Most research in this area has used the Child Feeding Questionnaire [47] or specific parenting style dimensions such as parents' perceived strictness as measures of parental monitoring [48,49]. In this study, however, another monitoring scale was used [35]. This scale did not include specific items related to their child's dietary behavior or food purchasing patterns in and around school, and therefore might have been too general. Likewise, this general monitoring scale might not have been sensitive enough to detect any differences between mothers. As this study is the first attempt to examine the association between maternal monitoring and adolescents' food purchasing behavior in and around school, our results should be replicated to assure that our measures and results are valid and reliable.

Strengths of the presents study include its relatively large sample size and the inclusion from multiple informants (mothers and adolescents) which enabled us to assess the variables of interest from the most relevant source. Also, we examined adolescents' frequency of food purchases in and around school, which is conceptually more directly linked to food environment exposure than dietary intake [50]. However, the present work also had limitations. First, data were cross-sectional, which limits us from drawing conclusions about the direction and temporality of the associations found. Future research is needed to examine the causal and longitudinal influence that perceived relationship support and monitoring might have on adolescents' food purchasing behaviors. Second, our measures were based on self-reports of bringing and purchasing food and drinks in and around school within four different food and drink categories. This method may be biased due to social desirability and lack of specificity [51]. As a result, this study does not give insight into which specific food and drink items are most frequently brought or purchased by adolescents in and around school. Novel smart technologies make it possible to overcome some of these limitations by incorporating functions such as global positioning (GPS) and ecological momentary assessment (EMA) (cf. [50]). Future research may benefit from using these methodologies to examine adolescents' actual food purchases, considering the accessible food environment in and around school by using a Geographical Information System (GIS) and on-site observations. This also makes it possible to examine socioeconomic differences in food outlet availability and its impact on adolescents' food purchasing behaviors. A final limitation is that our study relied on a healthy sample of well-educated adolescents and their mothers with a homogenous cultural background. Therefore, our findings may not generalize to adolescents with a more at-risk background, such as those with an ethnic background or those whose parents have a lower socioeconomic position. Further research is required to establish potential differences between these adolescent subgroups in their food purchasing behaviors.

In The Netherlands, there is no compulsory system of school meals. Instead, adolescents may choose to bring their own food and drinks and/or to purchase (supplementary) items in the school food environment. Although self-purchasing of food and drinks in and around school was not very prevalent in this age group, the associations found with sex, age and educational level indicate that the school food environment remains an important area for preventive programs aimed at stimulating healthy dietary intakes among adolescents. Indeed, a recent review and meta-analysis demonstrated the positive effects of specific school food environment policy interventions on adolescent's dietary intake behaviors [52]. Social norms regarding healthy eating may be a powerful mechanism underlying this effect [53,54]. It has been shown, for instance, that adolescents' snack and soft drink consumption are highly associated with that of their peers [55], particularly when these food and drinks are highly available and accessible in their school environment [56]. By increasing the accessibility and availability of healthy food (and subsequently decreasing the supply of unhealthy food), adolescents are nudged towards making healthy food choices in and around school [14–17]. As a result of these changes, social norms around eating in and around school may change, thereby further increasing the effectiveness of these preventive programs. The findings of this study, however, also indicate that parents have an important role in providing their children with healthy food during school hours. This suggests that family-home determinants of healthy and unhealthy eating are important factors to consider when examining the impact of the school food environment on adolescents' food purchasing patterns (cf. [57,58]).

Supplementary Materials: The following are available online at http://www.mdpi.com/2072-6643/12/3/733/s1, Table S1: Means and Standard Deviations by Sex in the Frequency of Bringing Food From Home and Purchasing Food (i.e., in the School Canteen, Vending Machines and Around School). Table S2: Means and Standard Deviations by Educational Level, Testing Differences in the Frequency of Bringing Food From Home and Purchasing Food (i.e., in the School Canteen, Vending Machines and Around School). The data and questionnaire used in this study are available from the corresponding author upon request.

Author Contributions: Conceptualization, R.C.J.H., L.V., K.S.; I.J.E.; methodology, R.C.J.H., K.S.; formal analysis, K.S., N.v.d.B.; investigation, R.C.J.H., N.v.d.B., K.S.; resources, R.C.J.H., K.S.; data curation, K.S.; writing—original draft preparation, R.C.J.H., N.v.d.B., K.S.; writing—review and editing, L.V., I.J.E.; visualization, K.S.; supervision, R.C.J.H.; project administration, K.S.; funding acquisition, K.S. All authors have read and agreed to the published version of the manuscript.

Funding: This research was funded by the Netherlands Organization for Scientific Research (NWO), VIDI grant 452-13-003 awarded to Emmanuel Kuntsche. The APC was funded by the Netherlands Nutrition Centre.

Acknowledgments: We would like to thank all adolescents and parents involved in this study for their participation. Further, we would like to thank Heleen Schuit-van Raamsdonk, Lisanne van der Kramer, and all members of the 'Healthy School Canteen Team' for their valuable input.

Conflicts of Interest: The authors declare no conflict of interest. The funders had no role in the design of the study; in the collection, analyses, or interpretation of data; in the writing of the manuscript, or in the decision to publish the results.

References

1. World Health Organization (WHO). Obesity and Overweight. Key Facts. Available online: https://www.who.int/news-room/fact-sheets/detail/obesity-and-overweight (accessed on 24 January 2020).
2. Statistics Netherlands (CBS). Kinderen Met Overgewicht en Obesitas Naar Leeftijd. 2018. Available online: https://www.volksgezondheidenzorg.info/onderwerp/overgewicht/cijfers-context/huidige-situatie#!node-overgewicht-kinderen (accessed on 24 January 2020).
3. World Health Organization (WHO). Healthy Diet. Available online: https://www.who.int/publications-detail/healthy-diet (accessed on 24 January 2020).
4. Diethelm, K.; Jankovic, N.; Moreno, L.A.; Huybrechts, I.; De Henauw, S.; De Vriendt, T.; Gonzalez-Gross, M.; Leclercq, C.; Gottrand, F.; Gilbert, C.C.; et al. Food intake of European adolescents in the light of different food-based dietary guidelines: Results of the HELENA (Healthy Lifestyle in Europe by Nutrition in Adolescence) Study. *Public Health Nutr.* **2012**, *15*, 386–398. [CrossRef] [PubMed]
5. Vereecken, C.; Pedersen, T.P.; Ojala, K.; Krølner, R.; Dzielska, A.; Ahluwalia, N.; Giacchi, M.; Kelly, C. Fruit and vegetable consumption trends among adolescents from 2002 to 2010 in 33 countries. *Eur. J. Public Health* **2015**, *25* (Suppl. S2), 16–19. [CrossRef] [PubMed]
6. National Institute for Public Health and the Environment (RIVM). Wat eet en Drinkt Nederland? Resultaten van de Voedselconsumptiepeiling 2012–2016. Available online: www.wateetnederland.nl (accessed on 24 January 2020).
7. Moreno, L.A.; Rodriguez, G.; Fleta, J.; Bueno-Lozano, M.; Lazaro, A.; Bueno, G. Trends of dietary habits in adolescents. *Crit. Rev. Food Sci. Nutr.* **2010**, *50*, 106–112. [CrossRef] [PubMed]

8. Hill, J.O.; Peters, J.C. Environmental contributions to the obesity epidemic. *Science* **1998**, *280*, 1371–1374. [CrossRef] [PubMed]
9. Story, M.; Kaphingst, K.M.; Robinson-O'Brien, R.; Glanz, K. Creating Healthy Food and Eating Environments: Policy and Environmental Approaches. *Annu. Rev. Public Health* **2008**, *29*, 253–272. [CrossRef] [PubMed]
10. Swinburn, B.; Egger, G.; Raza, F. Dissecting obesogenic environments: The development and application of a framework for identifying and prioritizing environmental interventions for obesity. *Prev. Med.* **1999**, *29 Pt 1*, 563–570. [CrossRef] [PubMed]
11. Driessen, C.E.; Cameron, A.J.; Thornton, L.E.; Lai, S.K.; Barnett, L.M. Effect of changes to the school food environment on eating behaviours and/or body weight in children: A systematic review. *Obes. Rev.* **2014**, *15*, 968–982. [CrossRef]
12. Gonzalez-Suarez, C.; Worley, A.; Grimmer-Somers, K.; Dones, V. School-based interventions on childhood obesity: A meta-analysis. *Am. J. Prev. Med.* **2009**, *37*, 418–427. [CrossRef]
13. Kubik, M.Y.; Lytle, L.A.; Hannan, P.J.; Perry, C.L.; Story, M. The association of the school food environment with dietary behaviors of young adolescents. *Am. J. Public Health* **2003**, *93*, 1168–1173. [CrossRef]
14. Frerichs, L.; Brittin, J.; Sorensen, D.; Trowbridge, M.J.; Yaroch, A.L.; Siahpush, M.; Tibbits, M.; Huang, T.T. Influence of school architecture and design on healthy eating: A review of the evidence. *Am. J. Public Health* **2005**, *105*, e46–e57. [CrossRef]
15. Kessler, H.S. Simple interventions to improve healthy eating behaviors in the school cafeteria. *Nutr. Rev.* **2016**, *74*, 198–209. [CrossRef] [PubMed]
16. Nornberg, T.R.; Houlby, L.; Skov, L.R.; Perez-Cueto, F.J. Choice architecture interventions for increased vegetable intake and behaviour change in a school setting: A systematic review. *Perspect. Public Health* **2016**, *136*, 132–142. [CrossRef] [PubMed]
17. Roy, R.; Kelly, B.; Rangan, A.; Allman-Farinelli, M. Food Environment Interventions to Improve the Dietary Behavior of Young Adults in Tertiary Education Settings: A Systematic Literature Review. *J. Acad. Nutr. Diet* **2015**, *115*, 1647–1681. [CrossRef] [PubMed]
18. He, M.; Tucker, P.; Gilliland, J.; Irwin, J.D.; Larsen, K.; Hess, P. The Influence of Local Food Environments on Adolescents' Food Purchasing Behaviors. *Int. J. Environ. Res. Public Health* **2012**, *9*, 1458–1471. [CrossRef] [PubMed]
19. Callaghan, M. Food for thought: Analysing the internal and external school food environment. *Health Educ.* **2015**, *115*, 152–170. [CrossRef]
20. Timmermans, J.; Dijkstra, C.; Kamphuis, C.; Huitink, M.; van der Zee, E.; Poelman, M. 'Obesogenic' School Food Environments? An Urban Case Study in the Netherlands. *Int. J. Environ. Res. Public Health* **2018**, *15*, 619. [CrossRef]
21. Hermans RC, J.; de Bruin, H.; Larsen, J.K.; Mensink, F.; Hoek, A.C. Adolescents' Responses to a School-Based Prevention Program Promoting Healthy Eating at School. *Front. Public Health* **2017**, *5*, 309. [CrossRef]
22. van Kleef, E. Moving towards a healthier assortment in secondary and vocational school food environments: Perspectives of Dutch students and school food policy professionals. *Br. Food J.* **2019**, *121*, 2052–2066. [CrossRef]
23. Costa, C.S.; Del-Ponte, B.; Assunção, M.C.F.; Santos, I.S. Consumption of ultra-processed foods and body fat during childhood and adolescence: A systematic review. *Public Health Nutr.* **2018**, *21*, 148–159. [CrossRef]
24. Larsen, J.K.; Hermans, R.C.; Sleddens, E.F.; Engels, R.C.; Fisher, J.O.; Kremers, S.P. How parental dietary behavior and food parenting practices affect children's dietary behavior. Interacting sources of influence? *Appetite* **2015**, *89*, 246–257. [CrossRef]
25. Yee, A.Z.H.; Lwin, M.O.; Ho, S.S. The influence of parental practices on child promotive and preventive food consumption behaviors: A systematic review and meta-analysis. *Int. J. Behav. Nutr. Phys. Act.* **2017**, *14*, 47. [CrossRef]
26. Blaine, R.E.; Kachurak, A.; Davison, K.K.; Klabunde, R.; Fisher, J.O. Food parenting and child snacking: A systematic review. *Int. J. Behav. Nutr. Phys. Act.* **2017**, *14*, 146. [CrossRef] [PubMed]
27. Sleddens, E.F.C.; Gerards, S.M.; Thijs, C.; De Vries, N.K.; Kremers, S.P.J. General parenting, childhood overweight and obesity-inducing behaviors: A review. *Int. J. Pediatr. Obes.* **2011**, *6*, e12–e27. [CrossRef] [PubMed]
28. Darling, N.; Steinberg, L. Parenting style as context. An integrative model. *Psychol. Bull.* **1993**, *113*, 487–496. [CrossRef]

29. Sleddens, E.F.C.; Kremers, S.P.J.; Stafleu, A.; Dagnelie, P.C.; De Vries, N.K.; Thijs, C. Food parenting practices and child dietary behavior. Prospective relations and the moderating role of general parenting. *Appetite* **2014**, *79*, 42–50. [CrossRef] [PubMed]
30. Gerards, S.M.; Sleddens, E.F.; Dagnelie, P.C.; de Vries, N.K.; Kremers, S.P. Interventions addressing general parenting to prevent or treat childhood obesity. *Int. J. Pediatr. Obes.* **2011**, *6*, e28–e45. [CrossRef] [PubMed]
31. Smit, K.; Voogt, C.; Otten, R.; Kleinjan, M.; Kuntsche, E. Exposure to Parental Alcohol Use Rather Than Parental Drinking Shapes Offspring's Alcohol Expectancies. *Alcohol. Clin. Exp. Res.* **2019**, *43*, 1967–1977. [CrossRef]
32. Smit, K.; Otten, R.; Voogt, C.; Kleinjan, M.; Engels, R.; Kuntsche, E. Exposure to drinking mediates the association between parental alcohol use and preteen alcohol use. *Addict. Behav.* **2018**, *87*, 244–250. [CrossRef]
33. Schönbeck, Y.; Talma, H.; van Dommelen, P.; Bakker, B.; Buitendijk, S.E.; HiraSing, R.A.; van Buuren, S. Increase in prevalence of overweight in Dutch children and adolescents: A comparison of nationwide growth studies in 1980, 1997 and 2009. *PLoS ONE* **2011**, *6*, e27608. [CrossRef]
34. Statistics Netherlands (CBS). Standaard Onderwijs Indeling (SOI). Available online: https://www.cbs.nl/nl-nl/onze-diensten/methoden/classificaties/onderwijs-en-beroepen/standaard-onderwijsindeling--soi--/standaard-onderwijsindeling-2016 (accessed on 2 March 2020).
35. Scholte, R.H.; Van Lieshout, C.F.; Van Aken, M.A. Perceived relational support in adolescence: Dimensions, configurations, and adolescent adjustment. *J. Res. Adolesc.* **2001**, *11*, 71–94. [CrossRef]
36. Kerr, M.; Stattin, H. What parents know, how they know it, and several forms of adolescent adjustment: Further support for a reinterpretation of monitoring. *Dev. Psychol.* **2000**, *36*, 366–380. [CrossRef] [PubMed]
37. Muthén, L.K.; Muthén, B.O. *Mplus User's Guide*, 8th ed.; Muthén & Muthén: Los Angeles, CA, USA, 1998.
38. Hu, L.T.; Bentler, P.M. Cutoff criteria for fit indexes in covariance structure analysis: Conventional criteria versus new alternatives. *Struct. Equ. Model. Multidiscip. J.* **1999**, *6*, 1–55. [CrossRef]
39. Hill, A.J. Developmental issues in attitudes to food and diet. *Proc. Nutr. Soc.* **2002**, *61*, 259–266. [CrossRef] [PubMed]
40. Brown, K. Nutritional awareness and food preferences of young consumers. *Nutr. Food Sci.* **2000**, *30*, 230–235. [CrossRef]
41. National Institute for Family Finance Information (NIBUD). Nibud Scholierenonderzoek 2016. Available online: https://www.nibud.nl/wp-content/uploads/Nibud-scholierenonderzoek_2016.pdf (accessed on 24 January 2020).
42. Ong, J.X.; Ullah, S.; Magarey, A.; Miller, J.; Leslie, E. Relationship between the home environment and fruit and vegetable consumption in children aged 6–12 years: A systematic review. *Public Health Nutr.* **2017**, *20*, 464–480. [CrossRef] [PubMed]
43. Newman, K.; Harrison, L.; Dashiff, C.; Davies, S. Relationships between parenting styles and risk behaviors in adolescent health: An integrative literature review. *Rev. Lat. Am. Enferm.* **2008**, *16*, 142–150. [CrossRef]
44. Vollmer, R.L.; Mobley, A.R. Parenting styles, feeding styles, and their influence on child obesogenic behaviors and body weight. A review. *Appetite* **2013**, *71*, 232–241. [CrossRef]
45. Elsayed, H.A.; Lissner, L.; Mehlig, K.; Thumann, B.F.; Hebestreit, A.; Pala, V.; Veidebaum, T.; Solea, T.; Moreno, L.; Molnár, D.; et al. Relationship between perception of emotional home atmosphere and fruit and vegetable consumption in European adolescents: Results from the I. Family survey. *Public Health Nutr.* **2020**, *23*, 53–62. [CrossRef]
46. Kremers, S.; Sleddens, E.; Gerards, S.; Gubbels, J.; Rodenburg, G.; Gevers, D.; van Assema, P. General and food-specific parenting: Measures and interplay. *Child Obes.* **2013**, *9* (Suppl. S1), S-22. [CrossRef]
47. Birch, L.L.; Fisher, J.O.; Grimm-Thomas, K.; Markey, C.N.; Sawyer, R.; Johnson, S.L. Confirmatory factor analysis of the Child Feeding Questionnaire: A measure of parental attitudes, beliefs and practices about child feeding and obesity proneness. *Appetite* **2001**, *36*, 201–210. [CrossRef]
48. Kremers, S.P.; Brug, J.; de Vries, H.; Engels, R.C. Parenting style and adolescent fruit consumption. *Appetite* **2003**, *41*, 43–50. [CrossRef]
49. van der Horst, K.; Kremers, S.; Ferreira, I.; Singh, A.; Oenema, A.; Brug, J. Perceived parenting style and practices and the consumption of sugar-sweetened beverages by adolescents. *Health Educ. Res.* **2006**, *22*, 295–304. [CrossRef] [PubMed]

50. Poelman, M.P.; van Lenthe, F.J.; Scheider, S.; Kamphuis, C.B. A Smartphone App Combining Global Positioning System Data and Ecological Momentary Assessment to Track Individual Food Environment Exposure, Food Purchases, and Food Consumption: Protocol for the Observational FoodTrack Study. *JMIR Res. Protoc.* **2020**, *9*, e15283. [CrossRef] [PubMed]
51. Subar, A.F.; Freedman, L.S.; Tooze, J.A.; Kirkpatrick, S.I.; Boushey, C.; Neuhouser, M.L.; Thompson, F.E.; Potischman, N.; Guenther, P.M.; Tarasuk, V.; et al. Addressing Current Criticism Regarding the Value of Self-Report Dietary Data. *J. Nutr.* **2015**, *145*, 2639–2645. [CrossRef] [PubMed]
52. Micha, R.; Karageorgou, D.; Bakogianni, I.; Trichia, E.; Whitsel, L.P.; Story, M.; Penalvo, J.L.; Mozaffarian, D. Effectiveness of school food environment policies on children's dietary behaviors: A systematic review and meta-analysis. *PLoS ONE* **2018**, *13*, e0194555. [CrossRef]
53. Cruwys, T.; Bevelander, K.E.; Hermans, R.C.J. Social modeling of eating: A review of when and why social influence affects food intake and choice. *Appetite* **2015**, *86*, 3–18. [CrossRef]
54. Higgs, S. Social norms and their influence on eating behaviours. *Appetite* **2015**, *86*, 38–44. [CrossRef]
55. Robinson, E.; Otten, R.; Hermans, R.C.J. Descriptive peer norms, self-control and dietary behaviour in young adults. *Psychol. Health* **2016**, *31*, 9–20. [CrossRef]
56. Wouters, E.J.; Larsen, J.K.; Kremers, S.P.; Dagnelie, P.C.; Geenen, R. Peer influence on snacking behavior in adolescence. *Appetite* **2010**, *55*, 11–17. [CrossRef]
57. Lloyd, J.; Creanor, S.; Logan, S.; Green, C.; Dean, S.G.; Hillsdon, M.; Abraham, C.; Tomlinson, R.; Pearson, V.; Taylor, R.S.; et al. Effectiveness of the Healthy Lifestyles Programme (HeLP) to prevent obesity in UK primary-school children: A cluster randomised controlled trial. *Lancet Child Adolesc. Health* **2018**, *2*, 35–45. [CrossRef]
58. Okely, A.D.; Hammersley, M.L. School-home partnerships: The missing piece in obesity prevention? *Lancet Child Adolesc. Health* **2018**, *2*, 5–6. [CrossRef]

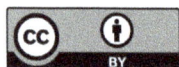 © 2020 by the authors. Licensee MDPI, Basel, Switzerland. This article is an open access article distributed under the terms and conditions of the Creative Commons Attribution (CC BY) license (http://creativecommons.org/licenses/by/4.0/).

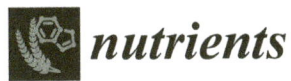

Article

Influence of Teaching Style on Physical Education Adolescents' Motivation and Health-Related Lifestyle

Rubén Trigueros [1,*], Luis A. Mínguez [2], Jerónimo J. González-Bernal [2], Maha Jahouh [2], Raul Soto-Camara [2] and José M. Aguilar-Parra [1,*]

[1] Department of Psychology, Hum-878 Research Team, Health Research Centre, University of Almeria, 04120 Almeria, Spain
[2] Department of Psychology, University of Burgos, 09001 Burgos, Spain; laminguez@ubu.es (L.A.M.); jejavier@ubu.es (J.J.G.-B.); mjx0002@alu.ubu.es (M.J.); rscamara@ubu.es (R.S.-C.)
* Correspondence: rtr088@ual.es (R.T.); jmaguilar@ual.es (J.M.A.-P.)

Received: 27 September 2019; Accepted: 24 October 2019; Published: 29 October 2019

Abstract: According to various WHO reports in 2018, a large number of adolescents worldwide are either overweight or obese. This situation is the result of not following a healthy and balanced diet, combined with a lack of practice of physical activity. In this sense, Physical Education classes could help to solve the problem. The present study seeks to analyze the relationship between the role of the teacher in relation to the structural dimensions of the PE teaching environment and the basic psychological needs and self-motivation of adolescents as determinants of their behaviors related to eating habits and the practice of physical activity. A total of 1127 secondary school adolescents between the ages of 13 and 18 participated in this study. Questionnaires were used: Perceived Autonomy Support Scale, Psychologically Controlling Teaching Scale, Basic Psychological Needs in Physical Education, Frustration of Psychological Needs in PE context, Physical Activity Class Satisfaction Questionnaire, Perceived Locus of Causality Revised, and WHO's Global school-based student health survey. A structural equations model was elaborated to explain the causal relationships between the variables. The results showed that autonomy support positively predicted the three structural dimensions of PE classes, while, in contrast, they were negatively predicted by psychological control. The three structural dimensions positively predicted the satisfaction of psychological needs and negatively predicted the thwarting of psychological needs. Self-determined motivation was positively predicted by the satisfaction of psychological needs and negatively predicted by the thwarting of psychological needs. Finally, self-determined motivation positively predicted healthy eating habits and the practice of physical activity and negatively predicted unhealthy eating habits. Certainly, the results obtained in this study support the postulates of the self-determination theory, demonstrating the predictability of PE class context towards the adoption of healthy lifestyle habits, such as a proper diet and the regular practice of physical activity.

Keywords: Physical Education; teacher; motivation; healthy habits; structural dimensions

1. Introduction

According to the WHO report [1], more than 276 million adolescents (12 to 19 years old) are overweight or suffer from obesity worldwide. This situation can be linked to the fact that our diets include more and more high-calorie foods that are also high in fat, compounded with a decrease in physical activity (PA) due to a more sedentary lifestyle. These data are even more alarming if we consider another WHO report [2], which reached the conclusion that 80% of the adolescent population does not practice in any type of physical sports activity on a regular basis. Indeed, a sedentary lifestyle combined with an unhealthy diet constitutes an important risk factor for the development of chronic diseases, obesity, depression, and anxiety, causing problems at psychological, physical, and emotional levels [3]. Therefore, PE classes represent the ideal medium for the education and overall training of adolescents, which helps them to consolidate active lifestyle habits that will last throughout the rest of their lives. In this regard, according to Spanish Education Law (LOMCE; Ley Organica de la Mejora de la Calidad Educativa), one of the basic objectives of PE classes is to consolidate healthy lifestyle habits, in terms of both diet and responsible PA [4]. Thus, the present study intends to analyze how PE classes can help to consolidate such habits during adolescence.

According to the Self-Determination Theory (SDT; [5]), individuals can be influenced by the social context that surrounds them via two completely different interpersonal styles: controlling style versus autonomy support. The former refers to the use of external pressures, impositions, threats, or punishments, among others, which are seen as the origin of the behaviors manifested by adolescents, negatively affecting personal response, self-knowledge, and effort [6]. In contrast, autonomy support deals with self-initiative, personal self-adjustment, and the mental and physical development of the adolescent [7]. However, SDT not only focuses on interpersonal styles but also on the structure of the environment, which ultimately determines how social agents provide clear, contingent, and coherent directions in the learning context [8]. With regard to PE, structure would involve the class lesson plan, class organization, how activities develop in class, the clarity and quality of teacher feedback, and the practical use of different abilities, among others. Therefore, if a teaching environment is well structured, it is more likely that adolescents will perceive they are learning concepts, improving their motor skills and health, and creating new bonds with classmates [9,10]. For this reason, during classes, it is necessary for the teacher to: (A) provide adolescents with a positive mastery experience, which implies the development and improvement of physical abilities; (B) foster their cognitive development, referring to the development and improvement of cognitive lessons; and (C) successfully execute teaching, which refers to the level of satisfaction with the teaching by the adolescents within the class content [11].

According to SDT, social context influences psychological needs that are defined as essential elements for well-being and personal development [12]. More specifically, there are three psychological needs: autonomy, competence, and relatedness [13]. Autonomy has been defined as the desire to feel that one is the origin and regulator of their own behavior. Competence is the individual's perception that they are capable of demonstrating effectiveness within a particular context. Finally, relatedness refers to the feeling one has of belonging to a specific social environment. However, very recent studies have incorporated novelty as another psychological need, defined as the individual's pursuit of new and different experiences and activities that promote personal development and well-being [14,15].

Essentially, adolescents feel autonomous when they make their own decisions, competent when their abilities meet the challenge, integrated into a given social group, and stimulated when activities are different and appealing. In these circumstances, adolescents will feel their psychological needs are satisfied, thereby allowing them to experience self-determined motivation, which is associated with acquiring new motor skills and contents, learning, improving relationships with classmates, and tuning and acquiring positive adaptive behaviors [5]. On the other hand, if in PE classes adolescents perceive a sense of neglect, excessively difficult or easy challenges, lack of control over their decisions, and tedious activities, adolescents will experience frustration of their psychological needs. As a result, they will tend to perceive non-autonomous motivation or even demotivation, which is associated with a lack of commitment, quitting an activity, a decrease in interpersonal relationships with classmates, and the adoption of negative behaviors [16].

Both social context and psychological needs can significantly influence the motivation of the adolescent towards PE classes [5,7]. According to SDT, motivation can be either non-autonomous or autonomous. The former is related to participation in activities due to acquired obligations or external pressures. Conversely, self-determined motivation is linked to behaviors based on personal initiative and choice. This second type of motivation facilitates the individual's adaptation because it leads to self-regulation of behavior as people tend to persevere due to the personal satisfaction that the activity produces. In contrast, non-autonomous motivation fosters maladaptive behavior as individuals tend to avoid an activity if they are not rewarded [13].

To date, existing studies in the field of PE classes have mainly focused on the clear perspective or, in other terms, the positive vertex of SDT. Such works have analyzed the influence of autonomy support on the satisfaction of psychological needs [17], self-motivation towards PE classes [18], and the influence of the latter on the adoption of healthy lifestyle habits [19]. Thus, in recent years, important lines of research have emerged that concentrate on the dark perspective of SDT or, in other words, the negative vertex [20]. This dark vertex has revealed that the controlling teaching style has negative effects on the satisfaction of psychological needs [21], self-determined motivation [22], resilience [23], and learning [24]; and positive effects on the frustration of psychological needs [21]. However, studies focusing on the dark perspective of SDT are rather scarce, and even more so are those investigations that analyze both types of teaching approaches (autonomy support versus controlling style). As for other research, studies which have analyzed the influence of social context have mainly focused on adolescents' perception of their teacher and not on their perceptions of the structured PE learning environment, when in fact the latter proves fundamental to gaining greater understanding of the relationships between behaviors and results achieved (e.g., healthy eating habits and regular practice of physical activity) by adolescents.

In this sense, it is important to highlight the importance of PE classes towards promoting a healthy and balanced diet and an active lifestyle through a learning climate and the participation of teachers [25]. In this sense, the PE curricula in different EU countries establish that adolescents should receive knowledge related to healthy living habits (diet and PA practice) and motor skills in the aim of improving their health and quality of life [26]. In this way, different studies in the context of Physical Education have shown their relationship with the adoption of active habits by adolescents outside the school context [27]. Similarly, different studies suggest that PE classes have a significant influence on the adoption of a healthy and balanced diet [28].

Taking into account the postulates of SDT and the previously-mentioned points, the present study aims to analyze the relationship between the role of the teacher in relation to the dimensions of the structured environment of PE teaching and the basic psychological needs and self-motivation of adolescents as determining factors of behaviors related to eating habits and the practice of physical activity. Thus, we propose the following hypotheses (see Figure 1): (1) autonomy-support by the teacher will positively predict teaching, cognitive development, and teaching experiences; (2) the controlling teaching style will negatively predict teaching, cognitive development, and teaching experience; (3) teaching, cognitive development, and mastery experiences will positively predict the satisfaction of psychological needs and negatively predict the thwarting of psychological needs; (4) the satisfaction of psychological needs will positively predict autonomous motivation; (5) the thwarting of psychological needs will negatively predict autonomous motivation; (6) autonomous motivation will positively predict healthy eating habits and participation in physical activity and negatively predict unhealthy eating habits.

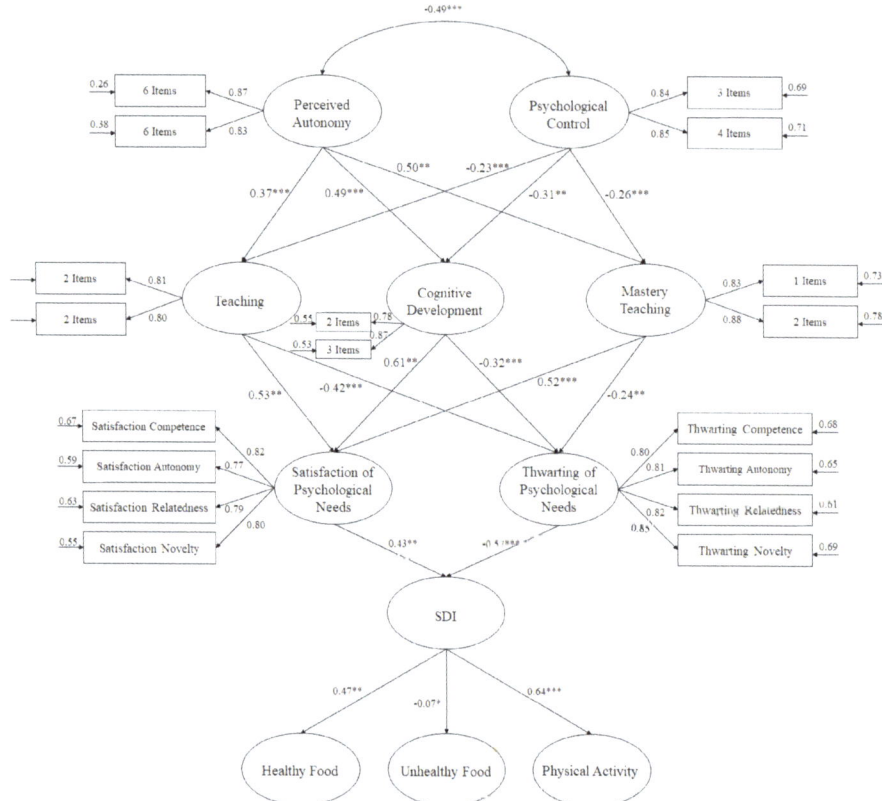

Figure 1. Hypothesized model, where all variables are related to one another. All parameters are statistically significant and are standardized. Note: * $p < 0.05$; ** $p < 0.01$; *** $p < 0.001$.

2. Method

2.1. Participants

A total of 1127 secondary school adolescents participated in this study, of whom 653 were male and 474 were female. The participants were between the ages of 13 and 18 (M = 15.27; SD = 1.35), and came from various secondary schools from the Spanish provinces of Burgos (45.78%) and Almeria (54.22%). The classes were carried out respecting the equal rights and duties of the adolescents. Participation in the study was voluntary but, in order to do so, written authorization from parents or legal guardians was required. Furthermore, all adolescents completed the questionnaires, as one of the criteria for inclusion in the study was to fill in each of the scales.

The sampling used was incidental non-probabilistic, based on those educational centers and adolescents to which access was obtained.

2.2. Instruments

2.2.1. Perceived Autonomy Support

The Spanish version of the Perceived Autonomy Support Scale for Exercise Settings by Hagger et al., [29], which was adapted and validated for the context of PE in Spain by Moreno, Parra, and González-Cutre [24]. There are 12 items that compose this scale, which evaluate only one factor of autonomy support (i.e., I am made to feel guilty when I disappoint my teacher). This tool scores responses using a Likert scale from totally disagree (1) to totally agree (7).

2.2.2. Psychological Control

This aspect was measured using the Psychologically Controlling Teaching Scale (PCTs; Soenens, et al., [30]), validated and adapted by Trigueros, Aguilar-Parra, González-Santos and Cangas [6] to the context of Physical Education. The scale featured the heading "My Physical Education teacher ... ". The questionnaire consisted of 7 items with one single factor (i.e., I am made to feel guilty when I disappoint my teacher). Adolescents had to respond according to a Likert scale, which ranged from totally disagree (1) to totally agree (5).

2.2.3. Satisfaction of Basic Psychological Needs

The tool used in this case was the version of Basic Psychological Needs in Physical Education (BPN-PE; [31]), adapted and validated to the Spanish PE context by Menéndez and Fernández-Río [32], to which Trigueros, Aguilar-Parra, Cangas, Álvarez, and González-Santos [33] integrated the items corresponding to novelty developed by González-Cutre et al., [15]. The scale is comprised of a total of 18 items divided among four factors: 4 correspond to autonomy, 4 correspond to competence, 4 items correspond to relatedness to others, and 6 items correspond to novelty. Adolescents responded according to a Likert scale from totally disagree (1) to totally agree (7).

2.2.4. Thwarting of Psychological Needs

In this case, the present adolescent utilized the version of the Scale for the Frustration of Psychological Needs in physical exercise by Sicilia, Ferriz and Sáenz-Álvarez [34], validated by and adapted to the Spanish PE context by Trigueros, Maldonado, Vicente, González-Bernal, and González-Santos [14]. The scale features the heading "In my PE classes ... " and consists of 17 items, which are divided among the scale factors as follows: 4 items for autonomy, 4 items for competence, 4 items for relatedness to others, and 5 items for novelty. Adolescents responded according to a Likert scale ranging from not true at all (1) to totally true (7).

2.2.5. Perceived Structured PE Teaching Environment

This aspect was measured using the version of the Physical Activity Class Satisfaction Questionnaire [10], adapted and validated to the Spanish PE context by Sicilia, Ferriz, Trigueros and González-Cutre [11]. The questionnaire consists of 45 items divided among 9 factors and features the heading: "Indicate your level of satisfaction with Physical Education classes you've received regarding ... ". However, to measure the satisfaction of adolescents with regard to knowledge of theory, acquired skills, and teaching style, only three factors were utilized: cognitive development, mastery experiences, and teaching. Adolescents indicated their responses according to a Likert scale from totally disagree (1) to totally agree (8).

2.2.6. Motivation

The instrument utilized was the version of the Perceived Locus of Causality Revised (PLOC-R) by Vlachopoulos et al. [35], adapted and validated to the Spanish PE context by Trigueros, Sicilia, Alcaraz and Dumitru [4]. The scale featured the heading "I participate in Physical Education class ... " and is comprised of 23 items grouped among six factors, which measure amotivation, external regulation, introjected regulation, identified regulation, integrated regulation, and intrinsic motivation. The pupils responded according to Likert scale that ranged between not true at all (1) and totally true (7).

Autonomous motivation was also evaluated using the self-determination index (SDI; [36]). The latter was calculated based on the following formula: 3 × intrinsic motivation, 2 × integrated regulation, 1 × identified regulation, −1 × introjected regulation, −2 × external regulation, and −3 × amotivation.

Various works have shown this index to be valid and reliable, and it is applied to obtain a value that facilitates quantifying that level of self-determination.thy and Unhealthy Eating Habits and Participation in Physical Activity

The tool utilized was the Spanish version [37] of the WHO's Global school-based student health survey [38]. For the purposes of this study, we selected indices related to healthy foods (such as fruit, fish, and vegetables) and unhealthy foods (such as candy, snacks, and pastries) consumed on a weekly basis. An index was calculated, which ranged from hardly ever (1) to every day (4). As for participation in physical activity, an index was calculated according to the number of days per week for each physical activity and the duration of each session. This index ranged from 1 to 6. For a more detailed explanation of these indices and their validity, see Balaguer [37].

2.3. Procedure

Firstly, the schools are contacted to ask for their collaboration. Later, the adolescents were asked for informed consent signed by their parents or legal guardians so that they could participate in the study. The PE teachers were then informed of the purpose of the study and that the questionnaires would be administered before the start of classes. Finally, the adolescents were informed that they would participate in research on motivation and healthy habits. This study was conducted according to the recommendations of the American Psychology Association. The experiment was carried out in compliance with the Declaration of Helsinki. Ethics approval was obtained (Ref. UALBIO 2019/014) from the Bioethics Committee for Human Research of the University of Almería.

2.4. Data Analysis

Analyses were performed on the descriptive statistics and the bivariate correlations, in addition to a reliability analysis, using the statistics program SPSS 25. Furthermore, Structural Equations Modelling (SEM) was constructed with the statistics program AMOS 20.

In order to develop the hypothesized model (Figure 1), a maximum likelihood estimation was utilized, along with a bootstrapping procedure. The estimators were not affected by the lack of normality, meaning they were considered robust. With the aim of assessing the tested model, various fit indices were considered: χ^2/df, Incremental Fit Index (IFI), Comparative Fit Index (CFI), Standardized Root Mean Square Residual (SRMR), and Root Mean Square Error of Approximation (RMSEA) plus its confidence interval (CI) at 90%. Values less than 3 for χ^2/df, values for CFI and IFI greater than or close to 0.95, and values for SRMR and RMSEA very close or less than to 0.06 and 0.08 were considered, respectively, as indicating a suitable fit of the model to the data [39].

However, these adjustment indices should be interpreted with caution, as they are too difficult and restrictive when analyzing complex models [40].

3. Results

3.1. Preliminary Analysis

Table 1 displays the bivariate correlations, the average and typical deviation and the reliability analysis conducted using Cronbach's alpha for each of the study variables: autonomy support, psychological control, teaching, cognitive development, mastery experiences, satisfaction of psychological needs, frustration of psychological needs, self-determination index, healthy eating habits, unhealthy eating habits, and physical activity.

Table 1. Correlations between all variables and descriptive statistics.

Factors	M	SD	α	1	2	3	4	5	6	7	8	9	10	11
1. Autonomy Support	4.11	0.68	0.89	-	−0.51 ***	0.62 ***	0.44 ***	0.37 ***	0.48 ***	−0.21 **	0.34 **	0.10 *	−0.14 *	0.23 **
2. Psychological Control	1.36	1.00	0.83		-	−0.26 **	−0.23 **	−0.31 **	−0.52 **	0.60 ***	−0.48 ***	−0.28 ***	0.12 **	−0.36 ***
3. Teaching	5.82	1.08	0.78			-	0.59 ***	0.70 ***	0.47 **	−0.22 ***	0.63 ***	0.34 **	−0.11 *	0.24 **
4. Cognitive Development	4.67	1.43	0.82				-	0.20 ***	0.45 ***	−0.31 **	0.64 ***	0.27 **	−0.23 **	0.42 ***
5. Mastery Experiences	5.23	1.97	0.80					-	0.28 **	−0.39 ***	0.54 **	0.29 *	−0.18 **	0.37 **
6. Satisfaction PN	5.32	0.81	0.87						-	−0.56 ***	0.75 ***	0.38 **	−0.13 *	0.49 ***
7. Thwarting PN	1.76	1.47	0.85							-	−0.37 ***	−0.19 **	0.27 ***	−0.38 **
8. SDI	12.95	13.62	-								-	0.51 ***	−0.14 **	0.67 ***
9. Healthy Food	2.79	0.77	-									-	−0.16 ***	0.69 ***
10. Unhealthy Food	1.92	0.87	-										-	−0.08 *
11. Prac. Physical Activity	3.79	1.24	-											-

Note: PN = Psychological Needs; SDI = Self-Determination Index; Prac. = Practice; *** $p < 0.001$; ** $p < 0.01$; * $p < 0.05$.

As for the correlation analyses, it can be observed that there was a positive correlation between autonomy support, teaching, cognitive development, teaching experiences, satisfaction of psychological needs, SDI, healthy eating habits, and physical activity. These analyses also revealed negative correlations between psychological control, frustration of psychological needs, and unhealthy eating habits. In addition, there was a positive correlation between psychological control, frustration of psychological needs, and unhealthy eating habits, while there was a negative correlation with autonomy support, teaching, cognitive development, teaching experiences, satisfaction of psychological needs, self-determination index, healthy eating habits, and physical activity.

3.2. Structural Equations Modelling Analysis

Due to the complexity of the model, the number of indicators was reduced by at least two to analyze the relationships between the model variables. Subsequently, through an SEM, the hypothesized model was tested [41]. More specifically, the existing variables used were: frustration of basic psychological needs, which included four indicators (frustration of competence, autonomy, relatedness to others, and novelty) [14]; satisfaction of basic psychological needs, which included four factors (satisfaction of competence, autonomy, relatedness to others, and novelty) [33]; and, finally, in the case of autonomy support, it was necessary to divide the 12 items on the scale into two indicators, as were the cases with the 7 items pertaining to psychological control, the 5 items of cognitive development, the four items of teaching, and the 3 items of teaching experiences. This procedure was followed to be able to identify the model [41].

The model for the hypothesized predictive relationships (Figure 1) revealed the following fit indices: χ^2 (215, N = 1127) = 641.35, CFI = 0.95, IFI = 0.95, χ^2/df = 2.98, $p < 0.001$, RMSEA = 0.053. (IC 90% = 0.049 – 057), SRMR = 0.046. The hypothesized model can be considered appropriate since the results are in compliance with the established parameters. In addition, the influence of each factor with respect to other variables was analyzed using standardized regression weights.

4. Discussion

The purpose of the present study was to analyze how the interpersonal style of the teacher influences the dimensions of the structured PE teaching environment and the basic psychological needs and self-motivation of adolescents as determinants of their behaviors related to eating habits and the practice of PA. This study is the first to consider the role of the teacher, in terms of the duality of autonomy support versus controlling style, in the three structural dimensions of PE classes and, in turn, the influence of the latter on psychological needs (satisfaction and frustration). This dual role of the teacher and of the structured teaching environment proves essential given the influence the teacher commands over the emotional, social, and psychological development of adolescents [7]. In addition, this influence is critical in determining how adolescents develop their abilities and knowledge based on a balance between discovery and past experiences, which allow them to make better decisions in their lives, both in the present and future [42]. Moreover, the present work analyzes the influence of PE classes on how adolescents make decisions related to specific aspects of their lifestyles, more specifically eating habits and the regular practice of physical activity. In this regard, the subject of PE is an ideal discipline for ensuring that adolescents develop knowledge and a set of abilities and attitudes which favor the adoption of healthy lifestyle habits.

The results demonstrate that autonomy support positively predicted the three structural dimensions of PE classes (teaching, cognitive development, and mastery experience). Conversely, psychological control negatively predicted the three structural dimensions. Results of studies similar to the present study conducted during the secondary school phase also showed that autonomy support is positively related to PE class structure [43,44]. However, there are hardly any examples of previous studies in the field of PE that link the controlling teaching style to the three structural dimensions of classes. In this sense, the present study sought to address certain limitations of past investigations that analyzed the influence of social context in the teaching field, more specifically, PE. In our case, a model was presented in which not only both roles of the teacher are included but also the structural dimensions and the existing relationships between the teacher's role and the structure. Thus, the results between the dual role of the teacher and PE class structures suggest that when teachers provide directions, rules, and comments necessary for guiding adolescent behavior, teachers tend to employ an autonomy support style. Furthermore, teachers who support autonomy try to respect their adolescents' internal frame of reference, and highly structured teachers try to promote feedback, assistance, knowledge about concepts and motor skills based on suitable challenges, which could explain why teachers who are perceived as partisan to autonomy support are also more prone to be highly structured [45]. The opposite would occur with psychological control by the teacher, given that when teachers tend to utilize unrealistic challenges and negative comments and feedback in their classes, they are not viewed by adolescents as structured.

The results also demonstrate that the three structural dimensions of PE classes positively predict the satisfaction of psychological needs and negatively predict the frustration of psychological needs. These findings are similar to those of previous studies in the field of PE, in particular, a study carried out by Ferriz, et al. [46] with PE adolescents in secondary school, which found that structure was positively related to the satisfaction of psychological needs. Nonetheless, hardly any research can be found that has related structure to the frustration of psychological needs. Thus, the present study aimed to address specific limitations of past investigations. In this sense, the frustration of psychological needs can generate a series of maladaptive behaviors among PE adolescents [47], which is why it is crucial to understand how these needs are generated in order to prevent them. The results of the present study on the relationship between PE class structures and the satisfaction and frustration of psychological needs reveal that those teachers who stimulate the learning of concepts, technical aspects, and fundamentals of PE and who increase adolescents' motor skills through integration and innovative methods make adolescents feel more autonomous, competent, and interested in their PE classes [44]. In this regard, adolescents with more knowledge and motor skills, and who have been exposed to enriching lessons, will perceive themselves as competent enough to carry out PE activities effectively. Possessing this attitude will motivate them to make their own decisions, both individually and in groups, and involve themselves more actively in the teaching-learning process, thereby fostering a greater perception of autonomy and connection to others [48]. In addition, the learning of new physical abilities and the utilization of innovative methods in teaching can be linked to the satisfaction of psychological needs, given that the various motor skills proposed during PE classes are practiced in groups and seek cooperative learning, thus increasing the satisfaction of competence, relatedness to others, and novelty [49].

The results also showed that the thwarting of psychological needs negatively predicted autonomous motivation, whereas the satisfaction of psychological needs positively predicted autonomous motivation. These results are similar to multiple previous studies [42,50,51], where feeling confident and competent during class exercises, feeling integrated and a good interpersonal relationships with classmates and/or with the teacher, feeling ownership of one's own destiny, and participating in original activities helps adolescents to feel an autonomous motivation towards PE classes [52]. Following this, autonomous motivation positively predicted healthy eating habits and the practice of physical activity and negatively predicted unhealthy eating habits. As for other results, autonomous motivation positively predicted healthy eating habits and participation in physical activity and negatively predicted unhealthy eating habits. These findings are similar to the studies conducted by Digelidis, Papaioannou, Laparidis, and Christodoulidis [53] and Hagger and Chatzisarantis [54] who established that motivation towards PE classes positively predicts the practice of physical activity with secondary school adolescents.

On the other hand, no studies were found that analyzed the relationship between autonomous motivation and unhealthy eating habits, yet there was a study that examined the relationship existing between the PE context and both healthy and unhealthy eating habits. However, a study conducted by Jiménez-Castuera, Cervelló, García-Calvo, Santos-Rosa, and Iglesias-Gallego [55] with adolescents showed that those who had a high level of involvement in Physical Education classes showed a greater predisposition towards the practice of physical activity outside the school context and the adoption of a healthy and balanced diet. Therefore, the results of this work suggest that if PE classes stimulate knowledge of theory and physical learning through methods that integrate, adolescents will be positively encouraged to engage in physical activity, maintain healthy eating habits, and reject unhealthy ones.

Finally, it should be noted that Pearson's analysis showed a strong correlation between PA and eating healthy food. This result is similar to multiple studies. In this sense, a study carried out by Pyper, Harrington, and Manson [56] showed that those adolescents who practice physical activity showed a greater predisposition towards a healthy and balanced diet and vice versa. These results can be explained by the fact that those adolescents who are engaged in regular physical activity in order to have a better quality of life showed a greater predisposition towards the adoption of a healthy and balanced diet based on the consumption of healthy foods that contribute to an improvement in physical and personal well-being.

As for the limitations of the present study, it should be noted that it is a correlational study whose results can be interpreted in a different way according to the reader's understanding so that cause-effect relations cannot be established. Therefore, in order to explain the relationships between the variables of the study, we have tried to present possibilities. Therefore, future research should analyze in detail the relationships established between the variables of the study, for example, through intervention studies. In addition, it would also be interesting to determine the influence of the teacher's pro-social skills on the structural dimensions and, in turn, their influence on adolescents' resilience and motivation, for the purpose of ascertaining their effect on the adoption of healthy adaptive behaviors.

5. Conclusions

The results obtained in the present study are in line with the postulates of SDT, demonstrating the importance and predictability of PE class context towards the adoption of healthy lifestyle habits, such as diet and the regular practice of physical activity.

Author Contributions: Conceptualization, R.T.; Methodology, R.T. and J.M.A.-P.; Project administration, L.A.M. and R.S.-C.; Resources, M.J.; Visualization, R.T. and J.J.G.-B.; Writing—original draft, L.A.M; Writing—review and editing, J.M.A.-P., R.T. and J.J.G.-B.

Funding: This research received no external funding.

Conflicts of Interest: The authors declare no conflict of interest.

References

1. Organización Mundial de la Salud. Obesidad y Sobrepeso. 2018. Available online: https://www.who.int/es/news-room/fact-sheets/detail/obesity-and-overweight (accessed on 6 August 2019).
2. Organización Mundial de la Salud. Actividad Física. 2018. Available online: http://www.who.int/es/news-room/fact-sheets/detail/physical-activity (accessed on 6 August 2019).
3. Standal, Ø.F.; Aggerholm, K. Habits, skills and embodied experiences: A contribution to philosophy of physical education. *Sport Ethics Philos.* **2016**, *10*, 269–282. [CrossRef]
4. Trigueros, R.; Sicilia, A.; Alcaraz-Ibáñez, M.; Dumitru, D.C. Spanish adaptation and validation of the Revised Perceived Locus of Causality Scale in physical education. *Cuad. Psicol. Deporte* **2017**, *17*, 25–32.
5. Deci, E.L.; Ryan, R.M. Optimizing students' motivation in the era of testing and pressure: A self-determination theory perspective. In *Building Autonomous Learners*; Springer: Singapore, 2016; pp. 9–29.
6. Trigueros, R.; Aguilar-Parra, J.M.; González-Santos, J.; Cangas, A.J. Validación y adaptación de la escala de control psicológico del profesor hacia las clases de educación física y su efecto sobre las frustraciones de las necesidades psicológicas básicas. *Retos* **2020**, *37*, 167–173.
7. Ricard, N.C.; Pelletier, L.G. Dropping out of high school: The role of parent and teacher self-determination support, reciprocal friendships and academic motivation. *Contemp. Educ. Psychol.* **2016**, *44*, 32–40. [CrossRef]

8. Ntoumanis, N. A self-determination theory perspective on motivation in sport and physical education: Current trends and possible future research directions. In *Advances in Motivation in Sport and Exercise*, 3rd ed.; Roberts, G.C., Treasure, D.C., Eds.; Human Kinetics: Champaign, IL, USA, 2012.
9. Jaakkola, T.; Washington, T.; Yli-Piipari, S. The association between motivation in school physical education and self-reported physical activity during finnish junior high school: A self-determination theory approach. *Eur. Phys. Educ. Rev.* **2012**, *19*, 127–141. [CrossRef]
10. Cunningham, G.B. Development of the physical activity class satisfaction questionnaire (PACSQ). *Meas. Phys. Educ. Exerc. Sci.* **2007**, *11*, 161–176. [CrossRef]
11. Sicilia, A.; Ferriz, R.; Trigueros, R.; González-Cutre, D. Spanish adaptation and validation of the Physical Activity Class Satisfaction Questionnaire (PACSQ). *Univ. Psychol.* **2014**, *4*, 1321–1332.
12. Vansteenkiste, M.; Ryan, R.M. On psychological growth and vulnerability: Basic psychological need satisfaction and need frustration as a unifying principle. *J. Psychother. Integr.* **2013**, *3*, 263. [CrossRef]
13. Ryan, R.M.; Deci, E.L. *Self-Determination Theory: Basic Psychological Needs in Motivation, Development, and Wellness*; Guilford Publications: New York, NY, USA, 2017.
14. Trigueros, R.; Maldonado, J.J.; Vicente, F.; González-Bernal, J.J.; Ortiz, L.; González-Santos, J. Adaptación y Validación al contexto de la Educación Física de la Escala de la Frustración de las Necesidades Psicológicas en el ejercicio físico, con la inclusión de la novedad como necesidad psicológica. *Revista Psicologia de Deporte.* **2019**. Manuscript accept.
15. González-Cutre, D.; Sicilia, Á.; Sierra, A.C.; Ferriz, R.; Hagger, M.S. Understanding the need for novelty from the perspective of self-determination theory. *Personal. Individ. Differ.* **2016**, *102*, 159–169. [CrossRef]
16. Standage, M.; Duda, J.L.; Ntoumanis, N. A test of self-determination theory in school physical education. *Br. J. Educ. Psychol.* **2005**, *75*, 411–433. [CrossRef] [PubMed]
17. Taylor, I.M.; Lonsdale, C. Cultural differences in the relationships among autonomy support, psychological need satisfaction, subjective vitality, and effort in British and Chinese physical education. *J. Sport Exerc. Psychol.* **2010**, *32*, 655–673. [CrossRef] [PubMed]
18. Yli-Piipari, S.; Watt, A.; Jaakkola, T.; Liukkonen, J.; y Nurmi, J.E. Relationships between physical education students' motivational profiles, enjoyment, state anxiety, and self-reported physical activity. *J. Sports Sci. Med.* **2009**, *8*, 327–338. [PubMed]
19. Bartholomew, K.J.; Ntoumanis, N.; Mouratidis, A.; Katartzi, E.; Thogersen-Ntoumani, C.; Vlachopoulos, S. Beware of your teaching style: A school-year long investigation of controlling teaching and student motivational experiences. *Learn. Instr.* **2018**, *53*, 50–63. [CrossRef]
20. Trigueros, R.; Aguilar-Parra, J.M.; Cangas, A.J.; Bermejo, R.; Ferrándiz, C.; López-Liria, R. Influence of emotional intelligence, motivation and resilience on academic performance and the adoption of healthy lifestyle habits among adolescents. *Int. J. Environ. Res. Public Health* **2019**, *16*, 2810. [CrossRef]
21. Trigueros, R.; Aguilar-Parra, J.M.; Cangas, A.J.; López-Liria, R.; Álvarez, J.F. Influence of physical education teachers on motivation, embarrassment and the intention of being physically active during adolescence. *Int. J. Environ. Res. Public Health* **2019**, *13*, 2295. [CrossRef]
22. Haerens, L.; Aelterman, N.; Vansteenkiste, M.; Soenens, B.; Van Petegem, S. Do perceived autonomy-supportive and controlling teaching relate to physical education students' motivational experiences through unique pathways? Distinguishing between the bright and dark side of motivation. *Psychol. Sport Exerc.* **2015**, *16*, 26–36. [CrossRef]
23. Trigueros, R.; Navarro, N.; Aguilar-Parra, J.M.; Ferrándiz, C.; Bermejo, C. Adaptación y Validación de la Escala de Resiliencia en el Contexto de la Actividad Física al Contexto de la Educación Física. *Apunts* **2019**. manuscript accept.
24. Moreno, J.A.; Parra, N.; González-Cutre, D. Influencia del apoyo a la autonomía, las metas sociales y la relación con los demás sobre la desmotivación en educación física. *Psicothema* **2008**, *20*, 636–641.
25. Erpič, S.C. The role of teachers in promoting students' motivation for physical education and physical activity: A review of the recent literature from a self-determination perspective. *Int. J. Phys. Educ.* **2013**, *2*, 2–11.
26. Eurydice. Physical Education and Sport at School in Europe. 2013. Available online: https://eacea.ec.europa.eu/national-policies/eurydice/content/physical-education-and-sport-school-europe_en (accessed on 15 October 2019).

27. Hagger, M.S.; Chatzisarantis, N.L.D. The trans-contextual model of motivation. In *Intrinsic Motivation and Self-Determination in Exercise and Sport*; Hagger, M.S., Chatisarantis, N.L.D., Eds.; Human Kinetics: Leeds, UK, 2007; pp. 53–70.
28. Simons-Morton, B.G.; Parcel, G.S.; Baranowski, T.; Forthofer, R.; O'Hara, N.M. Promoting physical activity and a healthful diet among children: Results of a school-based intervention study. *Am. J. Public Health* **1991**, *81*, 986–991. [CrossRef] [PubMed]
29. Hagger, M.S.; Chatzisarantis, N.L.D.; Hein, V.; Pihu, M.; Soós, I.; Karsai, I. The perceived autonomy support scale for exercise settings (PASSES): Development, validity and cross-cultural invariance in young people. *Psychol. Sport Exerc.* **2007**, *8*, 632–653. [CrossRef]
30. Soenens, B.; Sierens, E.; Vansteenkiste, M.; Dochy, F.; Goosens, L. Psychologically controlling teaching: Examining outcomes, antecedents, and mediators. *J. Educ. Psychol.* **2012**, *104*, 108–120. [CrossRef]
31. Vlachopoulos, S.P.; Katartzi, E.S.; Kontou, M.G. The basic psychological needs in physical education scale. *J. Teach. Phys. Educ.* **2011**, *30*, 263–280. [CrossRef]
32. Menéndez, J.I.; Fernández-Río, J. Versión española de la escala de necesidades psicológicas básicas en educación física. *Rev. Int. Med. y Cienc. Act. Fís. y Deporte* **2018**, *18*, 119–133.
33. Trigueros, R.; Mínguez, L.; González-Bernal, J.J.; Aguilar-Parra, J.M.; Padilla, D. Adaptación y Validación al contexto de la Educación Física de la Escala de la Satisfacción de las Necesidades Psicológicas en el ejercicio físico, con la inclusión de la novedad como necesidad psicológica. *Univ. Psychol.* **2019**. manuscript accept.
34. Sicilia, A.; Ferriz, R.; Sáez-Álvarez, P. Validación española de la escala de frustración de las necesidades psicológicas (EFNP) en el ejercicio físico. *Psychol. Soc. Educ.* **2013**, *1*, 1–19. [CrossRef]
35. Vlachopoulos, S.P.; Katartzi, E.S.; Kontou, M.G.; Moustaka, F.C.; Goudas, M. The revised perceived locus of causality in physical education scale: Psychometric evaluation among youth. *Psychol. Sport Exerc.* **2011**, *12*, 583–592. [CrossRef]
36. Vallerand, R.J. Intrinsic and extrinsic motivation in sport and physical activity. *Handb. Sport Psychol.* **2007**, *3*, 59–83.
37. Balaguer, I. Estilos de vida en la adolescencia. In *Lifestyles in Adolescence*; Promolibro: Valencia, Spain, 2002.
38. Wold, B. Health behavior in school-children: A WHO cross-national survey. *Resour. Package Quest.* **1993**, *94*. [CrossRef]
39. Hair, J.; Black, W.; Babin, B.; Anderson, R.; Tatham, R. *Multivariate Data Analysis*; Pearson/Prentice Hall: Upper Saddle River, NJ, USA, 2006.
40. Marsh, H.W.; Hau, K.T.; Wen, Z. In search golden rules: Comment on hypothesis-testing approaches to setting cutoff values for fit indexes and dangers in overgeneralizing Hu and Bentler's (1999) findings. *Struct. Equ. Model.* **2004**, *11*, 320–341. [CrossRef]
41. McDonald, R.P.; Ho, M.H.R. Principles and practice in reporting structural equation analyses. *Psychol. Methods* **2002**, *7*, 64. [CrossRef] [PubMed]
42. Trigueros, R.; Navarro, N. La influencia del docente sobre la motivación, las estrategias de aprendizaje, pensamiento crítico de los estudiantes y rendimiento académico en el área de Educación Física. *Psychol. Soc. Educ.* **2019**, *11*, 137–150. [CrossRef]
43. Sierens, E.; Vansteenkiste, M.; Goossens, L.; Soenens, B.; Dochy, F. The synergistic relationship of perceived autonomy support and structure in the prediction of self-regulated learning. *Br. J. Educ. Psychol.* **2009**, *79*, 57–68. [CrossRef]
44. Vansteenkiste, M.; Sierens, E.; Goossens, L.; Soenens, B.; Dochy, F.; Mouratidis, A.; Beyers, W. Identifying configurations of perceived teacher autonomy support and structure: Associations with self-regulated learning, motivation and problem behavior. *Learn. Instr.* **2012**, *6*, 431–439. [CrossRef]
45. González-Cutre, D.; Ferriz, R.; Beltrán-Carrillo, V.; Andrés-Fabra, J.A.; Montero-Carretero, C.; Cervelló, E.; Moreno-Murcia, J.A. Promotion of autonomy for participation in physical activity: A study based on the trans-contextual model of motivation. *Educ. Psychol.* **2014**, *34*, 367–384. [CrossRef]
46. Ferriz, R.; González-Cutre, D.; Sicilia, Á.; Hagger, M.S. Predicting healthy and unhealthy behaviors through physical education: A self-determination theory-based longitudinal approach. *Scand. J. Med. Sci. Sports* **2016**, *5*, 579–592. [CrossRef]
47. Hein, V.; Koka, A.; Hagger, M.S. Relationships between perceived teachers' controlling behaviour, psychological need thwarting, anger and bullying behaviour in high-school students. *J. Adolesc.* **2015**, *42*, 103–114. [CrossRef]

48. Ulstad, S.O.; Halvari, H.; Sørebø, Ø.; Deci, E.L. Motivation, learning strategies, and performance in physical education at secondary school. *Adv. Phys. Educ.* **2016**, *1*, 27. [CrossRef]
49. Dyson, B.P.; Linehan, N.; Hastie, P.A. The ecology of cooperative learning in elementary physical education classes. *J. Teach. Phys. Educ.* **2010**, *29*, 113–130. [CrossRef]
50. Xiang, P.; Ağbuğa, B.; Liu, J.; McBride, R.E. Relatedness need satisfaction, intrinsic motivation, and engagement in secondary school physical education. *J. Teach. Phys. Educ.* **2017**, *36*, 340–352. [CrossRef]
51. Cheon, S.H.; Reeve, J.; Lee, Y.; Ntoumanis, N.; Gillet, N.; Kim, B.R.; Song, Y.G. Expanding autonomy psychological need states from two (satisfaction, frustration) to three (dissatisfaction): A classroom-based intervention study. *J. Educ. Psychol.* **2019**, *4*, 685. [CrossRef]
52. De Meyer, J.; Tallir, I.B.; Soenens, B.; Vansteenkiste, M.; Aelterman, N.; Van den Berghe, L.; Haerens, L. Does observed controlling teaching behavior relate to students' motivation in physical education? *J. Educ. Psychol.* **2014**, *106*, 541–554. [CrossRef]
53. Digelidis, N.; Papaioannou, A.; Laparidis, K.; Christodoulidis, T. A one-year intervention in 7th grade physical education classes aiming to change motivational climate and attitudes towards exercise. *Psychol. Sport Exerc.* **2003**, *4*, 195–210. [CrossRef]
54. Hagger, M.S.; Chatzisarantis, N.L.D. Transferring motivation from educational to extramural contexts: A review of the trans-contextual model. *Eur. J. Psychol. Educ.* **2012**, *27*, 195–212. [CrossRef]
55. Jiménez-Castuera, R.; Cervelló, E.; García-Calvo, T.; Santos-Rosa, F.J.; Iglesias-Gallego, D. Estudio de las relaciones entre motivación, práctica deportiva extraescolar y hábitos alimenticios y de descanso en estudiantes de educación física. *Int. J. Clin. Health Psychol.* **2007**, *7*, 385–401.
56. Pyper, E.; Harrington, D.; Manson, H. The impact of different types of parental support behaviours on child physical activity, healthy eating, and screen time: A cross-sectional study. *BMC Public Health* **2016**, *16*, 568. [CrossRef]

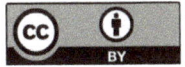

© 2019 by the authors. Licensee MDPI, Basel, Switzerland. This article is an open access article distributed under the terms and conditions of the Creative Commons Attribution (CC BY) license (http://creativecommons.org/licenses/by/4.0/).

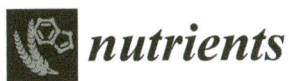

Article

Physical Education Classes as a Precursor to the Mediterranean Diet and the Practice of Physical Activity

Rubén Trigueros [1,*], Luis A. Mínguez [2], Jerónimo J. González-Bernal [2], José M. Aguilar-Parra [1,*], Raúl Soto-Cámara [2], Joaquín F. Álvarez [1] and Patricia Rocamora [3]

[1] Department of Psychology, Hum-878 Research Team, Health Research Centre, University of Almeria, 04120 Almeria, Spain; jalvarez@ual.es
[2] Department of Psychology, University of Burgos, 09001 Burgos, Spain; laminguez@ubu.es (L.A.M.); jejavier@ubu.es (J.J.G.-B.); rscamara@ubu.es (R.S.-C.)
[3] Department of Nursing, Physiotherapy and Medicine, Health Research Centre, University of Almería, 04120 Almería, Spain; rocamora@ual.es
* Correspondence: rtr088@ual.es (R.T.); jmaguilar@ual.es (J.M.A.-P.); Tel.: +34-950-015376 (R.T.); Tel.: +34-950-015376 (J.M.A.-P.)

Received: 22 November 2019; Accepted: 14 January 2020; Published: 16 January 2020

Abstract: Physical activity and a healthy, balanced diet are remaining unresolved issues among young people. According to the World Health Organization, young people do not get enough exercise during the week, and physical education classes are the best way to promote healthy habits. This study aims to analyze how the role of the teacher influences the frustration of psychological needs, coping strategies, motivation, and the adoption of healthy eating habits through the Mediterranean diet and the regular practice of physical activity. The study involved 1031 boys and 910 girls between the ages of 13 and 18. To explain the relationships between the different variables included in this study, a model of structural equations has been developed. The results showed that autonomy support negatively predicted the frustration of four psychological needs. The failure to meet four psychological needs negatively predicted resilience. Likewise, resilience positively predicted autonomous motivation, and this positively predicted the Mediterranean diet and the practice of physical activity. Thus, the results obtained in the present study are in line with those of various studies wherein physical education classes were seen to help consolidate healthy living habits.

Keywords: adolescence; mediterranean diet; physical activity; physical education; resilience; motivation

1. Introduction

Adolescence is a transitional stage in which there are important biological, psychological, and social changes that can affect young people's well-being [1]. It is during this period of life that young people begin to have greater independence and make their first independent decisions, establishing many of the behaviors that they will maintain during adulthood [2,3]. Thus, it is during adolescence that physical activity begins to decrease as they prefer to do other types of activities, and young people begin to eat unhealthy foods [4]. Therefore, in recent years, with the emergence of the science of positive psychology [5], new models have emerged that, starting from a deficit-based approach, move toward a new paradigm focused on the optimal functioning of adolescents [6]. These models of positive development attempt to determine the factors that promote healthy development during adolescence, with the adoption of healthy lifestyle habits and the regular practice of physical activity being two of the main aspects on which they focus [7].

1.1. Self-Determination Theory

Self-determination theory (SDT) is a social theory that tries to explain the influence of the social environment on people's adaptive and nonadoptive behaviors [8]. In this sense, the SDT affirms that the influence of the social context turns out to be key for the development of certain behaviors in individuals and that this can occur through two antagonistic interpersonal styles, controlling style versus autonomy support [9]. The first assumes that the social environment tries to influence the behavior of the person through the use of punishment, threats, obligations, abuses, and so forth, being observed by the individual as the cause of their behaviors [10]. This implies the loss of self-initiative and personal effort. On the other hand, autonomy support refers to the physical and mental self-development of the individual and to one's own initiative, with the support of the social environment and without eternal pressures [9]. Depending on the teacher, the choice of interpersonal style will influence the psychological needs of students in a significant way [8].

Starting from the postulates of SDT, psychological needs can be understood as essential elements that promote personal well-being [11]. These psychological needs include competence, which refers to feeling capable when performing any activity; autonomy, which is defined as the desire to feel that behavior originates with oneself; and relatedness, which refers to feeling integrated and understood by the social reference group [12]. In recent years, starting with the studies of González-Cutre et al. [13] and Trigueros et al. [14], it has been proposed that we incorporate a fourth psychological need called novelty, which is linked to the individual's search for new activities and experiences that will contribute to personal well-being.

In this way, students who feel autonomous and competent when they make the decision to participate in a given activity, and who feel integrated and supported by the social reference group and view the activities as interesting and different, will experience the satisfaction of their psychological needs, which, in turn, will significantly influence the autonomous motivation of the individual, which is related to learning new skills, psychological well-being, commitment, effort, and the adoption of adaptive behaviors [8,9]. On the other hand, if students feel controlled in their behaviors, experience a feeling of abandonment, or view the class challenges as complicated or repetitive, they will feel that their psychological needs are thwarted due to experiencing controlled motivation or even amotivation [10]. This type of motivation is generally linked to a lack of commitment to activity, abandonment, poor interpersonal relationships, and the adoption of nonadaptive behaviors [15].

In this way, psychological needs, as well as the social context, can have a significant influence on the student's motivation towards PE classes [16,17]. Following SDT, motivation can be controlled motivation or autonomous. The first is related to the acquisition of external obligations or rewards when performing an activity. On the contrary, autonomous motivation is linked to one's own choice and internal commitment when carrying out any activity. The latter leads to the self-regulation of the individual's behavior, remaining in the activity due to the internal satisfaction it produces. However, controlled motivation facilitates nonadaptive behaviors in that the student tends to move away from the activity if the obligation disappears and/or is not rewarded [18].

Current studies in the field of physical education classes are primarily interested in the clear perspective of SDT, examining the influence of autonomy support, the satisfaction of psychological needs, and autonomous motivation on the adoption of behaviors conducive to a healthy lifestyle [19]. Therefore, in recent years, a new line of research has emerged that has focused on the dark perspective of SDT, since PE classes can be an environment that can generate behaviors contrary to the adoption of healthy lifestyle habits if the controlling style of the teacher leads to the frustration of psychological needs [20], generating negative effects on autonomous motivation [21], learning [22], metacognitive strategies [23], and emotional intelligence [24]. Few studies have even looked at the dark side of SDT, or taken into consideration autonomy support versus the controlling style.

1.2. Resilience

Among the psychological factors affecting personal well-being is resilience, which refers to a set of positive psychological qualities linked to individual adaptation to adverse circumstances through the use of positive coping strategies [25]. In this sense, PE classes, unlike other academic areas, are characterized by continuous exposure to a series of adverse and stressful experiences that students must confront at some point (difficult situations, injuries, friction with classmates and/or teachers, etc.) [24]. In this way, the area of PE contributes to the development of human capacity to face, overcome, and come out stronger from those experiences of adversity.

These adverse situations and their overcoming were initially studied through the metatheory of resilience [26]. This theory affirms that resilience begins in a situation of physical, mental, and spiritual balance that is interrupted when a given situation arises where the individual does not possess sufficient resources or abilities to face adverse situations [27]. Over time, the individual will readjust and regain balance by raising his level of resilience or homeostasis. However, this metatheory suffers from a series of limitations since it considers resilience as a linear model, whereby the individual faces a single event. Furthermore, the model does not explain how emotions can affect the process of overcoming. This is especially important given the protective nature of emotions in the behavior of individuals [28] and the fact that those who show a capacity for resilience value emotions as facilitators to achieve it [29].

Because of these limitations, Fletcher and Sarkar [30] tried to reconceptualize the definition of resilience as being linked to the possession and presence of protective and vulnerability factors within and outside the people, which encourage the helpful adaptation to risk. Thus, the protective factors of resilience have been explored through numerous research trying to identify the qualities of resilient individuals in the fields of health [31], work [32], and sports [33], and there are a few studies in the educational field (e.g., [34]), focused mainly on external aspects of students rather than on what happens during classes and the influence it exerts with respect to the psychological responses it generates in students.

These resilience models propose a comprehensive representation of the process and outcome of resilience during the process of adaptation to difficulties. Furthermore, these models allow their application in psychoeducational interventions for the prevention of risk behaviors.

1.3. Objective and Hypothesis

As stated above, the aim of this study is to analyze how the role of the teacher influences the frustration of psychological needs, coping strategies, motivation, and the adoption of healthy eating habits through the Mediterranean diet and regular practice of physical activity. The following hypotheses have been formulated: (1) autonomy support will negatively predict the frustration of psychological needs, while psychological control will positively predict it; (2) frustration of psychological needs will negatively predict resilience; (3) resilience will positively predict autonomous motivation; (4) autonomous motivation will positively predict the adoption of a healthful Mediterranean diet and the practice of physical activity.

2. Materials and Methods

2.1. Participants

The secondary school students participating in the study were 1031 boys and 910 girls, for a total of 1941 students. The age of the students ranged from 13 to 18 years (M = 15.34; SD = 1.22). The PE classes were held with equal rights and duties between students belonging to various secondary educational centers in Almeria and Burgos.

Informed consent from parents or legal guardians as well as voluntary participation in the study were the criteria for the inclusion of students in the study.

2.2. Instruments

Perceived autonomy support. The Scale used was the Perceived Autonomy Support Scale for Exercise Settings (PASSES; [35]), validated for the Spanish PE context [36]. The scale evaluates a single factor called autonomy support through 12 items. The scale ranges from totally disagreed (1) to totally agreed (7).

Psychological controlling. The scale used was a version of the Psychologically Controlling Teaching Scale (PCTs; [37]), validated and adapted for the PE context [38]. The instrument consists of seven items with a single factor. The scale ranges from totally disagreed (1) to totally agreed (7).

Frustration of psychological needs: The scale utilized was the scale of Frustration of Psychological Needs, validated and adapted for the Spanish PE context [39]. The instrument consists of 17 items, distributed as follows among each of the factors that make up the scale: four items for competence, four items for relatedness, four items for autonomy, and five items for novelty. The scale ranges from not at all true (1) to totally true (7).

Resilience in PE. The instrument utilized was the Resilience Scale in PE classes [40]. This questionnaire consists of 25 items divided between two factors that measure acceptance of oneself and the context and personal competence. The scale ranges from total disagreement (1) to total agreement (7).

Motivation. The instrument utilized was the Perceived Locus of Causality Revised (PLOC-R; [41]), validated and adapted for the Spanish context of PE [42]. The questionnaire consists of 23 items divided into six factors that measure different kinds of motivation. The scale ranges from not at all true (1) to totally true (7).

For this study, the self-determination index (SDI) was calculated to quantify the level of self-determination [43] using the following formula: 3 × intrinsic motivation, 2 × integrated regulation, 1 × identified regulation, −1 × introjected regulation, −2 × external regulation, and −3 × demotivation.

Practice of physical activity. The Spanish version [44] of the WHO Health Behavior of Schoolchildren Survey [45] was used. For this study, we selected indices that referred to the practice of physical activity; an index was calculated based on the number of days per week of each physical activity and the duration of the sessions. For a more detailed explanation of the indices and their validity, see Balaguer [44].

Mediterranean diet. The kidmed scale [46], which measures dietary patterns related to the Mediterranean diet, was used. This scale has an index oscillating from 0 to 12 across 16 questions. Those questions with a negative connotation with respect to the Mediterranean diet were assigned a value of −1, and those with a positive connotation were assigned +1.

2.3. Procedure

Once the questionnaires were selected, several educational centers were contacted whose PE teachers were briefed of the aims of the present study in relation to resilience, motivation, and the adoption of healthy dietary patterns and the practice of physical activity. Subsequently, those students who wished to participate in the present study were required to obtain written authorization from their parents or legal guardians, since they were minors. The scales were given before the beginning of PE classes during the third week of February of the academic year 2018/2019, with the answers to the questionnaires being anonymous.

El estudio se llevó a cabo en cumplimiento de las directrices de la Asociación Psicológica Americana. The Research Ethics Committee of the University of Almeria, Spain, approved the present study (Ref. UALBIO 2019/014).

2.4. Data Analysis

In this study, the statistical program SPSS 25 was used to perform different analyses (e.g., mean, standard deviation, bivariate correlations, and reliability). In addition, the statistical program AMOS 20 was used to create a structural equation model (SEM).

With the purpose of analyzing the hypothetical model (Figure 1), the bootstrapping procedure was used, together with the maximum likelihood method. The estimators were considered robust despite the lack of normality. To judge the model tested, several adjustment rates were examined: values of χ^2/df lower than 3, comparative fit index (CFI) and incremental fit index (IFI) values close to or higher than 0.95, and root mean square error of approximation (RMSEA) and standardized root mean square residual (SRMR) values lower than or very close to 0.06 and 0.08, respectively [47], were considered indicative of the adequate fit of the model. However, for complex models these adjustment fit rates should be interpreted with care as it is very restrictive [48].

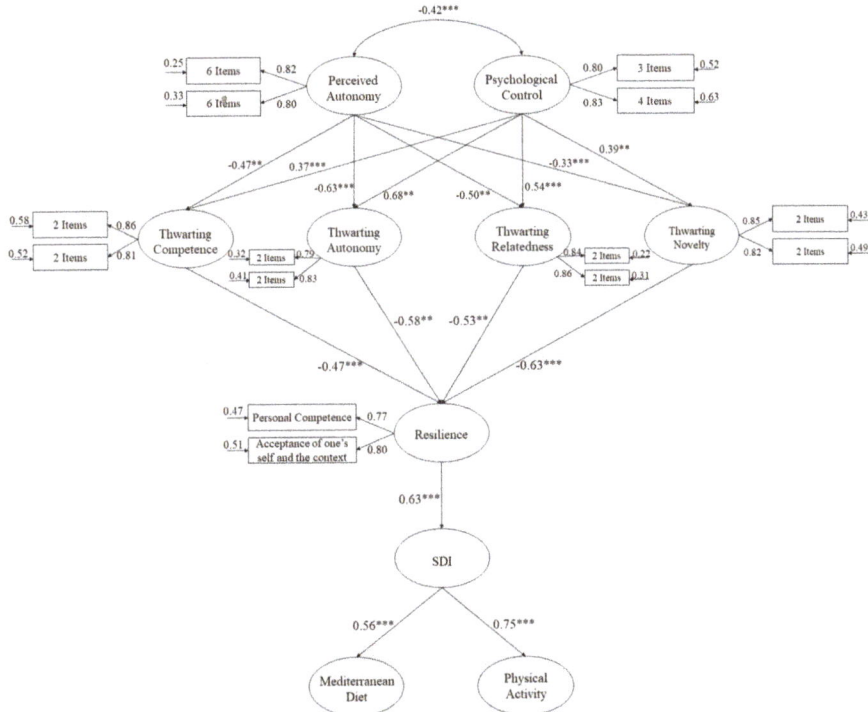

Figure 1. Hypothesized model, analizado a través de un SEM. All parameters are statistically significant. Note: *** $p < 0.001$; ** $p < 0.01$. SDI: self-determination index.

3. Results

3.1. Preliminary Analyses

Table 1 presents analyses of mean and standard deviation, bivariate correlations through Pearson, and reliability analysis through Cronbach's α of all variables supporting autonomy, psychological controlling, frustration of competition, relatedness, autonomy, novelty, resilience, SDI, adoption of the Mediterranean diet, and practice of physical activity.

Table 1. Preliminary analyses and correlations.

Factors	M	SD	α	1	2	3	4	5	6	7	8	9	10
1. Autonomy Support	4.65	0.98	0.84	—	−0.47 ***	−0.52 **	−0.75 ***	−0.31 ***	−0.38 ***	0.21 **	0.42 ***	0.30 **	0.17 **
2. Psychological Controlling	1.68	1.24	0.81		—	0.28 **	0.32 **	0.49 **	0.52 **	0.61 **	0.25 **	−0.37 ***	−0.52 ***
3. T. of Competence	5.23	0.78	0.80			—	0.71 ***	0.58 **	0.77 **	−0.72 ***	−0.23 ***	−0.31 **	−0.31 *
4. T. of Autonomy	5.41	0.43	0.83				—	0.56 ***	0.61 ***	−0.61 **	−0.51 **	−0.37 **	−0.42 ***
5. T. of Relatedness	5.01	0.94	0.88					—	0.53 **	−0.59 ***	−0.35 **	−0.22 *	−0.37 *
6. T. of Novelty	4.95	0.86	0.87						—	−0.36 ***	−0.42 ***	−0.25 **	−0.51 ***
7. Resilience	5.89	1.17	0.92							—	0.67 ***	0.59 **	−0.35 *
8. SDI	14.67	12.93	—								—	0.33 ***	−0.59 ***
9. Mediterranean Diet	8.52	1.77	—									—	−0.60 ***
10. Physical Activity	4.32	1.35	—										—

Note: T = Thwarting; SDI = Self-Determination Index; *** $p < 0.001$; ** $p < 0.01$; * $p < 0.05$.

As for the correlation analyses, these reflected a positive correlation between autonomy support, SDI, resilience, adoption of the Mediterranean diet, and physical activity practice, as well as negative correlations regarding psychological controlling, frustration of competition, relatedness, autonomy, novelty, and adoption of the Mediterranean diet.

3.2. Structural Equations Model

Due to the complexity of the hypothesized model (Figure 1), the number of indicators was reduced to at least two, in order to be able to analyze the relationships between the study variables [49]. In particular, the latent variables considered were resilience, which included two indicators (personal competence and acceptance of self and context) [39]; autonomy support, divided into the 12 items of the scale using two indicators, including the seven items of psychological control, the four items of frustration of competence, relatedness, autonomy, and novelty, all in order to identify the model [49].

The hypothesized predictive relationships model (Figure 1) showed that the adjustment indices were satisfactory: χ^2 (106, N = 1941) = 241.52, χ^2/df = 2.28, $p < 0.001$, IFI = 0.95, CFI = 0.95, RMSEA = 0.053 (Confidence interval 90% = 0.049–0.058), SRMR = 0.048. These results were adjusted to the established parameters, so the proposed model was accepted as adequate. In addition, the contribution of each of the factors to the prediction of other variables was examined through standardized regression weights.

4. Discussions

This study has attempted to analyze the way in which the interpersonal style of the teacher (autonomy support versus psychological controlling) influences the thwarting of psychological needs, resilience, autonomous motivation, and behaviors related to the adoption of balanced eating habits, which are typical of the Mediterranean diet, and the practice of physical activity.

This study examines for the first time the dual role of the teacher in each of the factors belonging to the thwarting of psychological needs, with special emphasis on the novelty factor as it is a psychological need of recent incorporation. In this sense, the studies that have analyzed the influence of the teacher based on the psychological needs of students have focused only on the bright side, that is, on the influence of autonomy support on the satisfaction of psychological needs, and the dark side is still under-represented in the literature [50,51]. On the other hand, the present study contemplates for the first time the influence of the dark side of SDT, that is, psychological control and the frustration of needs, on resilience in the field of Physical Education. In this sense, analyzing the dual role of the teacher is relevant given the influence it has on the social, emotional, and psychological development of students [52]. In addition, it is important to highlight the influence that teachers have on students' development of skills and knowledge based on a balance between discovery and previous experiences, which allows them to overcome difficulties and make the best decisions related to the adoption of behaviors that promote health [53,54]. In addition, PE is a discipline where students are exposed to continuous stressful situations and where, through the different proposed activities, they feel continually challenged, so success and failure are often present during classes [55–57]. Such circumstances can influence the opinion they have of PE classes, assuming a greater or lesser involvement of students during PE classes, affecting in the final stage the development of behaviors aimed at the adoption of healthy lifestyle habits.

The results of the present study showed how psychological control positively predicted the thwarting of the psychological needs of autonomy, competence, relatedness, and novelty; on the contrary, autonomy support negatively predicted each of the thwarting frustrations. These results cannot be compared with similar studies because we have no evidence of research that has analyzed this relationship in the context of physical education, especially in relation to the thwarting of novelty. However, there is evidence from studies that have analyzed the influence of autonomy support on the satisfaction of psychological needs, and in recent years, on novelty. A study with high school students conducted by Zhang, Solmon, Kosma, Carson, and Gu [58] showed that those students who had high levels of support for their autonomy were positively related to each of the factors of satisfaction of psychological needs, except novelty. However, a recent study by González-Cutre, Romero-Elías, Jiménez-Loaisa, Beltrán-Carrillo, and Hagger [59] showed how support for autonomy was positively related to each of the factors of psychological needs, including novelty. Similarly, different studies in the field of PE (i.e., [60–63]) have shown how support for autonomy predicted the thwarting of psychological needs in a negative way; on the contrary, psychological control predicted them in a positive way, but the thwarting of psychological needs was analyzed in a global way and not through the factors that compose it. Thus, the results of the present study are in line with the results shown in previous studies and within the postulates of SDT. The results on the dual role of the teacher and the frustrations of the psychological needs established in this study can be explained by the fact that if students feel coerced, rejected, and limited in their decision-making, they will feel frustrated in their perceived autonomy and competence, in their psychological well-being, and in their psychological needs.

The results also show that frustration of the four psychological needs of competence, autonomy, relatedness, and novelty negatively predicts resilience. These results are similar to those of various studies in the field of sports, where the negative effect of the frustration of psychological needs in relation to resilience has been observed, in contrast to the positive influence of satisfaction [64,65]. However, there is little evidence of research that has analyzed the influence of the four factors of frustration of psychological needs on student resilience in the context of PE. In this sense, the present study shows the importance of creating a climate where students feel their psychological needs are satisfied, in order to promote the adaptability of the students to the multiple vicissitudes that present themselves while participating in the different PE classes. To this end, it is essential that teachers try to instill in their students personal skills, social competence, autonomy, optimism, and hope [66].

Finally, the results revealed that resilience positively predicted autonomous motivation. However, studies on resilience in the field of PE classes are scarce, and there is little evidence of studies that have analyzed this relationship. Despite this situation, there are some studies in the university setting [67] that have analyzed the influence of resilience on autonomous motivation that indicated that those students who are psychologically resistant (resilient) use internal coping strategies that lead them to perceive, access, and precisely regulate their behaviors in order to achieve their objectives (autonomous motivation). Furthermore, in the sporting context, there are several studies that have explored this relationship. A study carried out by Sarkar and Fletcher [27] with semiprofessional athletes showed that those who had high levels of resilience showed a higher predisposition towards exercise merely for improving their own capacities and abilities through the overcoming of challenges. In addition, the present study has shown how autonomous motivation towards PE classes acted as a predictor of the adoption of a Mediterranean diet and regular physical activity. Although no studies have previously analyzed the relationship between motivation and the Mediterranean diet, a study by Jiménez, Cervelló, García, Santos, and Iglesias [68] with adolescents showed that those who actively participated in Physical Education classes were more predisposed to physical activity and a healthy, balanced diet. In such a way, the results of this work suggest that if physical education classes facilitate the adaptability and motivation of the students, they will feel more predisposed towards the assimilation of contents, abilities, and attitudes that focus on the carrying out of physical activity and maintaining a healthy and balanced diet typical of the Mediterranean [69].

There are several limitations to this study that must be highlighted. First, it is based primarily on self-reported measures. Secondly, it is a relational study that does not allow for the extrapolation of cause-effect relationships, so that the results obtained can be interpreted in different ways, based on the individual's viewpoint. On the other hand, future studies should analyze the influence of the social context on the resilience levels of students as well as on well-eating habits and regular practice of physical activity, given that it is a time of multiple changes for adolescents.

5. Conclusions

The results of the present study are in line with the theoretical postulates referring to the dark side of the SDT, demonstrating the importance and influence of the context of PE classes in the adoption of a Mediterranean diet and the regular practice of physical activity. In order to do so, teachers must create educational programs that focus on the achievement of basic objectives in the area of PE, based on positive experiences focused on the resolution of complex motor skills.

Author Contributions: Conceptualization, R.T., J.F.Á.; Methodology, R.T. and J.M.A.-P.; Formal analysis, R.T. and J.M.A.-P.; Investigation, L.A.M., and P.R.; Project administration, J.J.G.-B. and J.F.Á; Resources, P.R. and R.S.-C.; Visualization, R.T. and J.J.G.-B.; Writing—original draft, L.A.M., and R.T.; Writing—review and editing, J.M.A.-P., R.S.-C. and J.J.G.-B. All authors have read and agreed to the published version of the manuscript.

Funding: Convocatoria Ayudas a Transferencia de Investigación "Transfiere" 2018 (Ref. 001364).

Conflicts of Interest: The authors declare no conflict of interest.

References

1. Eryilmaz, A. A model for subjective well-being in adolescence: Need satisfaction and reasons for living. *Soc. Indic. Res.* **2012**, *3*, 561–574. [CrossRef]
2. Brassai, L.; Piko, B.F.; Steger, M.F. A reason to stay healthy: The role of meaning in life in relation to physical activity and healthy eating among adolescents. *J. Health Psychol.* **2015**, *5*, 473–482. [CrossRef]
3. Morris, B.; Lawton, R.; McEachan, R.; Hurling, R.; Conner, M. Changing self-reported physical activity using different types of affectively and cognitively framed health messages, in a student population. *Psychol. Health Med.* **2016**, *2*, 198–207. [CrossRef]
4. Organización Mundial De La Salud. Actividad Física. 2018. Available online: http://www.who.int/es/newsroom/fact-sheets/detail/physical-activity (accessed on 6 August 2019).
5. Seligman, M.E.; Csikszentmihalyi, M. Positive psychology: An introduction. In *Flow and the Foundations of Positive Psychology*; Springer: Dordrecht, The Netherlands, 2014; pp. 279–298.
6. Oliva, A.; Ríos, M.; Antolín, L.; Parra, A.; Hernando, A.; Pertegal, M. Más allá del déficit: Construyendo un modelo de desarrollo positivo adolescente. *Infanc. Y Aprendiz.* **2010**, *2*, 223–234. [CrossRef]
7. Geldhof, G.J.; Bowers, E.P.; Mueller, M.K.; Napolitano, C.M.; Callina, K.S.; Lerner, R.M. Longitudinal analysis of a very short measure of positive youth development. *J. Youth Adolesc.* **2014**, *6*, 933–949. [CrossRef] [PubMed]
8. Ryan, R.M.; Deci, E.L. *Self-Determination Theory: Basic Psychological Needs in Motivation, Development, and Wellness*; Guilford Publications: New York, NY, USA, 2017.
9. Reeve, J.; Jang, H.R.; Jang, H. Personality-based antecedents of teachers' autonomy-supportive and controlling motivating styles. *Learn. Individ. Differ.* **2018**, *62*, 12–22. [CrossRef]
10. Trigueros, R.; Fernández-Campoy, J.M.; Alías, A.; Aguilar-Parra, J.M.; Segura, M.C.L. Adaptación y validación española del Controlling Coach Behaviors Scale (CCBS). *Int. J. Dev. Educ. Psychol.* **2017**, *1*, 417–427. [CrossRef]
11. Chen, B.; Vansteenkiste, M.; Beyers, W.; Boone, L.; Deci, E.L.; Van der Kaap-Deeder, J.; Durize, B.; Lens, W.; Matos, L.; Ryan, R.M.; et al. Basic psychological need satisfaction, need frustration, and need strength across four cultures. *Motiv. Emot.* **2015**, *2*, 216–236. [CrossRef]
12. Núñez, J.L.; León, J. Autonomy support in the classroom: A review from self-determination theory. *Eur. Psychol.* **2015**, *4*, 275. [CrossRef]
13. González-Cutre, D.; Sicilia, Á.; Sierra, A.C.; Ferriz, R.; Hagger, M.S. Understanding the need for novelty from the perspective of self-determination theory. *Personal. Individ. Differ.* **2016**, *102*, 159–169. [CrossRef]
14. Trigueros, R.; Mínguez, L.A.; González-Bernal, J.J.; Aguilar-Parra, J.M.; Padilla, D.; Álvarez, J.F. Validation of the Satisfaction Scale of Basic Psychological Needs in Physical Education with the Incorporation of the Novelty in the Spanish Context. *Sustainability* **2019**, *22*, 6250. [CrossRef]
15. Escamilla-Fajardo, P.; Núñez-Pomar, J.M.; Prado-Gascó, V.J.; Calabuig-Moreno, F. Physical Education classes, sports motivation and adolescence: Study of some moderating variables. *Rev. De Psicol. Del Deporte* **2017**, *3*, 97–101.

16. Trigueros, R.; Aguilar-Parra, J.M.; Cangas, A.J.; López-Liria, R.; Álvarez, J.F. Influence of physical education teachers on motivation, embarrassment and the intention of being physically active during adolescence. *Int. J. Environ. Res. Public Health* **2019**, *13*, 2295. [CrossRef] [PubMed]
17. Kokkonen, J.; Yli-Piipari, S.; Kokkonen, M.; Quay, J. Effectiveness of a creative physical education intervention on elementary school students' leisure-time physical activity motivation and overall physical activity in Finland. *Eur. Phys. Educ. Rev.* **2019**, *3*, 796–815. [CrossRef]
18. García-González, L.; Sevil-Serrano, J.; Abós, A.; Aelterman, N.; Haerens, L. The role of task and ego-oriented climate in explaining students' bright and dark motivational experiences in Physical Education. *Phys. Educ. Sport Pedagog.* **2019**, *4*, 344–358. [CrossRef]
19. Pérez-González, A.M.; Valero-Valenzuela, A.; Moreno-Murcia, J.A.; Sánchez-Alcaraz, B.J. Systematic Review of Autonomy Support in Physical Education. *Apunt. Educ. Física I Esports* **2019**, *138*, 51–61.
20. Costa, S.; Cuzzocrea, F.; Gugliandolo, M.C.; Larcan, R. Associations between parental psychological control and autonomy support, and psychological outcomes in adolescents: The mediating role of need satisfaction and need frustration. *Child Indic. Res.* **2016**, *4*, 1059–1076. [CrossRef]
21. Patall, E.A.; Steingut, R.R.; Vasquez, A.C.; Trimble, S.S.; Pituch, K.; Freeman, J.L. Daily autonomy supporting or thwarting and students' motivation and engagement in the high school science classroom. *J. Educ. Psychol.* **2018**, *2*, 269. [CrossRef]
22. Trigueros, R.; Navarro, N. La influencia del docente sobre la motivación, las estrategias de aprendizaje, pensamiento crítico de los estudiantes y rendimiento académico en el área de Educación Física. *Psychol. Soc. Educ.* **2019**, *1*, 137–150. [CrossRef]
23. Trigueros, R.; Aguilar-Parra, J.M.; López-Liria, R.; Rocamora, P. The Dark Side of the Self-Determination Theory and Its Influence on the Emotional and Cognitive Processes of Students in Physical Education. *Int. J. Environ. Res. Public Health* **2019**, *16*, 4444. [CrossRef]
24. Trigueros, R.; Aguilar-Parra, J.M.; Cangas, A.J.; Bermejo, R.; Ferrandiz, C.; López-Liria, R. Influence of emotional intelligence, motivation and resilience on academic performance and the adoption of healthy lifestyle habits among adolescents. *Int. J. Environ. Res. Public Health* **2019**, *16*, 2810. [CrossRef] [PubMed]
25. Connor, K.M.; Davidson, J.R. Development of a new resilience scale: The Connor-Davidson resilience scale (CD-RISC). *Depress. Anxiety* **2003**, *2*, 76–82. [CrossRef] [PubMed]
26. Richardson, G.E. The metatheory of resilience and resiliency. *J. Clin. Psychol.* **2002**, *3*, 307–321. [CrossRef] [PubMed]
27. Sarkar, M.; Fletcher, D. Psychological resilience in sport performers: A review of stressors and protective factors. *J. Sports Sci.* **2014**, *15*, 1419–1434. [CrossRef]
28. Pekrun, R.; Lichtenfeld, S.; Marsh, H.W.; Murayama, K.; Goetz, T. Achievement emotions and academic performance: Longitudinal models of reciprocal effects. *Child Dev.* **2017**, *5*, 1653–1670. [CrossRef] [PubMed]
29. Pekrun, R.; Linnenbrink-Garcia, L. Academic emotions and student engagement. In *Handbook of Research on Student Engagement*; Springer: Boston, MA, USA, 2012; pp. 259–282.
30. Fletcher, D.; Sarkar, M. A grounded theory of psychological resilience in Olympic champions. *Psychol. Sport Exerc.* **2012**, *5*, 669–678. [CrossRef]
31. Heath, M.A.; Donald, D.R.; Theron, L.C.; Lyon, R.C. AIDS in South Africa: Therapeutic interventions to strengthen resilience among orphans and vulnerable children. *Sch. Psychol. Int.* **2014**, *3*, 309–337. [CrossRef]
32. MacEachen, E.; Polzer, J.; Clarke, J. "You are free to set your own hours": Governing worker productivity and health through flexibility and resilience. *Soc. Sci. Med.* **2008**, *5*, 1019–1033. [CrossRef]
33. Galli, N.; Vealey, R.S. "Bouncing back" from adversity: Athletes' experiences of resilience. *Sport Psychol.* **2008**, *3*, 316–335. [CrossRef]
34. Salavera, C.; Usán, P.; Jarie, L. Emotional intelligence and social skills on self-efficacy in Secondary Education students. Are there gender differences? *J. Adolesc.* **2017**, *60*, 39–46. [CrossRef]
35. Hagger, M.S.; Chatzisarantis, N.L.D.; Hein, V.; Pihu, M.; Soós, I.; Karsai, I. The perceived autonomy support scale for exercise settings (PASSES): Development, validity and cross-cultural invariance in young people. *Psychol. Sport Exerc.* **2007**, *8*, 632–653. [CrossRef]
36. Moreno, J.A.; Parra, N.; González-Cutre, D. Influencia del apoyo a la autonomía, las metas sociales y la relación con los demás sobre la desmotivación en educación física. *Psicothema* **2008**, *20*, 636–641.
37. Soenens, B.; Sierens, E.; Vansteenkiste, M.; Dochy, F.; Goosens, L. Psychologically controlling teaching: Examining outcomes, antecedents, and mediators. *J. Educ. Psychol.* **2012**, *104*, 108–120. [CrossRef]

38. Trigueros, R.; Aguilar-Parra, J.M.; González-Santos, J.; Cangas, A.J. Validación y adaptación de la escala de control psicológico del profesor hacia las clases de educación física y su efecto sobre las frustraciones de las necesidades psicológicas básicas. *Retos* **2020**, *37*, 167–173.
39. Trigueros, R.; Maldonado, J.J.; Vicente, F.; González-Bernal, J.J.; Ortiz, L.; González-Santos, J. Adaptación y Validación al contexto de la Educación Física de la Escala de la Frustración de las Necesidades Psicológicas en el ejercicio físico, con la inclusión de la novedad como necesidad psicológica. *Rev. Psicol. De Deporte* **2019**. (Manuscript Accept).
40. Trigueros, R.; Navarro, N.; Aguilar-Parra, J.M.; Ferrándiz, C.; Bermejo, C. Adaptación y Validación de la Escala de Resiliencia en el Contexto de la Actividad Física al Contexto de la Educación Física. *Sportis* **2020**. (Manuscript Accept).
41. Vlachopoulos, S.P.; Katartzi, E.S.; Kontou, M.G.; Moustaka, F.C.; Goudas, M. The revised perceived locus of causality in physical education scale: Psychometric evaluation among youth. *Psychol. Sport Exerc.* **2011**, *12*, 583–592. [CrossRef]
42. Trigueros, R.; Sicilia, A.; Alcaraz-Ibáñez, M.; Dumitru, D.C. Spanish adaptation and validation of the Revised Perceived Locus of Causality Scale in physical education. *Cuad. Psicol. Deporte* **2017**, *17*, 25–32.
43. Vallerand, R.J. Intrinsic and extrinsic motivation in sport and physical activity. *Handb. Sport Psychol.* **2007**, *3*, 59–83.
44. Balaguer, I. Estilos de vida en la adolescencia. In *Lifestylesin Adolescence*; Promolibro: Valencia, Spain, 2002.
45. Wold, B. *Health Behaviour in School Children: A Cross-National Survey*; Resource Package of Questions 1993-94; University of Bergen: Bergen, Norway, 1995.
46. Serra-Majem, L.; Ribas, L.; Ngo, J.; Ortega, R.M.; Garcia, A.; Perez-Rodrigo, C.; Aranceta, J. Food, Youth and the Mediterranean Diet in Spain. Development of KIDMED; Mediterranean Diet Quality Index in children and adolescents. *Public Health Nutr.* **2004**, *7*, 931–935. [CrossRef]
47. Hair, J.; Black, W.; Babin, B.; Anderson, R.; Tatham, R. *Multivariate Data Analysis*; Pearson/Prentice Hall: Upper Saddle River, NJ, USA, 2006.
48. Marsh, H.W.; Hau, K.T.; Wen, Z. In search golden rules: Comment on hypothesis-testing approaches to setting cutoff values for fit indexes and dangers in overgeneralizing Hu and Bentler's (1999) findings. *Struct. Equ. Model.* **2004**, *11*, 320–341. [CrossRef]
49. McDonald, R.P.; Ho, M.H.R. Principles and practice in reporting structural equation analyses. *Psychol. Methods* **2002**, *7*, 64. [CrossRef] [PubMed]
50. Haerens, L.; Aelterman, N.; Vansteenkiste, M.; Soenens, B.; Van Petegem, S. Do perceived autonomy-supportive and controlling teaching relate to physical education students' motivational experiences through unique pathways? Distinguishing between the bright and dark side of motivation. *Psychol. Sport Exerc.* **2015**, *16*, 26–36. [CrossRef]
51. Cannard, C.; Lannegrand-Willems, L.; Safont-Mottay, C.; Zimmermann, G. Brief report: Academic amotivation in light of the dark side of identity formation. *J. Adolesc.* **2016**, *47*, 179–184. [CrossRef]
52. Ricard, N.C.; Pelletier, L.G. Dropping out of high school: The role of parent and teacher self-determination support, reciprocal friendships and academic motivation. *Contemp. Educ. Psychol.* **2016**, *44*, 32–40. [CrossRef]
53. Harris, J. Physical education teacher education students' knowledge, perceptions and experiences of promoting healthy, active lifestyles in secondary schools. *Phys. Educ. Sport Pedagog.* **2014**, *5*, 466–480. [CrossRef]
54. Mitchell, F.; Gray, S.; Inchley, J. This choice thing really works ... Changes in experiences and engagement of adolescent girls in physical education classes, during a school-based physical activity programme. *Phys. Educ. Sport Pedagog.* **2015**, *6*, 593–611. [CrossRef]
55. Cecchini, J.; González, C.; Carmona, Á.; Arruza, J.; Escartí, A.; Balagué, G. The influence of the physical education teacher on intrinsic motivation, self-confidence, anxiety, and pre-and post-competition mood states. *Eur. J. Sport Sci.* **2001**, *4*, 1–11. [CrossRef]
56. Legey, S.; Aquino, F.; Lamego, M.K.; Paes, F.; Nardi, A.E.; Neto, G.M.; Mura, G.; Sancassiani, F.; Rocha, N.; Murillo-Rodríguez, E.; et al. Relationship Among Physical Activity Level, Mood and Anxiety States and Quality of Life in Physical Education Students. *Clin. Pract. Epidemiol. Ment. Health CP EMH* **2017**, *13*, 82. [CrossRef]
57. Kumar, S.; Bhukar, J.P. Stress level and coping strategies of college students. *J. Phys. Educ. Sport Manag.* **2013**, *1*, 5–11.

58. Zhang, T.; Solmon, M.A.; Kosma, M.; Carson, R.L.; Gu, X. Need support, need satisfaction, intrinsic motivation, and physical activity participation among middle school students. *J. Teach. Phys. Educ.* **2011**, *1*, 51–68. [CrossRef]
59. González-Cutre, D.; Romero-Elías, M.; Jiménez-Loaisa, A.; Beltrán-Carrillo, V.J.; Hagger, M.S. Testing the need for novelty as a candidate need in basic psychological needs theory. *Motiv. Emot.* **2019**. [CrossRef]
60. Hein, V.; Koka, A.; Hagger, M.S. Relationships between perceived teachers' controlling behaviour, psychological need thwarting, anger and bullying behaviour in high-school students. *J. Adolesc.* **2015**, *42*, 103–114. [CrossRef] [PubMed]
61. Lochbaum, M.; Jean-Noel, J. Perceived Autonomy-Support Instruction and Student Outcomes in Physical Education and Leisure-Time: A Meta-Analytic Review of Correlates. *Rev. Int. De Cienc. Del Deporte* **2015**, *43*, 29–47. [CrossRef]
62. Ulstad, S.; Halvari, H.; Sørebø, Ø.; Deci, E.L. Motivation, learning strategies, and performance in physical education at secondary school. *Adv. Phys. Educ.* **2016**, *1*, 27. [CrossRef]
63. Liu, J.; Bartholomew, K.; Chung, P.K. Perceptions of teachers' interpersonal styles and well-being and ill-being in secondary school physical education students: The role of need satisfaction and need frustration. *Sch. Ment. Health* **2017**, *4*, 360–371. [CrossRef]
64. González, L.; Castillo, I.; Balaguer, I. Análisis del papel de la resiliencia y de las necesidades psicológicas básicas como antecedentes de las experiencias de diversión y aburrimiento en el deporte femenino. *Rev. De Psicodidáctica* **2019**, *2*, 131–137. [CrossRef]
65. Trigueros, R.; Aguilar-Parra, J.M.; Cangas-Diaz, A.J.; Fernandez-Batanero, J.M.; Manas, M.A.; Arias, V.B.; Lopez-Liria, R. The influence of the trainer on the motivation and resilience of sportspeople: A study from the perspective of self-determination theory. *PLoS ONE* **2019**, *8*, e0221461. [CrossRef]
66. Trigueros-Ramos, R.; Gómez, N.N.; Aguilar-Parra, J.M.; León-Estrada, I. Influencia del docente de Educación Física sobre la confianza, diversión, la motivación y la intención de ser físicamente activo en la adolescencia. *Cuad. De Psicol. Del Deporte* **2019**, *1*, 222–232.
67. Magnano, P.; Craparo, G.; Paolillo, A. Resilience and Emotional Intelligence: Which role in achievement motivation. *Int. J. Psychol. Res.* **2016**, *1*, 9–20. [CrossRef]
68. Jiménez, R.; Cervelló, E.; García, T.; Santos, F.J.; Iglesias, D. Estudio de las relaciones entre motivación, práctica deportiva extraescolar y hábitos alimenticios y de descanso en estudiantes de educación física. *Int. J. Clin. Health Psychol.* **2007**, *7*, 385–401.
69. Trigueros, R.; Mínguez, L.A.; González-Bernal, J.J.; Jahouh, M.; Soto-Camara, R.; Aguilar-Parra, J.M. Influence of Teaching Style on Physical Education Adolescents' Motivation and Health-Related Lifestyle. *Nutrients* **2019**, *11*, 2594. [CrossRef] [PubMed]

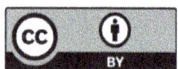

© 2020 by the authors. Licensee MDPI, Basel, Switzerland. This article is an open access article distributed under the terms and conditions of the Creative Commons Attribution (CC BY) license (http://creativecommons.org/licenses/by/4.0/).

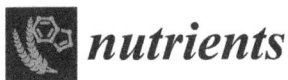

Article

Socioeconomic Inequalities in the Retail Food Environment around Schools in a Southern European Context

Julia Díez [1,*], Alba Cebrecos [1], Alba Rapela [1], Luisa N. Borrell [2,3], Usama Bilal [1,4,5] and Manuel Franco [1,2,6]

1. Public Health and Epidemiology Research Group, School of Medicine, Universidad de Alcalá, Alcalá de Henares, 28801 Madrid, Spain
2. Department of Surgery, Medical and Social Science, School of Medicine, Universidad de Alcalá, 28801 Madrid, Spain
3. Department of Epidemiology and Biostatistics, Graduate School of Public Health and Health Policy, The City University of New York, New York, NY 10027, USA
4. Urban Health Collaborative, Drexel Dornsife School of Public Health, Philadelphia, PA 19104, USA
5. Department of Epidemiology and Biostatistics, Drexel Dornsife School of Public Health, Philadelphia, PA 19104, USA
6. Department of Epidemiology, Johns Hopkins Bloomberg School of Public Health, Baltimore, MD 21205, USA
* Correspondence: julia.diez@uah.es; Tel.: +34-918-852-522

Received: 24 May 2019; Accepted: 2 July 2019; Published: 3 July 2019

Abstract: Across Europe, excess body weight rates are particularly high among children and adolescents living in Southern European contexts. In Spain, current food policies appeal to voluntary self-regulation of the food industry and parents' responsibility. However, there is no research (within Spain) assessing the food environment surrounding schools. We examined the association between neighborhood-level socioeconomic status (NSES) and the spatial access to an unhealthy food environment around schools using both counts and distance measures, across the city of Madrid. We conducted a cross-sectional study citywide (n = 2443 census tracts). In 2017, we identified all schools (n = 1321) and all food retailers offering unhealthy food and beverages surrounding them (n = 6530) using publicly available data. We examined both the counts of retailers (within 400 m) and the distance (in meters) from the schools to the closest retailer. We used multilevel regressions to model the association of neighborhood-level socioeconomic status (NSES) with both measures, adjusting both models for population density. Almost all schools (95%) were surrounded by unhealthy retailers within 400 m (median = 17 retailers; interquartile range = 8–34). After adjusting for population density, NSES remained inversely associated with unhealthy food availability. Schools located in low-NSES areas (two lowest quintiles) showed, on average, 29% (IRR (Incidence Rate Ratio) = 1.29; 95% CI (Confidence Interval) = 1.12, 1.50) and 62% (IRR = 1.62; 95% CI = 1.35, 1.95) more counts of unhealthy retailers compared with schools in middle-NSES areas (ref.). Schools in high-NSES areas were farther from unhealthy food sources than those schools located in middle-NSES areas (β = 0.35; 95% CI = 0.14, 0.47). Regulating the school food environment (within and beyond school boundaries) may be a promising direction to prevent and reduce childhood obesity.

Keywords: children; adolescents; schools; food environment; health inequalities; socioeconomic status; spatial exposure; Spain

1. Introduction

Childhood obesity is one of the most important public health challenges globally [1]. Globally, about 213 million children and adolescents (aged 5 to 19 years) are overweight, with 124 million being obese [2]. Across Europe, rates of excess body weight are particularly high among children and adolescents living in Southern European countries [3,4]. In Spain, about 27% of children (aged 2 to 14 years) and 19% of youth (aged 15 to 17 years) were overweight or obese in 2017, respectively [5]. Being obese in childhood increases the risk of illnesses in adulthood (e.g., cardiovascular diseases) and premature mortality [6,7]. Obesity may be shaped by the development of healthy eating behaviors during childhood and adolescence [8]. Eating behaviors are important because they could help prevent or promote weight gain.

In general, eating behaviors are shaped by different physical, sociocultural, economic, and political factors, such as the food environment [9–11]. The food environment defines the foods available and accessible to children and adolescents. Furthermore, the influence of physical environmental factors (e.g., healthy food availability) may be shaped by social environmental factors (e.g., socioeconomic status) [10–12]. Children and adolescents spend a significant amount of time at schools, and thus, the school food environment has been considered a key arena for obesity prevention [13,14]. Yet, for most of the school-based intervention trials on childhood obesity prevention and control, results are mixed and modest [15–17]. Thus, school surroundings are receiving increased attention because children and adolescents frequent food outlets on their way to and back from school, which may impact their food choices [17–19]. Indeed, adolescents leave school boundaries during breaks to buy foods and drinks [20].

Assessments of the food environment surrounding schools are common in the literature. However, most studies have been conducted in Anglo-Saxon settings such as the US, the UK, New Zealand, or Australia [21–24]. A study in the US found that adolescents obtained more than 90% of their total calories from outside the school setting [23]. Another study conducted in New Zealand showed that more than 60% of urban schools had an unhealthy food outlet within walking distance [22]. A recent UK longitudinal study found a positive association between the count of food retailers and adolescents' weight status [24]. Although effect sizes were small, these findings taken together highlight the potential impact of the food environment surrounding children's schools on children's food choices, diet quality, and body weight.

As a result, zoning policies to restrict unhealthy food retailing are being proposed and implemented [25]. Indeed, the New London Plan includes a new policy (Policy E9) stating that "hot food takeaways should not be permitted to be located within 400 m walking distance of an existing or proposed primary or secondary school" [26]. Similar to London, where 38% of children are overweight or obese, one in four children living in Madrid or Barcelona have excess body weight [5,26]. Adopting a Health in All Policies approach, Franco et al. identified a series of multisector policy changes that may help tackle childhood obesity in Spain [27]. Yet, the Spanish Strategy for Nutrition, Physical Activity, and the Prevention of Obesity (NAOS strategy) appeals to parents' responsibility and voluntary self-regulation of the food industry [28]. In addition, previous research has shown that, in regard to the nutritional quality of the products sold in vending machines within schools, compliance with NAOS recommendations is low [29].

Moreover, area-level socioeconomic status (SES) has been linked to spatial patterns of retailers' locations. Across the US, according to Zenk et al., schools located in more disadvantaged areas had 32% more fast food retailers than those located in more advantaged areas [30]. In New Zealand, unhealthy food access (within walking distance) was also greater from urban schools located in more deprived areas than from schools located in the leastdeprived areas [22]. Yet, studies conducted across European contexts have shown mixed results. For example, Timmermans et al. found that unhealthy options were the default around schools in the Netherlands [20]. Yet, they found few differences by area-SES level [20]. To date, no research assessing the environment surrounding children and adolescents (e.g., the food environment around schools) has been conducted in Spain. However, retail food environments have been shown to vary widely across geographical settings [31–33].

To fill this gap, our aim was to assess the spatial access to an unhealthy food environment around schools across the city of Madrid (Spain) and to examine its association with neighborhood-level socioeconomic status.

2. Materials and Methods

2.1. Study Design and Sample

This study was nested within the European-funded project "Heart Healthy Hoods", which assesses the association between the urban environment (including the food environment) and cardiovascular outcomes [34]. We did not require any institutional review board for this study because no human participants were involved.

Our study area comprised the entire city of Madrid, which was administratively divided into 21 Districts, 128 neighborhoods, and 2443 census tracts in 2017. For reference, census tracts are the smallest geographic units for which population data are released in Spain. Their average population size was 1323 residents in 2017 [35]. The city of Madrid covers a total area of 60,577 km^2, has a population density of 525,444 hab./km^2, and 14.2% of residents are of age between 3 and 18 years.

Schools were our spatial unit of analysis. We included all schools in the city, limiting the age range of children attending school to 3–18 years. We classified schools into (1) preschools, including children 3 to 6 years old; (2) primary schools, from the ages of 6 to 11 years (which may also offer preschool); and (3) secondary schools, including adolescents from 12 to 18 years, which may also offer preschool and primary education. We included public and private (including both independent private and partially publicly funded private) schools. The latter ("concerted" schools) are private schools receiving regional government support to provide education services, which follow the same rules as schools in the public system.

Data were obtained from the Department of Education of Madrid's Government (for 2017). Each school was mapped using the geographic x and y coordinates and entered into a Geographic Information System, using ArcGIS software 10.3. We then overlaid school points to census tract boundaries using a spatial join. The latter allowed us to identify the fitting census tract for each school.

2.2. Neighborhood-Level Socioeconomic Status

Our main exposure of interest was neighborhood-level socioeconomic status (NSES). Consistent with previous studies [36,37], we measured NSES using a composite index constructed at census tract level. This NSES index included seven indicators: (1) low education (% people above 25 years with primary studies or below); (2) high education (% people above 25 years with college or university studies); (3) part-time work (% workers in part-time jobs); (4) temporary work (% people aged 16 years or over in temporary jobs); (5) manual work (% of people aged 16 years or over working in manual or unqualified jobs with respect to the total employed population aged 16 or over); (6) unemployment (% of residents aged 16 years or over registered as unemployed among residents aged 16–64 years); and (7) average housing prices (€/m^2). These indicators relate to the four domains (education, occupation, living conditions, and wealth) suggested for the study of the effect of structural policies on health inequalities in Spain [38].

Further details on the development and use of this SES index have been previously published [36,37]. In brief, we collected data from a combination of administrative databases (the municipal census, social security, and employment services registries) and from a real estate company (IDEALISTA). All administrative data were freely available for the year 2017, except for the average housing prices, which were available for 2016.

For each indicator, we centered to the mean and divided it by the standard deviation (of all census tracts in Madrid) to obtain a z-score of each indicator. We then averaged z-scores of each indicator, resulting in a z-score for each domain (education, wealth, occupation, and living conditions); and finally, we calculated the composite index of NSES by summing the z-score of each of the four domains.

We operationalized the NSES measure as a categorical variable using quintiles based on the SES index score distribution across census tracts: Low (Q1), middle low (Q2), middle (Q3, reference category), middle high (Q4), and high (Q5).

2.3. Food Environment Assessment

Our main outcome was the spatial access to unhealthy retailers around schools in terms of (1) availability (counts) of retailers selling unhealthy foods and beverages within 400 m; and (2) distance to the nearest unhealthy retailer (in m).

We defined as unhealthy foods both energy-dense, nutrient-poor food products (e.g., potato chips, chocolate) and sugar-sweetened beverages (beverages containing caloric sweeteners). Although there is no universally accepted classification (or definition) of unhealthy food retailers, ours is consistent with previous studies examining food stores featuring unhealthy food [20,39].

Food retail data for 2017 came from a secondary database of the Department of Statistics of Madrid City Council (*Censo de Locales y Actividades*) covering all licensed premises citywide. This information is collected for statistical purposes, licensing, and inspections. It is freely available, yearly updated, and collects name, location, and type for each premise. Retailer types are coded following the statistical classification of economic activities in the European Community (NACE) [40]. For example, according to the NACE codes for food retail, any premise including retail sale (not for consumption on the premises) of bread, cakes, flour confectionery, and sugar confectionery in specialized stores is coded as a bakery.

Building on previous research using this dataset [39], we identified 6530 outlets within the scope of the study (selling any unhealthy food products): nonspecialized retailers (e.g., supermarkets or convenience stores), specialized retailers (e.g., bakeries), and food services (e.g., fast-food restaurants or take-away-only restaurants). We excluded full-service restaurants and outlets within closed facilities (e.g., airports) as children are unlikely to use them. Table S1 shows the food retailers considered for each category.

We defined unhealthy food availability by counting all unhealthy outlets within a 400 m Euclidian buffer surrounding each school, which reflects a 5 min walking distance. We also determined accessibility by calculating Euclidean distance measures (in meters) from school locations and the nearest "unhealthy" outlet, by performing a Near tool of ArcGIS (ArcGIS 10.3, ESRI). There is empirical evidence that suggests 400 m (or about a 5 min walk) [41] is the distance students are most likely to walk (on foot) during a short break. This small distance has previously been used in food environment research [20,42,43].

2.4. Population Density

Consistent with previous research [44,45] showing that certain types of food stores (e.g., fast-foods) are often co-located in areas of high residential density, we used population density to control for urban factors in our models. We specified population density, at the census tract level, by dividing the number of residents over the land area of the census tract. Population data came from the 2017 municipal registry. We downloaded the information for the administrative boundaries (including land area of the census tracts) from the Spanish National Mapping Agency.

2.5. Statistical Analysis

We used the Kruskal–Wallis test to compare medians for school characteristics (school type, funding, NSES, and population density) according to both count and distance measures. We then assessed the association between NSES and both dependent variables (counts of unhealthy outlets and distance to the nearest unhealthy outlet).

To model the counts of unhealthy food outlets, we used a multilevel negative binomial regression model. We used a negative binomial regression (instead of a Poisson regression) because the data were over-dispersed and zero-inflated [46]. To model the distance to the nearest unhealthy outlet, we log-transformed the variable and fit a multilevel linear mixed model. We transformed the distance variable because of its extreme right skewness, and thus, non-normal distribution. For all models, the unit of analysis was the school. To assess the need for random intercepts at different levels, we fit empty models and progressively added random intercepts for census tract ($n = 2443$), neighborhood ($n = 128$), and district ($n = 21$), and compared models using the AIC (Akaike Information Criterion). The final models had 4 levels, with random intercepts for the three administrative units. We then fit unadjusted models, with NSES quintiles as the main independent variable, and adjusted models with population density as a covariate.

In addition, we ran sensitivity analyses for both outcomes (counts of and distance to unhealthy retailers) without considering supermarkets. Supermarkets are difficult to categorize as unhealthy retailers because they offer a wide variety of both healthy (e.g., fresh fruits) and unhealthy food products (such as chips, unhealthy ready meals, sugar-sweetened beverages, etc.) [47,48]. We conducted all analyses using STATA/SE 15 (StataCorp., College Station, TX, USA).

3. Results

We identified 1321 schools. About a third of them were private (37%) or concerted (27.5%), while 35.4% were public schools. Preschools represented 45.6% of all schools, whereas 22.2% were primary schools and 32.2% were secondary schools. For reference, roughly 36% of all preschoolers and 37% of children attended public preschools and primary schools, respectively, during the academic year 2017–2018. Approximately 50% did so in secondary schools for the same year (data not shown).

3.1. Counts of Unhealthy Food Outlets and Neighborhood-level SES

We found that 94.9% of the schools had unhealthy outlets within 400 m. As shown in Table 1, there was a clear gradient in terms of NSES and the median number of unhealthy outlets per school. The median number of available unhealthy food outlets around the schools located in low-NSES areas was greater (median = 24) than those located in high-NSES ones (median = 8; $p = 0.0001$). We also found differences in terms of the type of school. Concerted schools had higher counts of unhealthy food outlets (median = 23) relative to those publicly-funded schools (median = 16; $p = 0.0001$).

Table 1. Counts (within 400 m) of and distance (m) to unhealthy retailers across schools ($n = 1321$) citywide (Madrid, 2017).

Characteristics	Availability		Distance	
	Median (IQR) [1]	p-Value [2]	Median (IQR) [1]	p-Value [2]
Type of school		0.0037		0.0011
Preschools	16 (8–31)		82 (48.10–151.85)	
Primary schools	18 (9–36)		90.07 (57.93–141.01)	
Secondary schools	17 (8–35)		100.80 (55.21–171.13)	
Funding		0.0001		0.0001
Public	16 (9–29)		100.78 (62.40–153.68)	
Private	14 (5–31)		90.41 (47.61–188.85)	
Concerted	23 (12–44)		74.16 (48.22–126.77)	
Neighborhood-level SES		0.0001		0.0001
Low-SES	24 (13–37)		77.09 (46.50–129.26)	
Middle-low	18 (13–30)		81.35 (54.65–128.57)	
Middle	16 (8–36)		77.52 (43.59–127.63)	
Middle-high	19 (7–43)		92.01 (52.83–162.77)	
High-SES	8 (3–16)		145.92 (77.48–254.71)	

Table 1. Cont.

Characteristics	Availability		Distance	
	Median (IQR) [1]	p-Value [2]	Median (IQR) [1]	p-Value [2]
Population density (10^3 residents/km^2)		0.0001		0.0001
Low	22 (13–39)		71.52 (44.85–125.07]	
Medium	21 (10–39)		83.99 (51.85–139.69]	
High	10 (4–21)		123.26 (69.24–193.26]	

[1] IQR=interquartile range, [2] p-values correspond to Kruskal–Wallis test. SES: socioeconomic status.

Figure 1a shows the spatial distribution of schools citywide, according to their availability of unhealthy retailers within a 400 m buffer. We found an east-west divide, with schools located in eastern parts of the city showing lower counts of retailers than schools located in the western part of the city. Schools located in suburban areas of the city also appeared to perform better (e.g., less unhealthy food sources around them) than those located in the city center.

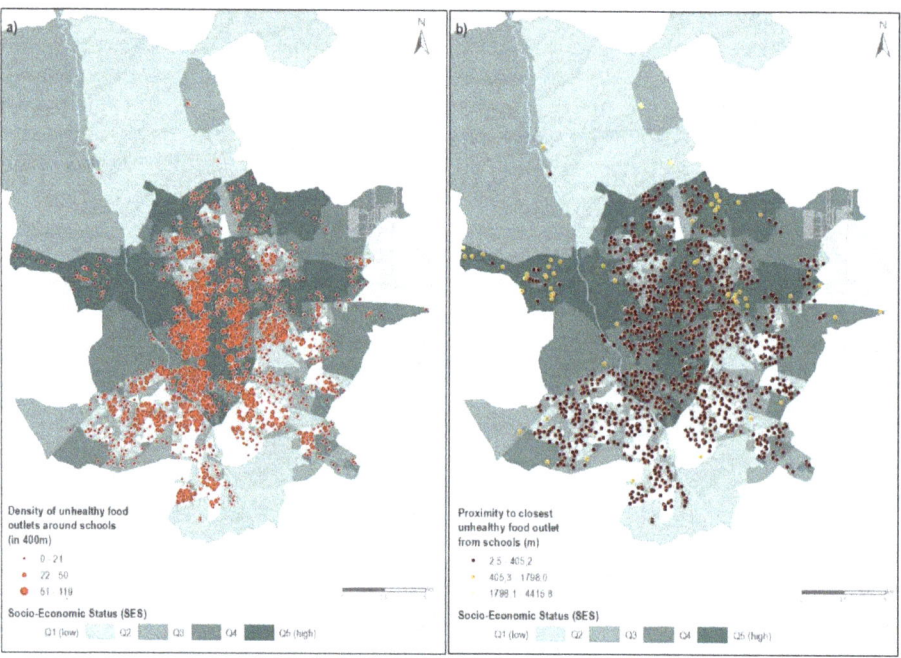

Figure 1. Schools in the city of Madrid (2017): (**a**) by availability of unhealthy outlets around schools; (**b**) by schools' proximity to the closest unhealthy food source.

Figure 2 shows the results from the binomial regression model assessing the socioeconomic correlates of unhealthy retailers' availability. As such, it depicts the results of the models on NSES, both adjusted (in red) and unadjusted (in blue) for population density. Figure 2 illustrates the relative availability: that is, the ratio of the count of food retailers (within 400 m) in each NSES category over the count of food retailers in the middle-NSES quintile.

Schools located in the most disadvantaged census tracts showed, on average, 67% more counts of unhealthy retailers (IRR (Incidence Rate Ratio) = 1.67; 95% CI (Confidence Interval) = 1.40, 1.99) than those located in middle-NSES areas (reference category). In contrast, schools located in more advantaged census tracts showed, on average, 41% fewer counts of unhealthy retailers (IRR = 0.59; 95% CI = 0.48, 0.72) than those in middle-NSES areas. After adjusting for population density, the effect of neighborhood-level socioeconomic status remained inversely associated with the counts of unhealthy retailers around schools (shown in red). For instance, schools located in low-NSES areas (two lowest Qs) were associated with greater counts, on average, of 29% (middle-low, IRR = 1.29; 95% CI = 1.12, 1.50) and 62% (low, IRR = 1.62; 95% CI = 1.35, 1.95) of retailers than those located in middle-NSES areas. Thus, population density did not change the NSES gradient observed in the unadjusted analyses. Table S2 shows further details of these results. In our sensitivity analysis, results remained the same when removing supermarkets from the counts of unhealthy retailers (see Table S3).

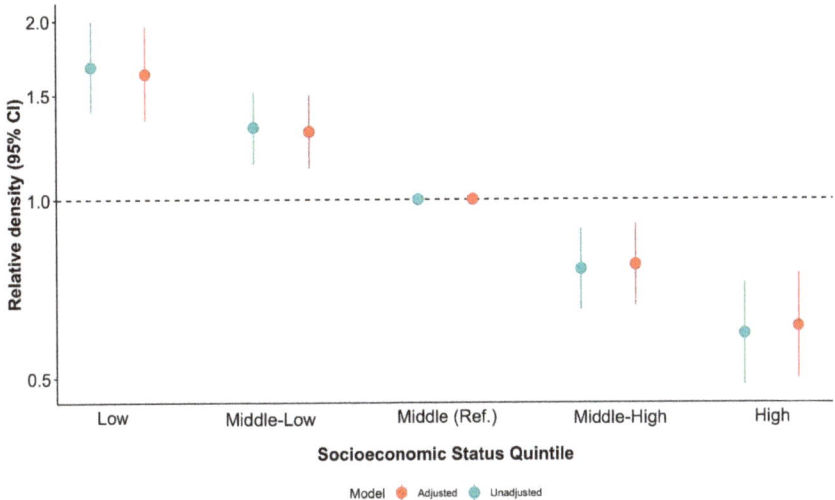

Figure 2. Multilevel negative binomial regression modelling neighborhood-level socioeconomic status with counts of unhealthy outlets around schools in Madrid (2017) before and after adjusting for population density.

3.2. Distance to the Nearest Unhealthy Outlet and Neighborhood-Level SES

As shown above, in Table 1, the median distance from schools located in more disadvantaged areas was smaller (77.09 m), relative to those located in more advantaged ones (145.92 m; p = 0.0001). On average, any school in Madrid was located within 88 m of an unhealthy retailer (median: 88.3 m; range: 2.53–4415 m). Figure 1b shows the spatial distribution of schools in the city, according to their proximity to the closest unhealthy food outlet. As shown in Figure 1b, we did not observe any clear spatial pattern in terms of distance to unhealthy retailers across the city.

Figure 3 presents the results of models of log (distance) on NSES (adjusted and unadjusted for population density). Therefore, it is a measure of relative distance: that is, the ratio of the distance to the closest unhealthy retailer in each NSES category over the distance to the closest unhealthy retailer in the middle-NSES category.

Schools located in more advantaged areas showed greater distances to the nearest unhealthy food retailer than those schools located in middle-NSES areas (unadjusted model shown in blue). Indeed, a unit change in the NSES represents an expected increase in the distance to the nearest unhealthy outlet of 41.9%. As we log-transformed the distance variable, the beta coefficients represent percentage changes.

The association remained nearly identical in direction and magnitude after controlling for population density (adjusted model shown in red). Having a school located in more disadvantaged areas (two lowest Qs) was negatively associated with the distance to unhealthy outlets, but results showed weak evidence (middle-low, β = 0.11; 95% CI = −0.06, 0.29; low, β = 0.05; 95% CI = −0.15, 0.26). Table S4 shows further details of these results. In our sensitivity analysis and as with counts of unhealthy food outlets, results remained the same after removing supermarkets from the distance metrics (see Table S5).

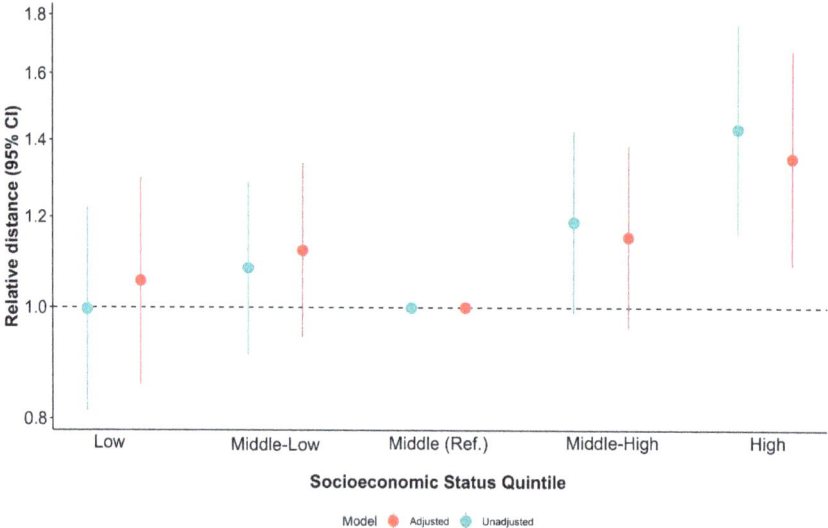

Figure 3. Multilevel linear regression modeling neighborhood-level socioeconomic status with distance to unhealthy retailers (in the log scale) from schools across Madrid (2017) before and after adjusting for population density.

4. Discussion

Our findings suggest that schools located in socioeconomic disadvantaged areas have a higher availability of unhealthy outlets in their immediate food environment than schools located in socioeconomic advantaged areas. Indeed, schools located in more disadvantaged areas showed, on average, 62.0% more counts of unhealthy retailers than those located in middle-NSES areas. When we excluded supermarkets, we still observed that schools located in more disadvantaged areas showed, on average, 69.0% more counts than those located in middle-NSES areas. Furthermore, and although not statistically significant, schools located in disadvantaged areas were closer to "unhealthy" outlets than school located in more advantaged areas.

By building on previous studies [3,4], these findings contribute to the literature by assessing the food environment around schools across a Southern European context, where children and adolescents present particularly high prevalence of overweight and obesity. To the best of our knowledge, this is the first study to examine the retail food environment surrounding schools across an entire Southern European city like Madrid. According to a recent systematic review by Bivoltsis et al. [49], there is no current consensus on the use of different exposure measures for food environment. Therefore, following their recommendations, we used a multimethod approach and decided to measure the effect of two dimensions of spatial access, availability and accessibility. These two measures of spatial access are the environmental correlates consistently found to be associated with children' and adolescents' dietary intake [50–53]. Further, they are interconnected and complementary.

Our measure of availability (counts) produced more important associations than our measure of accessibility (distance). These results are in line with the ones shown in the previous review [49], documenting effect sizes from accessibility measures to be smaller than effects from availability measures. Prior research has also shown different associations between neighborhood-level socioeconomic status and food access according to the accessibility dimension measured [54]. These two measures do also provide different insights from a policy perspective. Availability metrics (either raw counts or densities) are more relevant for implementing food policies, such as zoning policies. Across urban, dense, areas the number of unhealthy outlets (i.e., the concentration of these outlets) may have a greater influence on diet than the distance required to get to the closest unhealthy outlet.

In this study, we assessed multiple retailer types (supermarkets, convenience stores, bakeries, fast-food outlets, takeaways, etc.) to capture the wider experience of environmental features promoting unhealthier dietary intakes. Previous research has focused on whether specific food retailers (e.g., fast foods) were associated with youth excess weight risk [21]. However, children and adolescents interact with multiple types of retailers simultaneously. By including all sources of retailers offering unhealthy food products (including supermarkets), we help to better identify sources for purchasing unhealthy food and beverages options within schools' surroundings [55].

While supermarkets are often used as a proxy for "healthy" food options, they also stock a wide variety of unhealthy items. Indeed, previous studies (conducted in the US) have documented this wide availability of unhealthy options inside supermarkets, which leads to an increased intake of these energy-dense, nutrient-poor foods and beverages [56,57]. Moreover, Howard Wilsher et al. showed an association between supermarket sales of unhealthy foods and the prevalence of excess weight among children in the UK [58]. In other countries, as diverse as Brazil [59] and Switzerland [60], researchers have also documented how supermarkets are rapidly becoming the main source of ultra-processed foods. We found similar results when omitting supermarkets (see Tables S3 and S5).

Our findings support the "deprivation amplification" hypothesis, where socially disadvantaged individuals experience a further contextual disadvantage regarding their access to health-promoting resources due to their place of residence [61]. Indeed, our findings concur with previous studies [22,30,62,63] showing that unhealthy food options are the default around schools in urban settings, with this being more the case for schools located in more disadvantaged areas. For example, Soltero et al. examined the food environment around schools in three Mexican cities and showed that the food environment was saturated with unhealthy food stores (range 2–273 retailers) [63]. Regarding the socioeconomic gradient, the Soltero et al. study also found differences in all three cities by education and poverty levels. In Madrid, a recent study showed that youth living in more disadvantaged areas had greater odds of being obese compared with those living in more advantaged areas [64]. Yet, to date, there is no research for Southern European cities like Madrid, assessing whether these social disparities in obesity are associated with the food environment surrounding children and adolescents.

Moreover, prior studies have documented how supermarkets are becoming more prevalent in Spain, whereas traditional specialized food stores (e.g., fruit and vegetable stores) are disappearing [39,65]. These changes in the retail food environment might also impact dietary intake, and further, diet-related health outcomes. In Madrid, previous studies have documented that traditional stores provide urban residents with a greater ratio of fresh and/or healthy food, as compared with supermarkets [34,39]. In addition, Thornton et al. documented the ubiquity of unhealthy foods across supermarkets in Melbourne [66]. Furthermore, a recent study in Cape Town showed that socioeconomic status may play a role on the food available in supermarkets. This study showed that supermarkets in low-SES areas carried fewer healthy foods than supermarkets in higher-SES areas [67]. Thus, the potential implications that the proliferation of supermarkets may have on nutrition and health deserves attention.

The specific mechanisms by which the retail food environment influences children and adolescent food choices are not fully understood and may include different physical, sociocultural, economic, and political factors [9–11]. Physical factors (e.g., access to fast-food outlets) have been suggested to be positively associated with dietary behaviors or BMI (Body Mass Index) [68–70]. For instance, Cutumisu et al. found higher access to fast-food outlets around schools to be positively associated with higher intake of junk food [68]. In Finnland, Virtanen et al. found proximity to unhealthy retailers to be associated with eating snacks obtained from outside the school [69]. Baek et al. showed an increase (by 0.004 units) of children' BMI z-scores per each additional convenience store available within walking distance to public schools in California [70].

Our study findings underscore the need for examining childhood obesity from a social justice perspective. This need urges researchers, urban planners, and decision-makers to work together towards tackling the childhood obesity epidemic using a multiple systems approach. While the evidence is still inconsistent, several countries have introduced regulatory policies to restrict unhealthy food retailing [71–73]. Across the city of London, new hot food takeaways should not be permitted within 400 m walking distance of an existing school [26]. However, our findings showed that the median number of unhealthy retailers varied across schools located in high-, middle-, and low-SES neighborhoods (8, 16, and 24, respectively; Table 1). Thus, restricting only the location of new hot food takeaways may have little effect for those living in the most disadvantaged areas, compared with the effect for those living in the least disadvantaged areas. Developing food policies which promote healthier food environments, as well as considering wider health inequalities, may be more appropriate from a health-equity lens than restricting the location of new fast-food outlets. As shown in our results, and as also highlighted by Green et al., disadvantaged areas already have a level of saturation whereby restricting further outlets would likely have little impact [24]. This brings a further disadvantaged scenario for children and adolescents living in these areas. Thus, planning and zoning policies should include the existing retailers.

Our study has some limitations. We assumed that children attend schools within their neighborhood. However, this may or may not be the case. No conclusions about individuals can be drawn from this study. Another limitation is that we focused on unhealthy outlets within school surroundings, which is not fully representative of the school food environment, as vending machines and cafeterias within school boundaries are missing. While our unhealthy food environment measure is comprehensive, we assumed that food retailers are either healthy or unhealthy, which may be simplistic. Further, it is also important to account for other aspects of the retail food environment (such as the prices of food products or the opening hours of the retailers). Using administrative units to measure both SES and population density (at the census tracts in our study) also means results are subject to the modifiable areal unit problem [35]. Finally, it must be kept in mind that individuals residing in these areas would have additional exposure to fast-food restaurants beyond these areas. Taken together, these limitations may have underestimated our results. However, despite these limitations, our study has several strengths. This study is the first to assess the unhealthy food environment around schools in a Southern-European setting, characterized by the density of food retailers [31]. We have also used a validated neighborhood-level SES measure using an integrated composite index [35]. Our unhealthy food access measures include multiple types of food store types, yielding a more comprehensive picture of the food environment.

Future studies should try to extend our results by including individual-level data (e.g., dietary intake) to better understand how the food environment surrounding schools relates to actual food-purchasing practices and diet quality. Further, a wider range of spatial access dimensions should be assessed (e.g., affordability) to increase our understanding of how these spatial metrics are associated with food-purchasing practices.

5. Conclusions

Our study shows that schools located in more disadvantaged areas have a higher exposure to unhealthy outlets in their immediate food environment than schools located in more advantaged areas. Restricting policies (e.g., banning fast-food around schools) are warranted to protect children and adolescent from the harmful effects of unhealthy foods and beverages. Yet, it is important that public policy interventions consider the influence that socioeconomic inequalities have on the retail food environment.

Supplementary Materials: The following are available online at http://www.mdpi.com/2072-6643/11/7/1511/s1, Table S1: Unhealthy food retailers (by type) found within 400 m of schools (n = 6530) citywide (Madrid, 2017), Table S2: Association between neighborhood-level socioeconomic status and counts of unhealthy retailers, using multilevel negative binomial regression, Table S3: Sensitivity analysis: Association between neighborhood-level socioeconomic status and counts of unhealthy retailers (without including supermarkets), using multilevel negative binomial regression, Table S4: Association between neighborhood-level socioeconomic status and distance to the closest unhealthy retailer (logarithm), using multilevel linear regression. Table S5: Sensitivity analysis: Association between neighborhood-level socioeconomic status and distance (logarithm) to the closest unhealthy retailer (without including supermarkets), using multilevel linear regression.

Author Contributions: Conceptualization, J.D. and M.F.; methodology, J.D., A.C. and U.B.; software, J.D., A.R., A.C. and U.B.; formal analysis, J.D.; data curation, J.D., A.R., A.C. writing—original draft preparation, J.D.; writing—review and editing, J.D., A.R., A.C., L.N.B., U.B. and M.F.; visualization, J.D., A.C. and U.B.; supervision, L.N.B., U.B. and M.F.; funding acquisition, M.F.

Funding: J.D., A.C., and M.F. were funded by the European Research Council under the European Union's Seventh Framework Programme (FP7/2007-2013/ERC Starting Grant Heart Healthy Hoods Agreement no.336893). U.B. was supported by the Office of the Director of the National Institutes of Health under award number DP5OD26429.

Conflicts of Interest: The authors declare no conflict of interest. The funders had no role in the design of the study; in the collection, analyses, or interpretation of data; in the writing of the manuscript, or in the decision to publish the results.

References

1. Swinburn, B.A.; Kraak, V.I.; Allender, S.; Atkins, V.J.; Baker, P.I.; Bogard, J.R.; Brinsden, H.; Calvillo, A.; De Schutter, O.; Devarajan, R.; et al. The Global Syndemic of Obesity, Undernutrition, and Climate Change: The Lancet Commission report. *Lancet* **2019**, *393*, 791–846. [CrossRef]
2. Abarca-Gómez, L.; Abdeen, Z.A.; Hamid, Z.A.; Abu-Rmeileh, N.M.; Acosta-Cazares, B.; Acuin, C.; Adams, R.J.; Aekplakorn, W.; Afsana, K.; Aguilar-Salinas, C.A.; et al. Worldwide trends in body-mass index, underweight, overweight, and obesity from 1975 to 2016: A pooled analysis of 2416 population-based measurement studies in 128·9 million. *Lancet* **2017**, *390*, 2627–2642. [CrossRef]
3. Ahrens, W.; Pigeot, I.; Pohlabeln, H.; De Henauw, S.; Lissner, L.; Molnár, D.; Moreno, L.A.; Tornaritis, M.; Veidebaum, T.; Siani, A. Prevalence of overweight and obesity in European children below the age of 10. *Int. J. Obes.* **2014**, *38*, S99–S107. [CrossRef] [PubMed]
4. Lien, N.; Henriksen, H.B.; Nymoen, L.L.; Wind, M.; Klepp, K.-I. Availability of data assessing the prevalence and trends of overweight and obesity among European adolescents. *Public Health Nutr.* **2010**, *13*, 1680–1687. [CrossRef] [PubMed]
5. Ministerio de Salud, Consumo y Bienestar Social. Escuesta Nacional de Salud 2017. Available online: https://www.mscbs.gob.es/estadEstudios/estadisticas/encuestaNacional/encuesta2017.htm (accessed on 23 May 2019).
6. Owen, C.G.; Whincup, P.H.; Orfei, L.; Chou, Q.-A.; Rudnicka, A.R.; Wathern, A.K.; Kaye, S.J.; Eriksson, J.G.; Osmond, C.; Cook, D.G. Is body mass index before middle age related to coronary heart disease risk in later life? Evidence from observational studies. *Int. J. Obes.* **2009**, *33*, 866–877. [CrossRef] [PubMed]
7. Park, M.H.; Falconer, C.; Viner, R.M.; Kinra, S. The impact of childhood obesity on morbidity and mortality in adulthood: A systematic review. *Obes. Rev.* **2012**, *13*, 985–1000. [CrossRef] [PubMed]
8. Birch, L.L.; Fisher, J.O. Development of eating behaviors among children and adolescents. *Pediatrics* **1998**, *101*, 539–549. [PubMed]
9. Swinburn, B.A.; Sacks, G.; Hall, K.D.; McPherson, K.; Finegood, D.T.; Moodie, M.L.; Gortmaker, S.L. The global obesity pandemic: Shaped by global drivers and local environments. *Lancet* **2011**, *378*, 804–814. [CrossRef]
10. Story, M.; Kaphingst, K.M.; Robinson-O'Brien, R.; Glanz, K. Creating Healthy Food and Eating Environments: Policy and Environmental Approaches. *Annu. Rev. Public Health* **2008**, *29*, 253–272. [CrossRef]
11. Franco, M.; Bilal, U.; Díez, J. Food Environment. *Encycl. Food Health* **2016**, *4*, 22–26.
12. Glanz, K.; Sallis, J.F.; Saelens, B.E.; Frank, L.D. Healthy Nutrition Environments: Concepts and Measures. *Am. J. Health Promot.* **2005**, *19*, 330–333. [CrossRef] [PubMed]
13. Katz, D.L. School-Based Interventions for Health Promotion and Weight Control: Not Just Waiting on the World to Change. *Annu. Rev. Public Health* **2009**, *30*, 253–272. [CrossRef] [PubMed]
14. Bramante, C.T.; Thornton, R.L.J.; Bennett, W.L.; Zhang, A.; Wilson, R.F.; Bass, E.B.; Tseng, E. Systematic Review of Natural Experiments for Childhood Obesity Prevention and Control. *Am. J. Prev. Med.* **2019**, *56*, 147–158. [CrossRef] [PubMed]

15. Oosterhoff, M.; Joore, M.; Ferreira, I. The effects of school-based lifestyle interventions on body mass index and blood pressure: A multivariate multilevel meta-analysis of randomized controlled trials. *Obes. Rev.* **2016**, *17*, 1131–1153. [CrossRef] [PubMed]
16. Amini, M.; Djazayery, A.; Majdzadeh, R.; Taghdisi, M.H.; Jazayeri, S. Effect of school-based interventions to control childhood obesity: A review of reviews. *Int. J. Prev. Med.* **2015**, *6*, 68. [PubMed]
17. Gittelsohn, J.; Kumar, M.B. Preventing childhood obesity and diabetes: Is it time to move out of the school? *Pediatr. Diabetes* **2007**, *8*, 55–69. [CrossRef]
18. Lucan, S.C. Concerning Limitations of Food-Environment Research: A Narrative Review and Commentary Framed around Obesity and Diet-Related Diseases in Youth. *J. Acad. Nutr. Diet.* **2015**, *115*, 205–212. [CrossRef]
19. Engler-Stringer, R.; Le, H.; Gerrard, A.; Muhajarine, N. The community and consumer food environment and children's diet: A systematic review. *BMC Public Health* **2014**, *14*, 522. [CrossRef]
20. Timmermans, J.; Dijkstra, C.; Kamphuis, C.; Huitink, M.; van der Zee, E.; Poelman, M. "Obesogenic" School Food Environments? An Urban Case Study in The Netherlands. *Int. J. Environ. Res. Public Health* **2018**, *15*, 619. [CrossRef]
21. Williams, J.; Scarborough, P.; Matthews, A.; Cowburn, G.; Foster, C.; Roberts, N.; Rayner, M. A systematic review of the influence of the retail food environment around schools on obesity-related outcomes. *Obes. Rev.* **2014**, *15*, 359–374. [CrossRef]
22. Vandevijvere, S.; Sushil, Z.; Exeter, D.J.; Swinburn, B. Obesogenic Retail Food Environments Around New Zealand Schools. *Am. J. Prev. Med.* **2016**, *51*, e57–e66. [CrossRef] [PubMed]
23. Nielsen, S. Trends in Food Locations and Sources among Adolescents and Young Adults. *Prev. Med.* **2002**, *35*, 107–113. [CrossRef] [PubMed]
24. Green, M.A.; Radley, D.; Lomax, N.; Morris, M.A.; Griffiths, C. Is adolescent body mass index and waist circumference associated with the food environments surrounding schools and homes? A longitudinal analysis. *BMC Public Health* **2018**, *18*, 482. [CrossRef] [PubMed]
25. Nykiforuk, C.I.J.; Campbell, E.J.; Macridis, S.; McKennitt, D.; Atkey, K.; Raine, K.D. Adoption and diffusion of zoning bylaws banning fast food drive-through services across Canadian municipalities. *BMC Public Health* **2018**, *18*, 137. [CrossRef] [PubMed]
26. *Greater London Authority The London Plan, The Spatial Development Strategy for Greater London*; Greater London Authority: London, UK, 2017.
27. Franco, M.; Sanz, B.; Otero, L.; Domínguez-Vila, A.; Caballero, B. Prevention of childhood obesity in Spain: A focus on policies outside the health sector. SESPAS report 2010. *Gac. Sanit.* **2010**, *24*, 49–55. [CrossRef] [PubMed]
28. Neira, M.; de Onis, M. Preventing obesity: A public health priority in Spain. *Lancet* **2005**, *365*, 1386. [CrossRef]
29. Monroy-Parada, D.X.; Jácome-González, M.L.; Moya-Geromini, M.Á.; Rodríguez-Artalejo, F.; Royo-Bordonada, M.Á. Adherence to nutritional recommendations in vending machines at secondary schools in Madrid (Spain), 2014–2015. *Gac. Sanit.* **2018**, *32*, 459–465. [CrossRef]
30. Zenk, S.N.; Powell, L.M. US secondary schools and food outlets. *Health Place* **2008**, *14*, 336–346. [CrossRef]
31. Flavián, C.; Haberberg, A.; Polo, Y. Food retailing strategies in the European union. A comparative analysis in the UK and Spain. *J. Retail. Consum. Serv.* **2002**, *9*, 125–138. [CrossRef]
32. Pettinger, C.; Holdsworth, M.; Gerber, M. "All under one roof?" Differences in food availability and shopping patterns in Southern France and Central England. *Eur. J. Public Health* **2008**, *18*, 109–114. [CrossRef]
33. Diez, J.; Bilal, U.; Cebrecos, A.; Buczynski, A.; Lawrence, R.S.; Glass, T.; Escobar, F.; Gittelsohn, J.; Franco, M. Understanding differences in the local food environment across countries: A case study in Madrid (Spain) and Baltimore (USA). *Prev. Med.* **2016**, *89*, 237–244. [CrossRef] [PubMed]
34. Bilal, U.; Díez, J.; Alfayate, S.; Gullón, P.; Del Cura, I.; Escobar, F.; Sandín, M.; Franco, M. Population cardiovascular health and urban environments: The Heart Healthy Hoods exploratory study in Madrid, Spain. *BMC Med. Res. Methodol.* **2016**, *16*, 104. [CrossRef] [PubMed]
35. Cebrecos, A.; Domínguez-Berjón, M.F.; Duque, I.; Franco, M.; Escobar, F. Geographic and statistic stability of deprivation aggregated measures at different spatial units in health research. *Appl. Geogr.* **2018**, *95*, 9–18. [CrossRef]
36. Gullón, P.; Bilal, U.; Cebrecos, A.; Badland, H.M.; Galán, I.; Franco, M. Intersection of neighborhood dynamics and socioeconomic status in small-area walkability: The Heart Healthy Hoods project. *Int. J. Health Geogr.* **2017**, *16*, 21. [CrossRef] [PubMed]

37. Bilal, U.; Hill-Briggs, F.; Sánchez-Perruca, L.; Del Cura-González, I.; Franco, M. Association of neighbourhood socioeconomic status and diabetes burden using electronic health records in Madrid (Spain): The Heart Healthy Hoods study. *BMJ Open* **2018**, *8*, e021143. [CrossRef] [PubMed]
38. Borrell, C.; Malmusi, D.; Muntaner, C. Introduction to the "Evaluating the Impact of Structural Policies on Health Inequalities and Their Social Determinants and Fostering Change" (SOPHIE) Project. *Int. J. Health Serv.* **2017**, *47*, 10–17. [CrossRef]
39. Bilal, U.; Jones-Smith, J.; Diez, J.; Lawrence, R.S.; Celentano, D.D.; Franco, M. Neighborhood social and economic change and retail food environment change in Madrid (Spain): The heart healthy hoods study. *Health Place* **2018**, *51*, 107–117. [CrossRef]
40. *Eurostat Statistical Classification of Economic Activities in the European Community*; Eurostat: Luxembourg, 2008.
41. Zuniga-Teran, A.A.; Orr, B.J.; Gimblett, R.H.; Chalfoun, N.V.; Marsh, S.E.; Guertin, D.P.; Going, S.B. Designing healthy communities: Testing the walkability model. *Front. Archit. Res.* **2017**, *6*, 63–73. [CrossRef]
42. Elbel, B.; Tamura, K.; McDermott, Z.T.; Duncan, D.T.; Athens, J.K.; Wu, E.; Mijanovich, T.; Schwartz, A.E. Disparities in food access around homes and schools for New York City children. *PLoS ONE* **2019**, *14*, e0217341. [CrossRef]
43. Neckerman, K.M.; Bader, M.D.M.; Richards, C.A.; Purciel, M.; Quinn, J.W.; Thomas, J.S.; Warbelow, C.; Weiss, C.C.; Lovasi, G.S.; Rundle, A. Disparities in the Food Environments of New York City Public Schools. *Am. J. Prev. Med.* **2010**, *39*, 195–202. [CrossRef]
44. Mackenbach, J.D.; Charreire, H.; Glonti, K.; Bárdos, H.; Rutter, H.; Compernolle, S.; De Bourdeaudhuij, I.; Nijpels, G.; Brug, J.; Oppert, J.-M.; et al. Exploring the Relation of Spatial Access to Fast-food outlets with Body Weight: A Mediation Analysis. *Environ. Behav.* **2018**. [CrossRef]
45. Bader, M.D.M.; Schwartz-Soicher, O.; Jack, D.; Weiss, C.C.; Richards, C.A.; Quinn, J.W.; Lovasi, G.S.; Neckerman, K.M.; Rundle, A.G. More neighborhood retail associated with lower obesity among New York City public high school students. *Health Place* **2013**, *23*, 104–110. [CrossRef] [PubMed]
46. Lamb, K.E.; Thornton, L.; Cerin, E.; Ball, K. Statistical Approaches Used to Assess the Equity of Access to Food Outlets: A Systematic Review. *AIMS Public Health* **2015**, *2*, 358–401. [CrossRef] [PubMed]
47. Thornton, L.E.; Cameron, A.J.; McNaughton, S.A.; Waterlander, W.E.; Sodergren, M.; Svastisalee, C.; Blanchard, L.; Liese, A.D.; Battersby, S.; Carter, M.-A.; et al. Does the availability of snack foods in supermarkets vary internationally? *Int. J. Behav. Nutr. Phys. Act.* **2013**, *10*, 56. [CrossRef] [PubMed]
48. Charlton, E.L.; Kähkönen, L.A.; Sacks, G.; Cameron, A.J. Supermarkets and unhealthy food marketing: An international comparison of the content of supermarket catalogues/circulars. *Prev. Med.* **2015**, *81*, 168–173. [CrossRef] [PubMed]
49. Bivoltsis, A.; Cervigni, E.; Trapp, G.; Knuiman, M.; Hooper, P.; Ambrosini, G.L. Food environments and dietary intakes among adults: Does the type of spatial exposure measurement matter? A systematic review. *Int. J. Health Geogr.* **2018**, *17*, 19. [CrossRef] [PubMed]
50. Pearson, N.; Biddle, S.J.H.; Gorely, T. Family correlates of fruit and vegetable consumption in children and adolescents: A systematic review. *Public Health Nutr.* **2009**, *12*, 267–283. [CrossRef]
51. Van der Horst, K.; Oenema, A.; Ferreira, I.; Wendel-Vos, W.; Giskes, K.; van Lenthe, F.; Brug, J. A systematic review of environmental correlates of obesity-related dietary behaviors in youth. *Health Educ. Res.* **2006**, *22*, 203–226. [CrossRef]
52. Rasmussen, M.; Krølner, R.; Klepp, K.I.; Lytle, L.; Brug, J.; Bere, E.; Due, P. Determinants of fruit and vegetable consumption among children and adolescents: A review of the literature. Part I: Quantitative studies. *Int. J. Behav. Nutr. Phys. Act.* **2006**, *3*, 22. [CrossRef]
53. Verloigne, M.; Van Lippevelde, W.; Maes, L.; Brug, J.; De Bourdeaudhuij, I. Family- and school-based correlates of energy balance-related behaviours in 10–12-year-old children: A systematic review within the ENERGY (European Energy balance Research to prevent excessive weight Gain among Youth) project. *Public Health Nutr.* **2012**, *15*, 1380–1395. [CrossRef]
54. Ball, K.; Timperio, A.; Crawford, D. Neighbourhood socioeconomic inequalities in food access and affordability. *Health Place* **2009**, *15*, 578–585. [CrossRef] [PubMed]
55. Smith, D.; Cummins, S.; Clark, C.; Stansfeld, S. Does the local food environment around schools affect diet? Longitudinal associations in adolescents attending secondary schools in East London. *BMC Public Health* **2013**, *13*, 70. [CrossRef] [PubMed]

56. Shier, V.; An, R.; Sturm, R. Is there a robust relationship between neighbourhood food environment and childhood obesity in the USA? *Public Health* **2012**, *126*, 723–730. [CrossRef] [PubMed]
57. An, R.; Maurer, G. Consumption of sugar-sweetened beverages and discretionary foods among US adults by purchase location. *Eur. J. Clin. Nutr.* **2016**, *70*, 1396. [CrossRef] [PubMed]
58. Howard Wilsher, S.; Harrison, F.; Yamoah, F.; Fearne, A.; Jones, A. The relationship between unhealthy food sales, socio-economic deprivation and childhood weight status: Results of a cross-sectional study in England. *Int. J. Behav. Nutr. Phys. Act.* **2016**, *13*, 21. [CrossRef] [PubMed]
59. Machado, P.P.; Claro, R.M.; Martins, A.P.B.; Costa, J.C.; Levy, R.B. Is food store type associated with the consumption of ultra-processed food and drink products in Brazil? *Public Health Nutr.* **2018**, *21*, 201–209. [CrossRef] [PubMed]
60. Güsewell, S.; Floris, J.; Berlin, C.; Zwahlen, M.; Rühli, F.; Bender, N.; Staub, K. Spatial Association of Food Sales in Supermarkets with the Mean BMI of Young Men: An Ecological Study. *Nutrients* **2019**, *11*, 579. [CrossRef] [PubMed]
61. Macintyre, S. Deprivation amplification revisited; or, is it always true that poorer places have poorer access to resources for healthy diets and physical activity? *Int. J. Behav. Nutr. Phys. Act.* **2007**, *4*, 32. [CrossRef]
62. Thornton, L.E.; Lamb, K.E.; Ball, K. Fast food restaurant locations according to socioeconomic disadvantage, urban–regional locality, and schools within Victoria, Australia. *SSM-Popul. Health* **2016**, *2*, 1–9. [CrossRef]
63. Soltero, E.G.; Ortiz Hernández, L.; Jauregui, E.; Lévesque, L.; Lopez, Y.; Taylor, J.; Barquera, S.; Lee, R.E. Characterization of the School Neighborhood Food Environment in Three Mexican Cities. *Ecol. Food Nutr.* **2017**, *56*, 139–151. [CrossRef]
64. Villanueva, R.; Albaladejo, R.; Astasio, P.; Ortega, P.; Santos, J.; Regidor, E. Socio-economic environment, area facilities and obesity and physical inactivity among children. *Eur. J. Public Health* **2016**, *26*, 267–271. [CrossRef] [PubMed]
65. Díez, J.; Bilal, U.; Franco, M. Unique features of the Mediterranean food environment: Implications for the prevention of chronic diseases Rh: Mediterranean food environments. *Eur. J. Clin. Nutr.* **2018**, *28*, 1. [CrossRef] [PubMed]
66. Thornton, L.E.; Cameron, A.J.; McNaughton, S.A.; Worsley, A.; Crawford, D.A. The availability of snack food displays that may trigger impulse purchases in Melbourne supermarkets. *BMC Public Health* **2012**, *12*, 194. [CrossRef] [PubMed]
67. Battersby, J.; Peyton, S. The Geography of Supermarkets in Cape Town: Supermarket Expansion and Food Access. *Urban Forum* **2014**, *25*, 153–164. [CrossRef]
68. Cutumisu, N.; Traoré, I.; Paquette, M.-C.; Cazale, L.; Camirand, H.; Lalonde, B.; Robitaille, E. Association between junk food consumption and fast-food outlet access near school among Quebec secondary-school children: Findings from the Quebec Health Survey of High School Students (QHSHSS) 2010–11. *Public Health Nutr.* **2017**, *20*, 927–937. [CrossRef] [PubMed]
69. Virtanen, M.; Kivimäki, H.; Ervasti, J.; Oksanen, T.; Pentti, J.; Kouvonen, A.; Halonen, J.I.; Kivimäki, M.; Vahtera, J. Fast-food outlets and grocery stores near school and adolescents' eating habits and overweight in Finland. *Eur. J. Public Health* **2015**, *25*, 650–655. [CrossRef]
70. Baek, J.; Sanchez-Vaznaugh, E.V.; Sánchez, B.N. Hierarchical Distributed-Lag Models: Exploring Varying Geographic Scale and Magnitude in Associations between the Built Environment and Health. *Am. J. Epidemiol.* **2016**, *183*, 583–592. [CrossRef]
71. Sturm, R.; Hattori, A. Diet and obesity in Los Angeles County 2007–2012: Is there a measurable effect of the 2008 "Fast-Food Ban"? *Soc. Sci. Med.* **2015**, *133*, 205–211. [CrossRef]
72. Gittelsohn, J.; Rowan, M.; Gadhoke, P. Interventions in small food stores to change the food environment, improve diet, and reduce risk of chronic disease. *Prev. Chronic Dis.* **2012**, *9*, E59. [CrossRef]
73. Calancie, L.; Leeman, J.; Jilcott Pitts, S.B.; Khan, L.K.; Fleischhacker, S.; Evenson, K.R.; Schreiner, M.; Byker, C.; Owens, C.; McGuirt, J.; et al. Nutrition-Related Policy and Environmental Strategies to Prevent Obesity in Rural Communities: A Systematic Review of the Literature, 2002–2013. *Prev. Chronic Dis.* **2015**, *12*, 140540. [CrossRef]

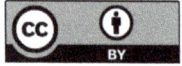

© 2019 by the authors. Licensee MDPI, Basel, Switzerland. This article is an open access article distributed under the terms and conditions of the Creative Commons Attribution (CC BY) license (http://creativecommons.org/licenses/by/4.0/).

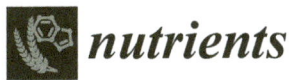

Article

We Don't Have a Lot of Healthy Options: Food Environment Perceptions of First-Year, Minority College Students Attending a Food Desert Campus

Jaapna Dhillon [1], L. Karina Diaz Rios [2,*], Kaitlyn J. Aldaz [1], Natalie De La Cruz [1], Emily Vu [1], Syed Asad Asghar [1], Quintin Kuse [1] and Rudy M. Ortiz [1]

1. School of Natural Sciences, University of California, Merced, CA 95343, USA; jdhillon5@ucmerced.edu (J.D.); kaldaz@ucmerced.edu (K.J.A.); ndelacruz2@ucmerced.edu (N.D.L.C.); evu2@ucmerced.edu (E.V.); sasghar@ucmerced.edu (S.A.A.); qkuse@ucmerced.edu (Q.K.); rortiz@ucmerced.edu (R.M.O.)
2. Division of Agriculture and Natural Resources, University of California, Merced, CA 95343, USA
* Correspondence: kdiazrios@ucmerced.edu; Tel.: +1-217-552-6336

Received: 19 February 2019; Accepted: 8 April 2019; Published: 11 April 2019

Abstract: First-year college students are at particular risk of dietary maladaptation during their transition to adulthood. A college environment that facilitates consistent access to nutritious food is critical to ensuring dietary adequacy among students. The objective of the study was to examine perceptions of the campus food environment and its influence on the eating choices of first-year students attending a minority-serving university located in a food desert. Focus group interviews with twenty-one first-year students were conducted from November 2016 to January 2017. Students participated in 1 of 5 focus groups. Most interviewees identified as being of Hispanic/Latino or Asian/Pacific Islander origin. A grounded theory approach was applied for inductive identification of relevant concepts and deductive interpretation of patterns and relationships among themes. Themes related to the perceived food environment included adequacy (i.e., variety and quality), acceptability (i.e., familiarity and preferences), affordability, and accessibility (i.e., convenience and accommodation). Subjective norms and processes of decisional balance and agency were themes characterizing interpersonal and personal factors affecting students' eating choices. The perceived environment appeared to closely interact with subjective norms to inform internal processes of decision-making and agency around the eating choices of first-year students attending a minority-serving university campus located in a food desert.

Keywords: barriers; college; diet quality; facilitators; qualitative research

1. Introduction

The transition from adolescence to adulthood is a critical period of increased autonomy and independence [1]. For about 20 million young adults in 2015, this represented the transition to college [2]. During this transition, students establish dietary independence and become vulnerable to unfavorable changes in diet and physical activity, which can lead to malnutrition and both acute and long-lasting behavioral and health outcomes [3]. According to the most recent data, adolescents aged 14 to 18 years consume lower than the recommended amount of fruits, vegetables, and whole grains and excessive amounts of calories from added sugar, solid fats, and alcohol [4]. A recent report indicates that adolescents in the lowest quartile of fruit and vegetable intake continue to have lower intake of those foods as young adults [5]. Poor diet quality during adolescence is associated with higher risk of developing cardiometabolic disorders later in life [6]. The prevalence of obesity among young adults is the greatest among those reporting some college education. At the same time, college and postsecondary education students are disproportionally affected by food insecurity [7–9].

The availability and access to nutritious food (e.g., fruits and vegetables) can facilitate nutritionally-sound food choices [10–15]. Because of their expected effects on diet quality and security, research on the impact of food systems on the availability and accessibility of nutritious food in vulnerable populations has been recently emphasized [16]. Decreased diet quality due to inadequate food access can lead to hampered academic performance, likely mediated by compromised mental health [17]. The significance of the food environment on eating behavior can be particularly critical in college campuses located in food deserts [18], where students have limited access to nutritious food due to physical and financial constraints [19]. Because perceptions are considered a core determinant of health behavior [20], the role of the perceived food environment in shaping dietary choices [13] has been emphasized in the literature. However, there is a paucity of evidence on the food environment perceptions of college students attending a food desert campus and whether and how these perceptions influence eating choices.

A food desert, as defined by the United States Department of Agriculture (USDA), is an urban area where at least 33% of its residents are located more than a mile away from a venue offering nutritious food (e.g., supermarkets) [21]. Despite being located at the heart of the most productive agricultural region in California, the university campus where this study was conducted is a food desert, i.e., about 4.5 miles from the nearest supermarket. The vast majority of students attending this campus are from underrepresented minorities and 60% come from low-income families [22]. Food insecurity, poor diet quality, higher risk of diet-related diseases, and inadequate access to health care are typically correlated with low socioeconomic status (SES) [23–25]. Reports indicate close to 60% of the students at this study site have experienced food insecurity, and the proportion of students reporting being food insecure widens with every year of enrollment [26]. According to the latest university census, most students living on campus are first-year students (72%) [27]. As food insecurity increases after the first year in college [28], first-year students represent a key target study population for early prevention of food insecurity and related acute and persistent dietary maladaptation.

The purpose of the present study was to examine perceptions on the campus food environment, the personal and interpersonal factors that interact with the perceived food environment, and their collective influence on the eating choices of first-year students attending a university located in a food desert. The identification of these factors will broaden the knowledge base in the area, providing the basis to explore their relevance in shaping eating choices in future qualitative studies. Ideas to improve the campus food environment were also explored.

2. Methods

Potential participants for focus group interviews were recruited from a pool of first-year college students participating in a parent clinical study (Clinical trials ID: NCT03084003). The objective of the parent study was to evaluate the effects of 8 weeks of different snacking options on glucoregulatory and cardiometabolic profiles of first-year college students [29]. Participants for the parent study were recruited via advertisements. Students were included if they were 18–19 years old and were newly enrolled, first-year college students living on campus. Participation in the focus groups was voluntary and was open to all participants in the parent study (n = 73). Twenty-one students consented to participate in focus group interviews, while others did not show an interest in participation. Students were monetarily compensated for participating in the parent study but did not receive additional compensation for participating in the focus groups. This study was approved by the Institutional Review Board of University of California, Merced. Signed written consent was obtained from all participants prior to the focus group sessions, and the data were kept confidential. A semistructured question guide was developed according to recommended methodology [30] to explore factors related to students' food choices and eating behavior in college, transition from home eating behaviors, perceived food environment, and barriers and facilitators to make nutritious choices. Questions were designed to probe constructs in the social cognitive theory (i.e., reciprocal determinism) [31] and the social ecological model [32]. Introductory and transition questions established the tone of the discussion and led to an in-depth discussion regarding the phenomenon of interest (i.e., eating choices and dietary behavior influences of first-year college students living in a low food-access campus environment). Closing questions explored students' opinions on solutions to improve the food environment on campus. The question guide was tested with a pilot focus group of first-year students meeting the inclusion criteria of the study ($n = 4$, focus group 1), and the data were later included in the final analysis because no substantial changes to the guide were made. The general question guide is depicted in Figure 1.

Opening	How is college life treating you?
Introduction	How does the way you eat today compare to the way you ate before college?
Transition	Do you think the way you were brought up influenced or shaped your food choices and preferences? How?
Key	Which factors have the most influence on your food choices as a college student? Please elaborate.
	What about [availability, variety, price, time, taste preferences, knowledge, skills, social influences]?
	What does the term 'healthy eating' means to you?
	Do you feel like you eat healthfully? Why or why not?
	What are some facilitators of eating healthfully on campus?
	What are some challenges of eating healthfully on campus?
Ending	Do you think the University has a role in facilitating the adoption of healthy eating practices? How?

Figure 1. Question guide for the focus group interviews of first-year college students.

Data were collected from November 2016 to January 2017. Focus groups were facilitated by a trained moderator and an assistant moderator (i.e., observer), who audio-recorded the session and took notes on nonverbal cues. The moderator led the discussion following the question guide, probing for in-depth information as needed. All focus group discussions were audio-recorded with permission from the participants. Audio-recordings were transcribed verbatim in Microsoft Word by trained scribes. Data were transferred to and organized in Microsoft Excel for analysis.

Data underwent a first round of preliminary coding done independently by 4 researchers under the supervision of an expert researcher. A codebook was developed in Microsoft Excel based on this preliminary analysis by identifying concepts from available literature [14,33] on the perceived environment and the health belief model (perceived barriers) [20], theory for planned behavior (subjective norms) [34], and the expectancy-value theory (decisional balance) [35]. A second round of coding using the codebook was done independently by 2 trained researchers to ensure reliability of data interpretations. Quotes were examined for recurrent patterns across the data set, assigned codes, and grouped into categories [36]. Similar codes were further divided into subcategories. Disagreements were resolved through further discussion with a third analyst and included contextualization based on theory and relevant literature. Codes were semiquantified to determine density and representativeness across focus groups and participants [37]. A grounded theory approach was applied for inductive identification of relevant concepts and deductive interpretation of patterns and relationships among themes and subthemes, seeking internal homogeneity and external heterogeneity [38]. A conceptual diagram was conceived to describe relationships among main themes and subthemes [39]. A negative case analysis was conducted for quotes that did not support emerging patterns [40]. Thematic saturation occurred at the third focus group (13 participants). Two additional focus groups were conducted (8 participants) to corroborate saturation and further probe salient themes.

For descriptive purposes, 2015 Healthy Eating Index (HEI-2015) scores [41] were computed from 2 24-hour food recalls spaced a week apart in the students' freshman year using a validated, automated, self-administered 24-h dietary assessment tool (ASA24) [42]. HEI 2015 scores were calculated using the per-person simple HEI scoring algorithm [43]. Sex differences were explored with the Kruskal–Wallis test. Significance was set at alpha ≤ 0.05.

3. Results

A total of 5 focus groups (n = 21) were conducted, lasting an average of 60 to 75 min. The majority (90.5%) of the participants were from an ethnic/racial minority, with the dominant groups being of Hispanic/Latino and Asian/Pacific Islander origin (Table 1).

Table 1. Characteristics of focus group participants, i.e., first-year college students attending a minority-serving university located in a food desert.

Characteristics	Males (n = 9)	Females (n = 12)
Age (years)	18.2 ± 0.4	18 ± 0
BMI (kg/m^2)	24.5 ± 3.8	25.2 ± 3.7
Race/Ethnicity, n (%)		
African American	1 (11.1%)	0 (0%)
Asian/Pacific Islander	3 (33.3%)	4 (33.3%)
Caucasian White	2 (22.2%)	1 (8.3%)
Hispanic	3 (33.3%)	7 (58.3%)

Values are means ± SDs or n (%).

According to HEI-2015 scores, participants had low fruit, vegetable, whole grain, and dairy intake, and high sodium intake. Male participants had a significantly lower fruit (total and whole) and higher sodium intake than females (P < 0.05, Table 2).

Table 2. 2015 Healthy Eating Index (HEI-2015) total and component scores for focus group participants, i.e., first-year college students attending a minority-serving university located in a food desert.

HEI-2015 Dietary Component	Males (n = 9)	Females (n = 11 *)
Total fruits (5)	1.2 ± 1.2	2.8 ± 1.8 **
Whole fruits (5)	1.3 ± 1.7	3.6 ± 1.5 **
Total vegetables (5)	3.3 ± 1.2	3.2 ± 1.3
Greens and beans (5)	3.1 ± 2.4	2.3 ± 2.3
Whole grains (10)	3.5 ± 2.4	3 ± 3.1
Dairy (10)	4.7 ± 2.4	4.4 ± 2.5
Total protein foods (5)	4.3 ± 1.7	4.2 ± 1.4
Seafood and Plant Proteins (5)	3 ± 2.5	4.1 ± 1.8
Fatty acids (10)	5.8 ± 3.3	6.8 ± 3.5
Refined grains (10)	4.1 ± 3.3	5.4 ± 3.4
Sodium (10)	1.8 ± 1.9	4.5 ± 2.7 **
Added sugars (10)	9.1 ± 0.9	7.7 ± 2.9
Saturated fats (10)	6.2 ± 2.3	5.6 ± 3.3
Total HEI 2015 score (100)	51.5 ± 10.9	57.6 ± 14.5

Values are means ± SDs. Numbers in parenthesis are maximum possible score values. * One participant did not complete 24-hour recalls. **, P < 0.05 using Kruskal–Wallis test. HEI 2015 scores were calculated using the per-person simple HEI scoring algorithm [43].

Six main themes were identified, four of which were related to the perceived food environment on campus: (1) Affordability, (2) acceptability, (3) accessibility, and (4) adequacy. Two additional themes were about the influence on eating choices of interpersonal and personal processes: (1) Subjective norms derived from family and peers, and (2) personal processes of decisional balance and agency. Solutions to improve their food environment and facilitate favorable eating behaviors were offered by participants. Figure 2 depicts a conceptual diagram devised to explain relationships among the main themes. Additional representative quotes for each theme are listed in Table S1.

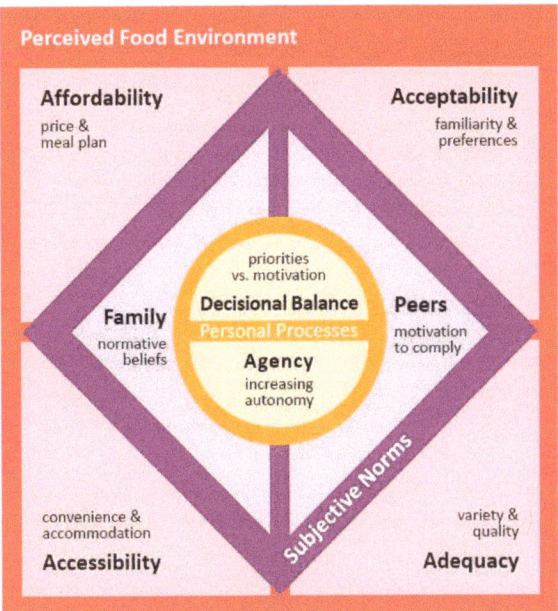

Figure 2. Schematic representation of the relationship among main themes, conceived upon an inductive, grounded theory analysis of focus groups with first-year college students. Personal processes of decisional balance and agency interact with four dimensions of the perceived food environment—affordability, acceptability, accessibility, and adequacy, —and with subjective norms—normative beliefs from family and motivation to comply with peers—to influence the food choices of students attending a food desert campus.

3.1. Perceived Affordability

The cost of foods on campus was consistently and most frequently brought up as having a major influence on eating choices. Participants perceived nutritious options as more expensive than less nutritious options, which often led them to opt for the latter:

"One of my major deciding factors when I buy food is how much the cost is, and the cost is usually lower with the unhealthy food"

(P19, G5)

"I would eat more fruits, so much more often if it wasn't so expensive; but, since it's so expensive I always get like burgers, which are cheaper."

(P12, G3)

Some participants considered their meal plan as an advantage to secure resources for food:

"[If I didn't have a meal plan], I would just spend the money that was dedicated for my food, I would probably spend it recklessly. So, I think it does help that I'm only able to spend that money on food on campus."

(P2, G1)

However, the meal plan was also perceived as restrictive for not allowing purchases from most outside food vendors, including some of the few located on campus:

"I only have [meal plan] dollars instead of real money; so, I can't really do anything about it and get food at the vendors on campus."

(P10, G3)

Overall, the limited affordability of nutritious options was consistently considered a barrier to healthy eating. Students' recommended solutions to minimize this barrier included allowing the use of their meal plan for purchasing food from third-party vendors on campus, making cheaper fruits and vegetables available on campus, and living off-campus after their freshman year for better access (e.g., proximity, transportation) to a greater variety of food options in terms of nutritional quality and price.

3.2. Perceived Acceptability

Students' food expectations appeared to be mostly related to their taste preferences and familiarity with available food. These expectations seemed to influence their perceptions on the quality of food on campus, which in turn led them to adjust their eating behavior. For some, the perceived negative organoleptic qualities of food were largely attributed to food preparation seen as inferior to that of familiar food:

" . . . when I eat the chicken here, it isn't like the chicken back home—it doesn't really taste like chicken to me. But, I usually don't eat at the [campus dining center]. If I do, I just get—if I'm desperate only and usually it's not appetizing—I get the peanut butter sandwich"

(P5, G2)

"I don't know if they make [the eggs] the day before or what, but, I wish it would taste like they were just made."

(P21, G5)

A few students contended familiar foods were not as available on campus:

"My family is White; so, the food that I'm used to eating is more plain, and the food that they have here has a lot of ethnic foods and I don't know what it is. So, I don't get it because I don't want to waste money on it if I don't like it."

(P10, G3)

Broadening the variety of food options and outlets on campus was among the ideas students offered to improve the campus food environment and, thus, their eating behavior. They also recommended a number of operational changes on the campus dining center, including posting menus in advance, making nutritional information of menu items readily available, and improving and varying food preparation techniques.

3.3. Perceived Accessibility

Factors related to the convenience of accessing food were saliently expressed as having a significant influence on eating behavior. Students indicated proximity to campus food outlets greatly influenced their eating choices. Proximity to places that offer energy-dense options and inconvenient location and schedule of fresh produce outlets were expressed as barriers to healthy eating:

"My first semester, it was bad—I eat all day, especially since I live in [a residence hall close to the dining center], I can just walk up to the cafeteria whenever I want. [The] first semester I probably ate more burgers and burritos than I should have."

(P14, G4)

"Occasionally there is the fresh fruit produce truck; but, they are only here on Wednesdays and occasionally it is hard to go up the hill and go there to get fruit."

(P8, G2)

Limited transportation options to off-campus grocery stores and food joints was also perceived as a barrier to accessing food, especially under the competing priorities imposed by academic demands:

"The bus takes too long; so, it cuts my day off and it cuts time off from studying and class—like, I would have to miss class. There's no point, I'm literally just on campus and [the campus dining center] is the main food access; so, I just stick to that."

(P20, G5)

Along with grocery shopping limitations, inconvenient access to cooking facilities was brought up as a factor affecting eating choices:

"If I had an option to cook and get groceries easily, I don't think I would rely on the [meal] plan so much."

(P1, G1)

"Reservations [for the campus kitchens] are always a hassle. So, there are days when I ... don't want to go to the [campus dining center]; but, knowing that you have to make [kitchen] reservations, just make you want to go to the [campus dining center]."

(P19, G5)

Several students indicated they often rely on food provided by their family to have enough and familiar food available. They reported bringing familiar foods from home, especially items that would conveniently withstand storage:

"As much as I can, I always try to bring stuff back [when I go home]. But, I never bring vegetables or fruits. I bring anything that's frozen, so that it can survive the trip and doesn't get nasty."

(P20, G5)

"I live an hour away, and my mom usually will freeze things and I'll put it in the freezer [sic]."

(P13, G3)

"I'm Nigerian, so I bring a lot of cultural food because I miss home. I also stock up on cereal like Costco bulk and mini snacks, like fruit snacks."

(P17, G4)

Potential solutions proposed by students to make accessing nutritious food more convenient included expanding the frequency and hours of operation and improving the location of produce outlets on campus, as well as better transportation options to off-campus food retailers.

3.4. Perceived Adequacy

According to participants' input, their food choices were generally influenced by on-campus availability of adequate options. As first-year students, most relied on the meal plan offered by the university to cover their dietary needs and indicated that the majority of their meals were consumed at the campus dining center. In general, they characterized the food and food establishments on campus as limited in number and lacking variety:

"There's only like 3 different places to eat around here [on-campus]."

(P13, G3)

"I eat whatever is available to me—like, whatever is at the [campus dining center]."

(P8, G2)

"I pretty much eat anything at the [campus dining center], even [if] I don't like it, because I don't really have a choice."

(P20, G5)

Most participants judged the food available on campus as nutritionally inadequate, with nutritious food options being scarce:

"I feel like we don't have a lot of healthy options [on-campus]."

(P2, G1)

"The only thing they have of fruit [at the campus convenience store] are the cups; and there really isn't anything healthy."

(P7, G2)

Conversely, a few students seemed content with the food options available on campus:

"The food overall here is a lot healthier than I had back in my hometown."

(P1, G1)

"They always have new things every day [at the campus dining center], and I'm willing to try new things."

(P11, G3)

3.5. Subjective Norms

Norms that governed their eating behavior before college, along with new normative beliefs acquired by being immersed in a new social environment, appeared to mediate students' perception of and interaction with their food environment. In terms of pre-college influences, students indicated health history and eating practices at home were ways their family influenced their eating choices:

"We have like a pretty bad history with health. Something shifted in my parents' way of thinking and then they went super healthy. I've been trying to move towards the healthier side."

(P1, G1)

"[My siblings and I] we all like to eat a lot, and our parents never told us we should slow down. They always told us 'you need to grow and eat a lot.' So, it kind of influenced what I eat here. Like, when I first came here I was like 'oh, look at these options,' right? And I was like eating like $30 a day for like the first 2 or 3 weeks. After that, I was realizing that I should probably slow down on this."

(P17, G4)

Other comments alluded to the role of fellow students in shaping new normative beliefs around their food choices:

"My roommate tried to get me to eat healthier, in a way, by having me get like cereal from the [campus convenience store] and stuff."

(P20, G5)

"I remember there was time when [I wanted to] eat healthy and just eat salad every day. But, my friends said that salad was more expensive; so, I agreed. So, it's cheaper to just get pizza. She kind of influenced me to not get salads because it's more expensive."

(P12, G3)

3.6. Personal Processes

Along with environmental and normative factors, personal decision-making processes requiring self-evaluation and introspection were also raised by participants when discussing eating choices. Students often described going through an internal conflict of choice, particularly when deciding between more and less nutritious food options:

"You have a healthy option and a non-healthy option, like a burger and fries or veggies. And you must decide if you want to eat healthy or not—the internal conflict of being healthy."

(P14, G4)

Participants mentioned competing priorities with respect to time, money, and academic demands importantly weighing in, sometimes to the detriment of their eating choices:

"We have to find something to eat in a certain amount of time. It doesn't matter if you like it or not, you kind of just have to eat it."

(P13, G3)

"I was always more focused on saving money [than eating healthy]."

(P4, G1)

"[Healthy eating] starts becoming less important around finals."

(P2, G1)

Lack of motivation to comply with the expectations of maintaining a healthy lifestyle was also expressed:

"I would get milk and food and stuff [from a grocery store]. But, it's too much work and I don't think it's important enough."

(P10, G3)

Notably, some comments alluded to a conflict arising when pondering options. This was compounded by an awareness of increased autonomy, which required students to assert agency over their diet:

"[It was] my mom who always was like 'here you go, eat this.' Here, I have all these options. And I'm free to choose. And sometimes I don't want to choose. And sometimes I do want to choose. So, it's like I didn't want to have that responsibility—to buy it, cook it, and choose it."

(P15, G4)

Taking better advantage of available resources (e.g., making kitchen reservations), developing and/or deploying skills (e.g., portion control, mindful eating), as well as earning more money and living off-campus were some ideas students mentioned they could pursue to improve their diets.

4. Discussion

This qualitative inquiry revealed four aspects of the perceived food environment: (1) Affordability, (2) acceptability, (3) accessibility, and (4) adequacy. These four aspects appear to influence the food choices and eating behavior of first-year minority students attending a university campus, located in a USDA-defined food desert. These aspects seem to closely interact with subjective norms from family and peers to inform students' internal processes of decision-making (i.e., decisional balance) and agency. These findings illustrate how multiple factors at several levels of influence interact to inform eating choices by preventing the continuation and adoption of desirable eating behaviors and/or reinforcing maladaptive dietary practices. Findings from this study echo the literature on the role of the physical, economic, and sociocultural environment to affect the ability to secure nutritious food [13,14,16,44,45], and notably, it is the first to extend the knowledge on how this phenomenon is expressed in first-year college students exposed to a food desert, an environment deprived of a consistent variety of nutritious options.

Affordability of available options was a major factor affecting students' food choices. The perceived higher price of nutritious food on campus compared to food of poor nutritional value was recurrently mentioned as a deterrent to choose the former. Economic factors are main drivers of food choices for both low-income populations and college students [33,46–49]. Given the socioeconomic background of this study's informants, economic factors were expectedly central when discussing their food choices. The majority of the students in this study were from low-income backgrounds. The cost of attendance for these students living on campus is 27% to 34% higher than that for those living off-campus, mostly due to higher cost of housing [50]; most first-year students live on campus (72%) [27]. Although a significant proportion of students in this campus are eligible for and do receive financial aid, their disposable income is seemingly low. In fact, recent reports [26] indicate the majority of the students attending this university struggle to cover their basic needs, especially when it comes to having consistent access to nutritious food. To alleviate these disparities, the university has appointed a taskforce of students, staff, and academics to execute a plan [26] that includes establishing and expanding food distribution programs (e.g., food pantries, food banks, electronic meal donations), supporting infrastructure (e.g., meal preparation facilities, transportation), financial and nutrition education, and guidance on food assistance applications. Monitoring the effectiveness and relevance of these activities is paramount to identifying best practices and areas of improvement. Ultimately attaining a campus food environment that allows for adequate and consistent access to nutritious food is essential, especially among students at the greatest risk of malnutrition due to limited access to resources.

As emphasized by students in this study, a meal plan program can help to mitigate some of the food access challenges faced by first-year students living on campus. Having a meal plan can mean regular access to convenient meals [51]. In addition, and according to some students, having a budget committed to food may help to lessen the possibility of competing spending priorities to affect their ability to secure the food they needed in a given period. Students also revealed disadvantages to the meal plan, including poor acceptability of the food offered at approved venues and its restricted use to only designated dining locations (and not outside food or produce trucks) on campus. Internal reports indicate students have a choice between one of three meal plans, two of which are recommended for students who consume less than 3 meals per day. Thus, these meal plans may be insufficient to meet their dietary needs, especially considering all meal options offered are à la carte. Given their socioeconomic status and in an effort to maximize their food budget, these students may choose the limited meal plans and make food choices based on taste preferences and convenience rather than nutritional value, as expressed by many in this study. Access to and greater consumption of food of low nutritional quality as related to meal plans has been reported by others [51]. In this study, students' HEI-2015 scores corroborate poor alignment with dietary recommendations [52]. Incentivizing the consumption of nutritious food by making it more ubiquitous, affordable, and appealing has been proposed to prevent dietary maladaptation in college students [45]. Some evidence suggests that eating behavior worsens with each semester in college [53] and that first-year students living on campus may be more responsive to interventions that incentivize nutritious food purchases than older students and students living off-campus [54].

Aspects of the physical environment, such as availability and accessibility, are expected to be particularly restricting to the food choices of those living in food deserts [11,14]. Availability of a variety of nutritious options is the dimension of the perceived food environment most consistently associated with positive dietary outcomes [14,33]. Mixed results are reported in the literature for the accessibility dimension, with some evidence indicating proximity to nutritious food outlets is secondary to the quality, variety, and price of available food [14,48]. However, most of available evidence is not specific to college settings. Moreover, in this inquiry, low variety and poor quality of available options on campus did appear to inform student food choices in favor of a less nutritious diet but not independently of and as prominently as price. For instance, although quality and variety were valued attributes, cost was described as a decisive factor in choosing one food over another. At the time this study was conducted, food outlets on campus included the campus dining center, one cold-food cafeteria, a convenience store, a few alternating food trucks from local restaurants, one produce truck visiting campus once a week, and vending machines. Although a systematic environmental mapping of food outlets to triangulate student perceptions was beyond the scope of this study, it was apparent that consistent access to affordable nutritious food was questionable, at best, in this university campus.

Unlike reports from noncollege populations [14], convenient access to nutritious food was also deemed an important determinant of eating choices by this study's informants. Convenience was mostly expressed as the time required to acquire and prepare food, and it was regarded in terms of proximity to food outlets and access to kitchen facilities. Based on the input from this study's informants and similar to what others have reported [45,55], the combination of academic demands and lack of access to consistent transportation appears to be a circumstance unique to college students that makes convenience a major barrier to accessing food that affect the quality of their food choices.

Relying on food provided by family was a coping strategy to obtain desired food. In the case of this study, this process is assumed to be facilitated by geography, as the majority of students come from local communities, which allow them to visit home often. Meals provided by family seemed to have the key advantage of being convenient, acceptable (i.e., familiarity and taste preferences), and free. Family food provision has been associated with greater consumption of fruits and vegetables in European college populations [56,57]. However, evidence on the prevalence of this practice and its effects on the diet quality of college students in the US is sparse. Along with the tangible value of food provisions, sharing meals at a distance may also represent a means for preserving family connections during the transition to independence of members leaving for college. Future research may explore the significance of using food to maintain such connections, especially during the developmental milestone that is the transition to adulthood and its potential consequences on the physical and emotional health of the students and their families.

Beyond food provisions, students' insight suggests that norms and beliefs acquired at home and new normative beliefs shaped by fellow students influenced the way they interact with their new food environment. On one hand, the quality of available food on campus was judged against the perceived quality of meals consumed before college. On the other hand, food choices were often made after views were expressed by fellow students. The way these normative beliefs interact to inform the process of making food decisions may depend on the motivation to align with norms imposed by family and peers [45,58]. In turn, motivation to comply with norms can be influenced by the intrinsic, extrinsic, and cost–opportunity value ascribed to acting on them [35,59]. Increasing the cost–opportunity value of nutritious options through a food environment that provides for affordable and consistent variety of such options may reinforce and/or help to establish normative beliefs that elicit sound dietary choices, which could be carried onto life after college.

To support the translation into action and the sustainability of positive normative beliefs acquired or reinforced in college, developing relevant skills is necessary [34,60,61]. In this inquiry, students consistently alluded to their agency at selecting and preparing food, under the circumstances of their new environment, as a determining factor for their eating choices. Comments from informants suggested that for many first-year students, a newly acquired independence and resulting increased autonomy can be a burden if skills needed to successfully navigate their new physical, economic, and sociocultural environment are underdeveloped or absent. In fact, student informants in this study consistently suggested that education-related solutions would improve the way they navigate their food environment and thus improve their eating choices. Interventions targeting nutrition knowledge and self-efficacy have been successful at improving eating behavior among college populations in the short term [62], especially when combined with environmental facilitators [33,45,63,64]. However, research on solutions that allow for sustained, long-term changes is needed. Actively offering nutrition education resources to students entering college appears to be a sensible way to mitigate barriers and amplify the impact of environmental and interpersonal facilitators to sustain a healthy diet. However, for educational interventions to be effective, they must be participatory, and framed on theory and evidence-based behavior change methods [65].

Findings from this study need to be pondered in light of its strengths and limitations. A key strength of this study is the ethnic makeup of the student informants, the majority of whom were from groups traditionally underrepresented in research [66]. Given the increasing incidence of food insecurity [28] and diet-related cardiometabolic disorders among ethnic/racial minority groups [25], studying these groups advances the understanding of this phenomenon for more inclusive practice and policy [67]. Limitations pertain to the bias risk inherent to the qualitative design [68] and informants being recruited from a nutrition study, which may indicate their interest in nutrition and diet beyond that of those who did not participate. To mitigate these risks, efforts to ensure trustworthiness were made, including the application of well-established methods by experienced and trained researchers, having analysts from the population of interest (i.e., undergraduate students), and considering theory and evidence in the interpretation of the results. Additionally, student informants were encouraged to be as open and thorough as possible. Moreover, all interviews were conducted by the same trained moderator, who applied recommended techniques to create a safe, nonjudgmental atmosphere.

5. Conclusions

The focus of this study was on first-year college students because of the potential for early prevention of eating behavior maladaptation, such as skipping breakfast, increased snacking, and low intake of fruits and vegetables [69] which can be tracked forth into adulthood [5] and increase the risk of weight gain and other cardiometabolic disorders. Adequacy (i.e., variety and quality), acceptability (i.e., familiarity and preferences), affordability, and accessibility (i.e., convenience and accommodation) are the aspects of the perceived environment that appeared to closely interact with subjective norms to inform internal processes of decision-making (i.e., decisional balance) and agency around the eating choices of first-year students. Perceptions are a core determinant of health behavior; thus, characterizing the perceived food environment is necessary to understand its influence on eating choices. This is particularly critical for those exposed to a nutritionally deprived food environment and simultaneously transitioning to independence. Future research should explore how these factors of the perceived environment are expressed in representative samples of college populations attending food desert campuses, and examine how student perceptions on the food environment manifest into action and transform as they become more acquainted to life in college. Although the influence of emotional health on food choices was discussed by only a minority of students in this inquiry, it deserves further examination as it has been found relevant by others [70,71]. Future robust empirical research should explore whether or not these findings hold among college students from a variety of demographic, socioeconomic, cultural, academic, and living conditions.

Supplementary Materials: The following are available online at http://www.mdpi.com/2072-6643/11/4/816/s1, Table S1: Additional representative quotes from focus group participants within thematic categories.

Author Contributions: Conceptualization, J.D., L.K.D.R. and R.M.O.; Formal analysis, J.D., L.K.D.R., K.J.A., N.D.L.C., E.V., S.A.A. and Q.K.; Funding acquisition, R.M.O.; Methodology, J.D. and L.K.D.R.; Project administration, J.D. and L.K.D.R.; Resources, R.M.O.; Supervision, J.D. and L.K.D.R.; Writing—original draft, J.D. and L.K.D.R.; Writing—review and editing, J.D., L.K.D.R. and R.M.O.

Funding: The research was partially funded through a grant from the Almond Board of California (PI: R.M.O.). J.D. is supported by the National Institute on Minority Health and Health Disparities of the National Institutes of Health under award number K99MD012815. The content is solely the responsibility of the authors and does not necessarily represent the official views of the funder. The funder had no role in the study conception, design and implementation, data collection, data analysis, or interpretation of results.

Conflicts of Interest: The authors declare no conflict of interest.

References

1. Nelson, M.C.; Story, M.; Larson, N.I.; Neumark-Sztainer, D.; Lytle, L.A. Emerging Adulthood and College-aged Youth: An Overlooked Age for Weight-related Behavior Change. *Obesity* **2008**, *16*, 2205–2211. [CrossRef] [PubMed]
2. Snyder, T.; de Brey, C.; Dillow, S. *Digest of Education Statistics 2016*, 52nd ed.; NCES 2017-094; National Center for Education Statistics: Jessup, MD, USA, 2018.
3. Vadeboncoeur, C.; Townsend, N.; Foster, C. A meta-analysis of weight gain in first year university students: Is freshman 15 a myth? *BMC Obes.* **2015**, *2*, 22. [CrossRef] [PubMed]
4. Banfield, E.C.; Liu, Y.; Davis, J.S.; Chang, S.; Frazier-Wood, A.C. Poor adherence to U.S. dietary guidelines for children and adolescents in the NHANES population. *J. Acad. Nutr. Diet.* **2016**, *116*, 21–27. [CrossRef] [PubMed]
5. Christoph, M.J.; Larson, N.I.; Winkler, M.R.; Wall, M.M.; Neumark-Sztainer, D. Longitudinal trajectories and prevalence of meeting dietary guidelines during the transition from adolescence to young adulthood. *Am. J. Clin. Nutr.* **2019**, *109*, 656–664. [CrossRef]
6. Dahm, C.C.; Chomistek, A.K.; Jakobsen, M.U.; Mukamal, K.J.; Eliassen, A.H.; Sesso, H.D.; Overvad, K.; Willett, W.C.; Rimm, E.B.; Chiuve, S.E. Adolescent Diet Quality and Cardiovascular Disease Risk Factors and Incident Cardiovascular Disease in Middle-Aged Women. *J. Am. Heart Assoc.* **2016**, *5*, e003583. [CrossRef]
7. Mokdad, A.H.; Serdula, M.K.; Dietz, W.H.; Bowman, B.A.; Marks, J.S.; Koplan, J.P. The spread of the obesity epidemic in the United States, 1991-1998. *JAMA* **1999**, *282*, 1519–1522. [CrossRef]
8. Bruening, M.; Argo, K.; Payne-Sturges, D.; Laska, M.N. The Struggle Is Real: A Systematic Review of Food Insecurity on Postsecondary Education Campuses. *J. Acad. Nutr. Diet.* **2017**, *117*, 1767–1791. [CrossRef]
9. Nazmi, A.; Martinez, S.; Byrd, A.; Robinson, D.; Bianco, S.; Maguire, J.; Crutchfield, R.M.; Condron, K.; Ritchie, L. A systematic review of food insecurity among US students in higher education. *J. Hunger Environ. Nutr.* **2018**, 1–16. [CrossRef]
10. Chen, X.; Yang, X. Does food environment influence food choices? A geographical analysis through "tweets.". *Appl. Geogr.* **2014**, *51*, 82–89.
11. Bivoltsis, A.; Cervigni, E.; Trapp, G.; Knuiman, M.; Hooper, P.; Ambrosini, G.L. Food environments and dietary intakes among adults: Does the type of spatial exposure measurement matter? A systematic review. *Int. J. Health Geogr.* **2018**, *17*, 19. [CrossRef] [PubMed]
12. Glanz, K.; Basil, M.; Maibach, E.; Goldberg, J.; Snyder, D. Why Americans Eat What They Do: Taste, Nutrition, Cost, Convenience, and Weight Control Concerns as Influences on Food Consumption. *J. Am. Diet. Assoc.* **1998**, *98*, 1118–1126. [CrossRef]
13. Alber, J.M.; Green, S.H.; Glanz, K. Perceived and Observed Food Environments, Eating Behaviors, and BMI. *Am. J. Prev. Med.* **2018**, *54*, 423–429. [CrossRef]
14. Caspi, C.E.; Sorensen, G.; Subramanian, S.V.; Kawachi, I. The local food environment and diet: A systematic review. *Health Place* **2012**, *18*, 1172–1187. [CrossRef]
15. Lacaille, L.J.; Dauner, K.N.; Krambeer, R.J.; Pedersen, J. Psychosocial and environmental determinants of eating behaviors, physical activity, and weight change among college students: A qualitative analysis. *J. Am. Coll. Health* **2011**, *59*, 531–538. [CrossRef]
16. Holben, D.H.; Marshall, M.B. Position of the Academy of Nutrition and Dietetics: Food Insecurity in the United States. *J. Acad. Nutr. Diet.* **2017**, *117*, 1991–2002. [CrossRef]
17. Martinez, S.M.; Frongillo, E.A.; Leung, C.; Ritchie, L. No food for thought: Food insecurity is related to poor mental health and lower academic performance among students in California's public university system. *J. Health Psychol.* **2018**. [CrossRef]
18. Calvez, K.; Miller, C.; Thomas, L.; Vazquez, D.; Walenta, J. The university as a site of food insecurity: Evaluating the foodscape of Texas A&M University's main campus. *Southwest. Geogr.* **2016**, *19*, 1–14.
19. Conceptualizing College Campuses as Food Deserts | Abstract Gallery | AAG Annual Meeting 2018. Available online: https://aag.secure-abstracts.com/AAG%20Annual%20Meeting%202018/abstracts-gallery/731 (accessed on 5 July 2018).
20. Janz, N.K.; Becker, M.H. The Health Belief Model: A decade later. *Health Educ. Q.* **1984**, *11*, 1–47. [CrossRef]
21. USDA ERS—Go to the Atlas. Available online: https://www.ers.usda.gov/data-products/food-access-research-atlas/go-to-the-atlas/ (accessed on 28 April 2017).

22. UC Merced Institutional Planning & Analysis ~ Student Statistics. Available online: http://irds.ucmerced.edu/student.htm (accessed on 17 April 2018).
23. Link, C.L.; McKinlay, J.B. Disparities in the prevalence of diabetes: Is it race/ethnicity or socioeconomic status? Results from the Boston Area Community Health (BACH) survey. *Ethn. Dis.* **2009**, *19*, 288–292.
24. Karlamangla, A.S.; Merkin, S.S.; Crimmins, E.M.; Seeman, T.E. Socioeconomic and ethnic disparities in cardiovascular risk in the United States, 2001-2006. *Ann. Epidemiol.* **2010**, *20*, 617–628. [CrossRef]
25. Lancaster, K.J.; Bermudez, O.I. Beginning a discussion of nutrition and health disparities. *Am. J. Clin. Nutr.* **2011**, *93*, 1161S–1162S. [CrossRef]
26. *UC Global Food Initiative: Food and Housing Security at the University of California*; University of California Office of the President: Oakland, CA, USA, 2017; Available online: https://www.ucop.edu/global-food-initiative/_files/food-housing-security.pdf (accessed on 6 September 2018).
27. Quick Facts | Housing & Residence Life. Available online: https://housing.ucmerced.edu/about/quick-facts (accessed on 6 September 2018).
28. Martinez, S.M.; Webb, K.; Frongillo, E.A.; Ritchie, L.D. Food insecurity in California's public university system: What are the risk factors? *J. Hunger Environ. Nutr.* **2018**, *13*, 1–18. [CrossRef]
29. Dhillon, J.; Thorwald, M.; De La Cruz, N.; Vu, E.; Asghar, S.A.; Kuse, Q.; Diaz Rios, L.K.; Ortiz, R.M. Glucoregulatory and Cardiometabolic Profiles of Almond vs. Cracker Snacking for 8 Weeks in Young Adults: A Randomized Controlled Trial. *Nutrients* **2018**, *10*, 960. [CrossRef]
30. Krueger, R. *Developing Questions for Focus Groups*; SAGE Publications, Inc.: Thousand Oaks, CA, USA, 1998; ISBN 978-0-7619-0819-7.
31. Bandura, A. Social Cognitive Theory: An Agentic Perspective. *Annu. Rev. Psychol.* **2001**, *52*, 1–26. [CrossRef]
32. McLeroy, K.R.; Bibeau, D.; Steckler, A.; Glanz, K. An ecological perspective on health promotion programs. *Health Educ. Q.* **1988**, *15*, 351–377. [CrossRef]
33. Roy, R.; Kelly, B.; Rangan, A.; Allman-Farinelli, M. Food Environment Interventions to Improve the Dietary Behavior of Young Adults in Tertiary Education Settings: A Systematic Literature Review. *J. Acad. Nutr. Diet.* **2015**, *115*, 1647.e1–1681.e1. [CrossRef]
34. Ajzen, I. The theory of planned behavior. *Organ. Behav. Hum. Decis. Process.* **1991**, *50*, 179–211. [CrossRef]
35. Wigfield, A.; Eccles, J.S. Expectancy-Value Theory of Achievement Motivation. *Contemp. Educ. Psychol.* **2000**, *25*, 68–81. [CrossRef]
36. Maykut, P.; Morehouse, R. *Beginning Qualitative Research: A Philosophical and Practical 403 Guide*; Psychology Press: London, UK, 1994.
37. Sandelowski, M. Real qualitative researchers do not count: The use of numbers in qualitative research. *Res. Nurs. Health* **2001**, *24*, 230–240. [CrossRef]
38. Patton, M. *How to Use Qualitative Methods in Evaluation*, 2nd ed.; SAGE Publications: Newbury Park, CA, USA, 1987; Volume 4.
39. Strauss, A.; Corbin, J. Grounded theory methodology: An overview. In *Handbook of Qualitative Research*; Sage Publications, Inc.: Thousand Oaks, CA, USA, 1994; pp. 273–285. ISBN 978-0-8039-4679-8.
40. Lincoln, Y.; Guba, E. *Naturalistic Inquiry*; SAGE Publications: Newbury Park, CA, USA, 1985.
41. Krebs-Smith, S.M.; Pannucci, T.E.; Subar, A.F.; Kirkpatrick, S.I.; Lerman, J.L.; Tooze, J.A.; Wilson, M.M.; Reedy, J. Update of the Healthy Eating Index: HEI-2015. *J. Acad. Nutr. Diet.* **2018**, *118*, 1591–1602. [CrossRef]
42. Automated Self-Administered 24-Hour (ASA24®) Dietary Assessment Tool. Available online: https://epi.grants.cancer.gov/asa24/ (accessed on 6 September 2018).
43. Healthy Eating Index: Choosing a method and SAS code website. Available online: https://epi.grants.cancer.gov/hei/sas-code.html (accessed on 8 October 2018).
44. Sleddens, E.F.; Kroeze, W.; Kohl, L.F.; Bolten, L.M.; Velema, E.; Kaspers, P.J.; Brug, J.; Kremers, S.P. Determinants of dietary behavior among youth: An umbrella review. *Int. J. Behav. Nutr. Phys. Act.* **2015**, *12*, 7. [CrossRef] [PubMed]
45. Deliens, T.; Clarys, P.; De Bourdeaudhuij, I.; Deforche, B. Determinants of eating behaviour in university students: A qualitative study using focus group discussions. *BMC Public Health* **2014**, *14*, 53. [CrossRef] [PubMed]
46. Burns, C.; Cook, K.; Mavoa, H. Role of expendable income and price in food choice by low income families. *Appetite* **2013**, *71*, 209–217. [CrossRef]

47. Steenhuis, I.H.M.; Waterlander, W.E.; de Mul, A. Consumer food choices: The role of price and pricing strategies. *Public Health Nutr.* **2011**, *14*, 2220–2226. [CrossRef]
48. Ghosh-Dastidar, B.; Cohen, D.; Hunter, G.; Zenk, S.N.; Huang, C.; Beckman, R.; Dubowitz, T. Distance to store, food prices, and obesity in urban food deserts. *Am. J. Prev. Med.* **2014**, *47*, 587–595. [CrossRef] [PubMed]
49. Tam, R.; Yassa, B.; Parker, H.; O'Connor, H.; Allman-Farinelli, M. University students' on-campus food purchasing behaviors, preferences, and opinions on food availability. *Nutr. Burbank Los Angel. Cty. Calif* **2017**, *37*, 7–13. [CrossRef]
50. Cost of Attendance | Financial Aid. Available online: https://financialaid.ucmerced.edu/cost-attendance (accessed on 6 September 2018).
51. Gonzales, R.; Laurent, J.S.; Johnson, R.K. Relationship Between Meal Plan, Dietary Intake, Body Mass Index, and Appetitive Responsiveness in College Students. *J. Pediatr. Health Care Off. Publ. Natl. Assoc. Pediatr. Nurse Assoc. Pract.* **2017**, *31*, 320–326. [CrossRef]
52. Healthy Eating Index (HEI) | Center for Nutrition Policy and Promotion. Available online: https://www.cnpp.usda.gov/healthyeatingindex (accessed on 20 December 2017).
53. Small, M.; Bailey-Davis, L.; Morgan, N.; Maggs, J. Changes in eating and physical activity behaviors across seven semesters of college: Living on or off campus matters. *Health Educ. Behav. Off. Publ. Soc. Public Health Educ.* **2013**, *40*, 435–441. [CrossRef] [PubMed]
54. McComb, S.; Jones, C.; Smith, A.; Collins, W.; Pope, B. Designing Incentives to Change Behaviors: Examining College Student Intent Toward Healthy Diets. *West. J. Nurs. Res.* **2016**, *38*, 1094–1113. [CrossRef]
55. Pelletier, J.E.; Laska, M.N. Balancing healthy meals and busy lives: Associations between work, school and family responsibilities and perceived time constraints among young adults. *J. Nutr. Educ. Behav.* **2012**, *44*, 481–489. [CrossRef]
56. Winpenny, E.M.; van Sluijs, E.M.F.; White, M.; Klepp, K.-I.; Wold, B.; Lien, N. Changes in diet through adolescence and early adulthood: Longitudinal trajectories and association with key life transitions. *Int. J. Behav. Nutr. Phys. Act.* **2018**, *15*, 86. [CrossRef]
57. El Ansari, W.; Stock, C.; Mikolajczyk, R.T. Relationships between food consumption and living arrangements among university students in four European countries—A cross-sectional study. *Nutr. J.* **2012**, *11*, 28. [CrossRef]
58. Reicks, M.; Banna, J.; Cluskey, M.; Gunther, C.; Hongu, N.; Richards, R.; Topham, G.; Wong, S.S. Influence of Parenting Practices on Eating Behaviors of Early Adolescents during Independent Eating Occasions: Implications for Obesity Prevention. *Nutrients* **2015**, *7*, 8783–8801. [CrossRef]
59. Cook, D.A.; Artino, A.R. Motivation to learn: An overview of contemporary theories. *Med. Educ.* **2016**, *50*, 997–1014. [CrossRef]
60. Bandura, A. Health promotion by social cognitive means. *Health Educ. Behav. Off. Publ. Soc. Public Health Educ.* **2004**, *31*, 143–164. [CrossRef]
61. Bandura, A.; Adams, N.E.; Beyer, J. Cognitive processes mediating behavioral change. *J. Pers. Soc. Psychol.* **1977**, *35*, 125–139. [CrossRef]
62. Kelly, N.R.; Mazzeo, S.E.; Bean, M.K. Systematic review of dietary interventions with college students: Directions for future research and practice. *J. Nutr. Educ. Behav.* **2013**, *45*, 304–313. [CrossRef]
63. Yahia, N.; Brown, C.A.; Rapley, M.; Chung, M. Level of nutrition knowledge and its association with fat consumption among college students. *BMC Public Health* **2016**, *16*, 1047. [CrossRef]
64. Plotnikoff, R.C.; Costigan, S.A.; Williams, R.L.; Hutchesson, M.J.; Kennedy, S.G.; Robards, S.L.; Allen, J.; Collins, C.E.; Callister, R.; Germov, J. Effectiveness of interventions targeting physical activity, nutrition and healthy weight for university and college students: A systematic review and meta-analysis. *Int. J. Behav. Nutr. Phys. Act.* **2015**, *12*, 45. [CrossRef]
65. Kok, G.; Peters, L.W.H.; Ruiter, R.A.C. Planning theory- and evidence-based behavior change interventions: A conceptual review of the intervention mapping protocol. *Psicol. Reflex. E Crítica* **2017**, *30*, 19. [CrossRef]
66. Erves, J.C.; Mayo-Gamble, T.L.; Malin-Fair, A.; Boyer, A.; Joosten, Y.; Vaughn, Y.C.; Sherden, L.; Luther, P.; Miller, S.; Wilkins, C.H. Needs, Priorities, and Recommendations for Engaging Underrepresented Populations in Clinical Research: A Community Perspective. *J. Community Health* **2017**, *42*, 472–480. [CrossRef] [PubMed]
67. Johnson-Askew, W.L.; Gordon, L.; Sockalingam, S. Practice paper of the American Dietetic Association: Addressing racial and ethnic health disparities. *J. Am. Diet. Assoc.* **2011**, *111*, 446–456. [CrossRef] [PubMed]

68. Mays, N.; Pope, C. Qualitative Research: Rigour and qualitative research. *BMJ* **1995**, *311*, 109–112. [CrossRef] [PubMed]
69. Stok, F.M.; Renner, B.; Clarys, P.; Lien, N.; Lakerveld, J.; Deliens, T. Understanding Eating Behavior during the Transition from Adolescence to Young Adulthood: A Literature Review and Perspective on Future Research Directions. *Nutrients* **2018**, *10*, 667. [CrossRef] [PubMed]
70. Ashurst, J.; van Woerden, I.; Dunton, G.; Todd, M.; Ohri-Vachaspati, P.; Swan, P.; Bruening, M. The Association among Emotions and Food Choices in First-Year College Students Using mobile-Ecological Momentary Assessments. *BMC Public Health* **2018**, *18*, 573. [CrossRef] [PubMed]
71. Meza, A.; Altman, E.; Martinez, S.; Leung, C.W. "It's a Feeling That One Is Not Worth Food": A Qualitative Study Exploring the Psychosocial Experience and Academic Consequences of Food Insecurity Among College Students. *J. Acad. Nutr. Diet.* **2018**. [CrossRef] [PubMed]

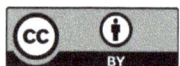

© 2019 by the authors. Licensee MDPI, Basel, Switzerland. This article is an open access article distributed under the terms and conditions of the Creative Commons Attribution (CC BY) license (http://creativecommons.org/licenses/by/4.0/).

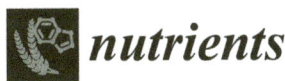

Article

Tracking Kids' Food: Comparing the Nutritional Value and Marketing Appeals of Child-Targeted Supermarket Products Over Time

Charlene Elliott

Department of Communication, Media, and Film, and Faculty of Kinesiology, University of Calgary, Calgary, AB T2N 1N4, Canada; celliott@ucalgary.ca; Tel.: +1-403-220-3180

Received: 25 June 2019; Accepted: 7 August 2019; Published: 9 August 2019

Abstract: Marketing unhealthy foods negatively impacts children's food preferences, dietary habits and health, prompting calls for regulations that will help to create an "enabling" food environment for children. One powerful food marketing technique is product packaging, but little is known about the nature or quality of child-targeted food products over time. This study assesses how child-targeted supermarket foods in Canada have transformed with respect to nutritional profile and types of marketing appeals (that is, the power of such marketing). Products from 2009 ($n = 354$) and from 2017 ($n = 374$) were first evaluated and compared in light of two established nutritional criteria, and then compared in terms of marketing techniques on packages. Overall, child-targeted supermarket foods did not improve nutritionally over time: 88% of child-targeted products (across both datasets) would not be permitted to be marketed to children, according to the World Health Organization (WHO) criteria, and sugar levels remained consistently high. Despite this poor nutritional quality, the use of nutrition claims increased significantly over time, as did the use of cartoon characters and appealing fonts to attract children's attention. Character licensing—using characters from entertainment companies—remained consistent. The findings reveal the critical need to consider packaging as part of the strategy for protecting children from unhealthy food marketing. Given the poor nutritional quality and appealing nature of child-oriented supermarket foods, food product packaging needs to be included in the WHO's call to improve the restrictions on unhealthy food marketing to children.

Keywords: Children; nutrition; food marketing; food packaging; power; Canada; time trends; policy

1. Introduction

"See it, want it, buy it, eat it!" Such was the title of a 2018 Cancer Research UK-funded study on the impact of food advertising on children's diets [1]—and, in many respects, this title sums up the prevailing concerns related to food marketing to children writ large. Unhealthy food and beverage marketing has been shown to negatively impact children's food choice and diet-related health [2–7], and is implicated in the rising rates of childhood obesity [8].

Recognizing the need to protect children from the marketing of foods high in sugar, fat and/or salt, in 2010, the World Health Organization (WHO) developed a set of recommendations on the topic [9]. Nearly a decade later, such calls for protection are especially pressing. A recent systematic review on the influence of food marketing on children's attitudes, preferences and consumption concluded that food marketing had "significant detrimental effects" on children's food preferences and tastes [10] (pp. 1).

Food marketing entails a range of commercial communication strategies designed to promote a product. Techniques include advertising (on broadcast media, print media, online or outdoors), product placement and branding, sponsorship, direct marketing (such as text messages to mobile phones or promotion of foods in schools), point of sale (such as on-shelf displays, or free samples), and product design and packaging [9] (pp. 10). Product packaging is of particular interest, here, because it is a key promotional technique for capturing the attention of children and parents [9] (pp. 10), [11] (pp. 9), [12,13]. Food products have been packaged with cartoon characters, fun appeals (including promoting unusual shapes, flavors or qualities), and licensed characters from children's television programs, merchandise and films in order to amplify their appeal to, and for, children [14–17]. However, these products have also been criticized for their poor nutritional quality [18–23].

Despite the importance of food packaging in our contemporary foodscape and to children's health, very little is known about the nature or quality of child-targeted food products over time. Studies are typically cross-sectional in nature, providing little insight into the transformations of child-targeted foods over time, both nutritionally and in terms of marketing appeals. This study aims to fill this research gap. The purpose of this study is to assess how child-targeted supermarket foods in Canada have transformed over time—between 2009 and 2017—with respect to nutritional profile and types of marketing appeals. The findings not only speak to the extent to which the food industry has embraced its promise to improve the nutritional profile of children's food, but also provide valuable insight into the changing landscape of supermarket foods targeted to children in Canada.

2. Materials and Methods

Data collection of child-targeted food products in 2009 [21,24] and 2017 [23] was similar, and has been detailed elsewhere. In brief, all child-targeted food and drink products were purchased from two grocery stores in Calgary, Alberta in the years 2009 and 2017. The Real Canadian Superstore and Safeway were selected as data collection sites because they represent Canada's two leading retail grocery and food distributors (Loblaws Companies Ltd. and Sobeys Inc). Child-targeted foods were defined as products containing: the word 'child' or 'kid' in the brand or product name; appeals to fun or play on the package; links with children's popular culture; or child-friendly graphics or games. Excluded from the study were baby and toddler foods (which are their own separate category). Also excluded were "junk food" products (such as sodas, potato chips, and confectionary products), because these items are typically viewed as of poor nutritional value and extraneous to one's diet. Instead, the study focused on how 'regular' food (items in the dairy, dry goods, produce, meat, refrigerated and frozen) and beverage categories have been repackaged to appeal to children. Two trained graduate students photographed and coded each product for multiple nutritional and packaging variables. Drawing from previous research [14], a codebook was developed for product coding. The codebook explicitly described how to code each variable: for example, an unusual product shape was defined as foodstuff having a non-traditional physical form (e.g., pasta shaped like Scooby Doo or Star Wars characters), while an unusual package shape was defined as packaging or individual food packets having a non-traditional physical form (e.g., pudding in a tube, yogurt drink in an hourglass-shaped container). Prior to coding, the products collected were reviewed, and additional variables were added to the codebook as necessary. Any questions and clarifications were discussed with the study lead and decisions were documented in the codebook.

2.1. Nutritional Criteria

The nutritional value of products were assessed using two evaluative criteria: the US Centre for Science in the Public Interest (CSPI) criteria for Poor Nutritional Quality (PNQ) with a modified criteria to evaluate sugar [25] (to represent an established nutritional standard at the time of the first data collection in 2009) and the WHO Regional Office for Europe Model (to represent current standards) [26].

The CSPI's PNQ criteria use nutrient content thresholds per serving size to determine the nutritional value of a product. According to the CSPI, a product is of PNQ if it meets one of the following criteria:

- >35% of total calories from fat, excluding nuts, seeds, and peanut or other nut butters;
- >35% added sugars by weight;

- >230 mg sodium per serving for chips, crackers, cheeses, baked goods, French fries, or other snacks;
- >480 mg sodium per serving for cereals, soups, pastas and meats;
- >600 mg sodium for pizza, sandwiches and main dishes;
- >770 mg sodium for meals

As mentioned, unique criteria were used to assess sugar levels. Drawing from previous research [18,27] and the American Heart Association recommendations, we classified foods as of poor nutritional quality if more than 20% of their calories derive from sugar per 200-calorie serving. This approach allows for a more nuanced analysis because it assesses the percentage of sugars (instead of an absolute cut-off regardless of portion size) [18] (pp. 370).

The WHO model, in contrast, represents current thinking when it comes to evaluating the nutritional quality of foods for children: it classifies products regarding their suitability for marketing to children. Products are first classified into one of 17 food categories. Chocolate and confectionery products, cakes, cookies and other sweet baked goods, juices, energy drinks, and edible ices are not permitted to be marketed to children regardless of their nutrient content. Products in the remaining categories are then assessed based on category-specific nutrient content thresholds per 100 gram (or mL) servings for total fat, saturated fat, total sugar, added sugar, non-sugar sweetener, salt, and energy (see Annex 1 of the WHO Regional Office for Europe Nutrient Profile Model Report [26] for a detailed description of nutrient criteria). Products that exceed one or more nutrient thresholds are deemed unsuitable for marketing to children.

2.2. Approaches to Assessing the 2009 and 2017 Datasets

Child-targeted products from the 2009 and 2017 datasets were assessed using four approaches. First, we compared the nutritional value of products using the PNQ and WHO criteria (detailed above). Next, we selected a subsample ($n = 14$) of identical products from 2009 and 2017 and compared the content of sugar, sodium, and fat per serving size and per 100 g. The subsample of identical products provides a snapshot of changes over time (but the list is not exhaustive). Standardized comparisons per 100 g are more valid and interpretable in this context to account for varying serving sizes. We then assessed differences in nutritional claims made on product packaging, such as "low in nutrient", "source of nutrient", and organic, among others. Finally, we compared the marketing appeals used for products in each year, including references to fun, cartoon images, unusual product or package shapes, and parent appeal, among others. Frequencies were used to summarize the data. Chi-square tests or Fisher's exact tests were used for all proportion comparisons (i.e., nutritional value, nutritional claims, marketing appeals). Identical product comparisons were not appropriate for bivariate analysis given that single products were compared in 2009 and 2017, but rather nutrient differences were assessed descriptively. All data cleaning and analysis were completed using SPSS (IBM Corp, Armonk, NY, USA) [28] and Stata (StataCorp, College Station, TX, USA) [29].

3. Results

3.1. Child-Targeted Food Products in 2009 and 2017

Overall, the number of child-targeted supermarket foods increased over time—from 354 products in 2009 to 374 products in 2017 (See Table 1). The proportion of children's food in the Dry Goods category increased moderately from 63.8% in 2009 to 77.5% in 2017: Cookies and Biscuits and Fruit Snacks and Applesauce were the most common food types at both time points. Within this category, the largest increase was with Granola/Cereal bars, which jumped from 4.0 to 12.6% of products between 2009 and 2017. Cereal products also increased over the 8-year span—from 8.8 to 15.8% of the dataset. With respect to the other broad categories, Refrigerated and Frozen Foods increased slightly (from 8.5% in 2009 to 10.4% in 2017), generally due to a small increase in Ice Cream and Frozen Ices and Popsicles products. Dairy represented 14.7% of the products in 2009, but fell to 7.8% in 2017, with Cheese, Milk, and Yogurt products in particular decreasing across the time periods. Refrigerated and Frozen Meal products also dropped from 10.2% in 2009 to 2.9% in 2018. Produce and Meat were consistently the smallest food categories, with approximately 1–2% of products (See Table 1).

Table 1. Frequency of children's foods in 2009 and 2017 by category.

Category	2009 n (%)	2017 n (%)
Dry goods	226 (63.8)	290 (77.5)
Cereal	31 (8.8)	59 (15.8)
Crackers	11 (3.1)	18 (4.8)
Cookies and Biscuits	52 (14.7)	59 (15.8)
Fruit Snacks and Applesauce	47 (13.3)	46 (12.3)
Granola/Cereal Bars	14 (4.0)	47 (12.6)
Pasta (Boxed/Canned) and Soups	17 (4.8)	25 (6.7)
Drinks and Drink boxes	19 (5.4)	29 (7.8)
Drink Syrups, Crystals, and Powders	22 (6.2)	0 (0)
Puddings and Jell-Os	5 (1.4)	2 (0.5)
Dressing, Sauces, Condiments, and Toppings	1 (0.3)	4 (1.1)
Peanut Butters, Jams, and Spreads	7 (2.0)	1 (0.3)
Meat	6 (1.7)	3 (0.8)
Chicken	5 (1.4)	2 (0.5)
Beef	1 (0.3)	0 (0)
Fish	0 (0)	1 (0.3)
Produce	4 (1.1)	2 (0.5)
Fruit	2 (0.6)	1 (0.3)
Vegetable	2 (0.6)	1 (0.3)
Refrigerated and Frozen Foods	30 (8.5)	39 (10.4)
Fries and Potatoes	3 (0.8)	1 (0.3)
Frozen Breakfast Foods and Strudels	9 (2.5)	7 (1.9)
Frozen Ices and Popsicles	13 (3.7)	19 (5.1)
Ice Cream	5 (1.4)	9 (2.4)
Refrigerated Cookies	0 (0)	3 (0.8)
Refrigerated and Frozen Meals	36 (10.2)	11 (2.9)
Packaged Lunch	15 (4.2)	10 (2.7)
Frozen Dinners and Meals	5 (1.4)	0 (0)
Pizza and Pogos	16 (4.5)	1 (0.3)
Dairy	52 (14.7)	29 (7.8)
Milk	16 (4.5)	6 (1.6)
Yogurt	15 (4.2)	9 (2.4)
Milk and Yogurt Drinks	1 (0.3)	8 (2.1)
Cheese	20 (5.6)	6 (1.6)
Total	354 (100)	374 (100)

3.2. Nutritional Value

Child-targeted supermarket products have overall poor nutritional quality, irrespective of the evaluative criteria used (see Table 2). Using the CSPI criteria, 88.7% of products in 2009 and 86.9% of products in 2017 would be classified as poorly nutritious. Using the WHO model, 88% of these child-targeted products (in both years tracked) would *not* be permitted to be marketed to children.

Table 2. Comparison of the nutritional value of children's food products from 2009 and 2017.

Nutritional Criteria	2009 n (%)	2017 n (%)	p-value
CPSI Criteria for Poor Nutritional Quality			
High in sugar [1]	258 (72.9)	289 (77.3)	0.171
High in fat	57 (16.1)	62 (16.6)	0.862
High in sodium	43 (12.1)	20 (5.3)	0.001 *
High in sugar, fat, or sodium	314 (88.7)	325 (86.9)	0.458
Low in sugar, sodium, and fat	40 (11.3)	49 (13.1)	
WHO Nutrient Profile Model for Marketing to Children			
Permitted for marketing to children	42 (11.9)	44 (11.8)	0.967
Not permitted for marketing to children	312 (88.1)	330 (88.2)	

CPSI = The US Center for Science in the Public Interest. WHO = World Health Organization. * statistically significant.
[1] Over 20% calories from sugar.

By far, the most common nutrient threshold exceeded was sugar, with 72.9 and 77.3% of products having excess sugar in 2009 and 2017, respectively; this difference was not significant. Approximately 16% of products were high in fat in each dataset. Products with excess sodium per serving size dropped over time, and this was statistically significant, with 12.1% of products in 2009 compared to 5.3% of products in 2017 ($p = 0.001$). Overall, no significant difference exists in the share of nutritionally poor products in 2009 versus 2017, with nearly nine out of every 10 products exceeding the sugar, sodium, or fat threshold at both time points. Furthermore, the proportion of products deemed suitable for marketing to children (based on nutritional value) was not significantly different, remaining at approximately 12% over time.

3.3. Product Comparison

Of the 14 identical products we compared, none had the same serving size and nutrient content in 2009 and 2017. Kellogg's Pop Tarts (Frosted Strawberry) changed the least from 2009 to 2017, with equal serving size, sodium, and fat but decreased sugar. Six of the 14 products decreased their serving size, which was always accompanied by an increase in at least one of sugar, sodium, or fat per 100 g even if the respective nutrient content per serving size did not change or decreased. For example, Quaker's Kid's Oatmeal (Dino Eggs) decreased in serving size from 46 g in 2009 to 38 g in 2017. The fat content per serving size is 3 g in both years. However, the fat content per 100 g increased from 6.5 g in 2009 to 7.9 g in 2017. Irrespective of serving size, four products had no change or a decrease in sugar, sodium, and fat content per 100 g, whereas no products had an increase in all three nutrients per 100 g. Ten products had a combination of nutrient changes per 100 g over time. For example, Dare Bear Paws Soft Cookies (Banana Bread) had an increase in sugar but a decrease in sodium and fat in 2017 compared to 2009. The most common nutrient to change in products per 100 g was sodium (12 products) followed by sugar (11 products) and fat (10 products). General Mills Lucky Charms was the only product that had reduced sugar, sodium, and fat per 100 g from 2009 to 2017 (see Table 3).

Table 3. Comparison in serving size and nutrient content for identical children's food products from 2009 and 2017.

Product Name	Serving Size (SS) [1]		Sugar			Sodium			Fat		
			Per SS	Per 100 g		Per SS	Per 100 g		Per SS	Per 100 g	
Dare Bear Paws Soft Cookies (Banana Bread)											
2009	50	↓	14	28	↑	230	460	↓	7	14	↓
2017	45		13	28.9		170	377.8		5	11.1	
Betty Crocker Dunkaroos (Vanilla Frosting and Rainbow Sprinkles)											
2009	28	↓	12	42.9	↑	75	267.9	↑	4.5	16.1	↓
2017	26		12	46.2		75	288.5		3.5	13.5	
Betty Crocker Fruit Gushers (Gushin' Grape and Tropical Flavors)											
2009	26	↓	13	50	↓	40	153.8	↑	1	3.8	↑
2017	23		9	39.1		40	173.9		1	4.3	
Pepperidge Farm Goldfish (Xplosive Pizza)											
2009	20	=	1	5.0	=	160	800	↑	4.5	22.5	↓
2017	20		1	5.0		200	1000		3.5	17.5	
Quaker Kid's Oatmeal (Dino Eggs)											
2009	46	↓	16	34.8	↓	280	608.7	↓	3	6.5	↑
2017	38		12	31.6		170	447.4		3	7.9	
Quaker Kid's Oatmeal (Cookies 'n Crème)											
2009	38	=	10	26.3	↓	230	605.3	↓	3.5	9.2	=
2017	38		9	23.7		190	500		3.5	9.2	
General Mills Lucky Charms Cereal											
2009	25	↑	11	44.0	↓	180	720	↓	1	4	↓
2017	28		10	35.7		180	642.9		1	3.6	
General Mills Chocolate Lucky Charms Cereal											
2009	25	↑	11	44.0	↓	130	520	↑	1	4	↓
2017	29		10	34.5		160	551.7		1	3.4	
Schneiders LunchMate Nachos (Cheese and Salsa)											
2009	121	↓	17	14.0	=	670	553.7	↑	17	14.0	=
2017	100		14	14.0		560	560.0		14	14.0	
Saputo Milk 2 Go (Chillin' Chocolate)											
2009	250	=	26	10.4	=	270	108	↓	3	1.2	↓
2017	250		26	10.4		180	72		2.5	1	
Kellogg's Pop Tarts (Frosted Strawberry)											
2009	50	=	18	36	↓	160	320	=	5	10	=
2017	50		16	32		160	320		5	10	
Kellogg's Rice Krispies (Vanilla)											
2009	32	=	9	28.1	↑	190	593.8	↓	0	0	=
2017	32		10	31.25		160	500		0	0	
Yoplait Yogurt Tubes (Peach and Blueberry)											
2009	60	=	5	8.3	↑	30	50	=	1.5	2.5	↓
2017	60		6	10		30	50		1	1.7	
President's Choice Zookies Animal Cookies											
2009	35	↓	6	17.1	↓	160	457.1	↓	5	14.3	↑
2017	30		5	16.7		90	300		4.5	15	

[1] SS = serving size.

3.4. Nutritional Claims

Products with any front of package nutrition claim increased dramatically, from 31.4% in 2009 to 86.6% in 2017 ($p < 0.001$), while back or side of package claims did not differ significantly across time (see Table 4). Both gluten-free claims and peanut/nut-free claims were four times more common in 2017 compared to 2009 increasing from 2.8 to 13.1% ($p < 0.001$) and from 5.7 to 21.1% ($p < 0.001$). Claims of no artificial flavors/colors also jumped significantly, from 11.6 to 35.3% ($p < 0.001$). Conversely, "source of" (e.g., vitamin D, iron, calcium) claims and organic claims have generally become significantly less common in 2017 compared to 2009. A number of nutrient and ingredient claims—such as no added sugar, low in saturated fat, and source of essential nutrients—remained stable and low in usage (roughly between 1 and 3% of products) over time. With respect to nutrition symbols or seals, the Health Check (developed by the Heart and Stroke Foundation of Canada) was labelled on very few products in 2009 (4.8%), and discontinued by 2017, respectively. In the 2009 dataset, we did not code specifically for industry-created nutrition symbols (with the exception of PepsiCo's Smart Spot, a green symbol ostensibly designed to help consumers identify brands that can contribute to "healthier lifestyles" [30]—as that was the prevalent symbol at the time). Yet in 2017, industry-created nutrition symbols or claims were prevalent (these include marketing taglines that communicate "better" brand choices to consumers, such as Annie's Made with Goodness! claim, Kellogg's Simply Good! claim or Dare's Made Better! claim). Such claims were found on more than one of every three products—35.6%—in 2017.

Table 4. Comparison of nutrition claims on children's food products from 2009 and 2017.

Nutrition Claim	2009 n (%)	2017 n (%)	p-value
Any front of package nutrition claim	111 (31.4)	324 (86.6)	<0.001 *
Any back or side of package nutrition claim	164 (46.3)	158 (42.3)	0.268
"No" claims			
No artificial flavors/colors	41 (11.6)	132 (35.3)	<0.001 *
No trans-fat	46 (13.0)	22 (5.9)	0.001 *
No preservatives	11 (3.1)	35 (9.4)	0.001 *
No added sugar	10 (2.8)	8 (2.1)	0.551
No artificial sweeteners	5 (1.4)	0 (0)	0.027 *
"Low" claims			
Low sodium	3 (0.9)	5 (1.3)	0.726
Low fat	18 (5.1)	11 (2.9)	0.139
Low sugar	8 (2.3)	1 (0.3)	0.018 *
Low in saturated fat	10 (2.8)	9 (2.4)	0.723
"Source of" Claims			
Whole grain OR source of fiber	30 (8.5)	38 (10.2)	0.435
Source of iron	22 (6.2)	7 (1.9)	0.003 *
Source of calcium	41 (11.6)	23 (6.2)	0.010 *
Source of essential nutrients	6 (1.7)	6 (1.6)	0.924
Source of Vitamin D	23 (6.5)	10 (2.7)	0.013 *
Source of Vitamin C	36 (10.2)	0 (0)	<0.001 *
Source of protein	7 (2.0)	1 (0.3)	0.034 *
"Free" claims			
Peanut/nut free	20 (5.7)	79 (21.1)	<0.001 *
GMO free	0 (0)	8 (2.1)	0.008 *
Gluten free	10 (2.8)	49 (13.1)	<0.001 *
Fat free	11 (3.1)	6 (1.6)	0.180

Table 4. Cont.

Nutrition Claim	2009 n (%)	2017 n (%)	p-value
Other nutrition claims			
Organic	28 (7.9)	12 (3.2)	0.005 *
Non-hydrogenated oil	6 (1.7)	1 (0.3)	0.062
Nutritionist-endorsed	1 (0.3)	0 (0)	0.486
Health Check	17 (4.8)	0 (0)	—
Smart Spot	3 (0.9)	NA	—
Industry created nutrition symbol/seal	NA	133 (35.6)	—

NA = Data not available. * Statistically significant. All items refer to front of package claims, unless indicated otherwise. GMO, Genetically Modified Organism.

3.5. Marketing Appeals

Several types of marketing appeals remained consistent between the 2009 and 2017 datasets. These include character licensing, emphasizing product portability, unique qualities (e.g., product changes color, glows in the dark), unusual product shapes, and premium claims (e.g., urging children to collect points, enter a contest, offering a free download/access with a code or providing a coupon for another product (such as LEGO or Star Wars)). Other marketing appeals differed in use from 2009 to 2017. For example, the two most common marketing appeals in 2009 and 2017 were the same—child-appealing fonts (bubble fonts and fonts that look like crayoned handwriting) and cartoon images on the front of the package. However, child-appealing fonts increased from 86.4 to 94.7% ($p < 0.001$), while cartoon images (front of package) jumped from 69.2 to 85.6% ($p < 0.001$). Appealing to parents was the marketing technique that increased the most on child-targeted foods (from 65.3% in 2009 to 85.3% in 2017), whereas the use of unusual product names dropped the most from 54.5 to 12.3%. Kid-size products and/or packaging, the use of games or activities (e.g., mazes, word searches) on packaging, and references to fun also decreased in use to varying degrees (see Table 5).

Table 5. Comparison of marketing appeals used with children's food products from 2009 and 2017.

Marketing Appeals	2009 n (%)	2017 n (%)	p-value
Fun reference	78 (22.0)	59 (15.6)	0.031 *
Character licensing	60 (17.0)	59 (15.8)	0.669
Cartoon image (front of package)	245 (69.2)	320 (85.6)	<0.001 *
Child font (cartoonish, chalk, etc.)	306 (86.4)	354 (94.7)	<0.001 *
Unusual product names/flavors	193 (54.5)	46 (12.3)	<0.001 *
Portability	196 (55.4)	201 (53.7)	0.660
Unique qualities			
Interactivity	13 (3.7)	44 (11.8)	<0.001 *
Changes color	4 (1.1)	0 (0)	0.055
Transforms	1 (0.3)	1 (0.3)	0.999
Unusual package shape	93 (23.3)	67 (17.9)	0.006 *
Unusual product shape	121 (34.2)	126 (33.7)	0.889
Kid-size product			
Product	57 (16.1)	22 (5.9)	<0.001 *
Package	61 (17.2)	14 (3.7)	<0.001 *
Product and package	90 (25.4)	16 (4.3)	<0.001 *
Games or activities on package	105 (29.7)	43 (11.5)	<0.001 *
Premium claim	52 (14.7)	54 (14.4)	0.924
Parent appeal	231 (65.3)	319 (85.3)	<0.001 *

* statistically significant.

4. Discussion

In 1999, James McNeal published The Kids Market, which called for manufacturers to "kidize" packaging to attract children [31] (pp. 88). In particular, McNeal explained how marketers could shift from the "A to K" (adult to kid) in package design, so as to better serve the "end user" (i.e., the child) [31] (pp. 88). Implicit in this call to kidize packaging is the recognition that children matter as consumers. Indeed, the very notion of pester power—also known as the "nag factor"—pivots on the idea that children can influence family purchasing by nagging their parents to buy products, and studies have documented the significant influence children have on parental food choices [32,33].

As our study reveals, "K"-style packaging was commonplace in the Canadian supermarket by 2009, with 354 products spanning all food categories. Rising to 374 products by 2017, such numbers reveal how pervasive, and embedded, child-targeted food has become in the supermarket. "Kidized" food in Canada is also quite consistent, insomuch as the majority of the products were found in the Dry Goods category across both time points, with Cookie and Biscuits and Fruit Snacks and Applesauces as the most common food types. Growth in the number of kid-oriented Cereals and Granola/Cereal Bars in 2017—representing roughly one of every six products, and one of every eight products, respectively—reveals the importance of breakfast and lunchbox fare/portable snacks to the Canadian market. Interestingly, the number of frozen meals designed for children, represented in the 2009 dataset by products such as Bobo Kids Secret Agent Pasta or Secret Agent Stew and Pizza Pops, dropped over the 8 years tracked, from 10.2% of the products to 2.9%. This drop is partly due to discontinued brands (e.g., the Bobo Kids brand is no longer available), but also occurred because of changing packaging strategies, in which products previously using techniques to attract children become more 'serious' over time. This is a positive trend—although it is tempered by the fact that only 1% of the products in both datasets were fruits or vegetables (such as "packaged" bagged salads with Disney character licensing).

4.1. The Problem of Nutritional Quality

Let us return, for a moment, to McNeal's notion that "kidized" packaging better serves the "end user" of the child [31]. Certainly, kids' packaging attracts children, but this study questions how well served the "end user" is, both in terms of nutrition and marketing techniques. Child-targeted supermarket foods were found in this study to be consistently of poor nutritional quality across time, irrespective of the evaluative criteria used, with roughly 87%–89% of the products exceeding thresholds for sugar, salt and/or fat. Especially striking is that the products in the study were selected because they were child-targeted products—and yet, according to the WHO criteria, 88% the products 'designed' for children (from both years tracked) would not be permitted to be marketed to children. From a nutritional standpoint, then, children are not well served by 'kidized' packaged foods at all. While the decrease in sodium over time is promising, no improvement was observed with respect to fat, and sugar levels remained consistently high. Over seven out of every 10 products had high sugar levels at both time points. Previous studies also document the dubious nutritional quality of supermarket foods targeted at children [17,18,21–23,34–36]; yet only one other study examined changes in nutritional quality over time, and for a much shorter time period. In this US-based study, food products with child-targeted cross-promotions were purchased on three occasions between 2006 and 2008: researchers found that the nutritional quality of products "worsened" over the two years studied [17] (pp. 414), and underscored the lack of a "meaningful improvement in the food environment that surrounds young people" [17] (pp. 416).

Our analysis of the 14 identical products over time provides key insight into how "meaningful" some of the changes really are—as well as the challenges for parents in terms of understanding the Nutrition Facts table. All of the products changed in some way with respect to serving size, sugar, sodium, or fat content. Many of these changes were minimal. For example, the pre-packaged serving size was reduced from 28 to 26 g for Betty Crocker Dunkaroos and fat content per 100 g increased from 14.3 to 15 g for President's Choice Zookies from 2009 to 2017. Such changes, perhaps, result from more precise measurement techniques when it comes to assessing nutritional value. For four products, changes appear to reflect efforts to improve (or maintain) the nutritional quality of the food product, given that serving sizes and nutrient densities per 100 g either stayed the same or (one or more of these elements) decreased between time periods. For the remaining 10 products assessed, changes in the nutrition facts table may reflect modifications of product ingredients, or a more troubling strategy to improve the optics of the product's nutritional value.

This might be about optics, not health, because a decrease in serving size (6/14 products) was always observed with an increase in at least one nutrient per 100 g—even if the respective nutrient content per serving size did not change or decreased. Several instances of this were found in products with pre-portioned packets, whereby parents may be reassured by smaller single portion sizes. Consider Schneiders LunchMate Nachos: if parents could compare the Nutrition Facts tables on the 2009 and 2017 versions of this product, they might reasonably conclude that it has become "healthier" because the serving size, sugar, sodium, and fat have all been reduced. This conclusion is erroneous, however, as it is based on an unstandardized amount of food (per serving size). Our standardized comparison (calculated per 100 g) reveals that this product has in fact become less "healthy". While the serving size decreased, sugar and fat content did *not* change, and the sodium content increased. This type of standardized comparison is not readily available to consumers, who typically look for low values of selected nutrients on the Nutrition Facts tables (in combination with packaging claims) to discern the nutritional value of a product [37].

4.2. The Problem of Nutrition and Health Claims

Despite the overall poor nutrition (particularly when it comes to sugar) of the products analyzed, the marketing of value via front-of-package (FOP) nutrition claims has become much more aggressive over time. This trend reflects what can be understood as the co-consumption model [38] (pp. 235), which recognizes that parents buy items for their children and shop with them in mind. Parents think about, care for, and react to their children's desires [38] (pp. 235) within the context of wanting to provide healthy foods [39]: nutrition and health claims provide one way to communicate a product's healthful qualities. This increased parental demand for providing healthy, packaged food choices is signaled by the ubiquitous FOP claims in the study: in 2009, three out of 10 products had a FOP claim; by 2017, almost nine of 10 products did. Shifts in types of claims being made further reveal current trends when it comes to nutrition and health. For instance, the substantial jump in gluten-free claims and peanut/nut-free claims over time aligns with trends in pediatric health (notably, the increasing prevalence and awareness of nut allergies and celiac disease [40–42]). Joining these claims are the no artificial flavors or no artificial colors claims emblazoning 35% of products by 2017. Such claims represent what the trade literature calls the free-from trend [43] that reflects consumer demands for "more natural and simple ingredients rather than artificial ones" [43].

Free-from claims are also part of what is known as the broader clean label [43,44] approach to products, in which consumers want to know what is in their foods (often represented by easily identifiable ingredients) and strive to avoid artificial ingredients. These trends are positive movements forward. However, research also reveals that "better for you" claims and claims like gluten free do not necessarily signal a healthier product nutritionally [21,45]; indeed, a comprehensive analysis of food and beverage products sold in Canadian supermarkets found that almost 42% of the 6990 products with nutrition claims were "less healthy" and, therefore, would be ineligible to carry such claims according to the international profiling system used (i.e., The Food Standards Australia New Zealand Nutrient Profiling Scoring Criterion) [46]. Other studies similarly document the presence of nutrition claims on food products with lower nutritional quality [47,48].

Further complicating the matter are the unregulated, industry-created nutrition claims, which (in this study) adorned 35.6% of products in 2017. Claims like Made with Goodness! Simply Good! and Made Better! trumpeted from packages ranging from fruit snacks and cookies to cereal and boxed macaroni. Not only are these claims nebulous, they are also (in some cases) misleading. For instance, a box of fruit snacks with the Made Better! tagline listed corn syrup as the first ingredient and derived 65% of the calories from sugar. The question thus arises: Made Better than what?

4.3. The Power of Child Targeted Packaged Foods: The Problem of Marketing Techniques

Tracking the evolving marketing techniques of child-targeted foods is particularly compelling because it shifts the discussion from nutrition content (the focal point of most discussions on children's food marketing) toward the particulars of what makes these products appealing to children. Such techniques can be understood as part of what the WHO, in its discussion of the marketing of foods and beverages to children, defines as the power of marketing communications [49] (pp. 10). Power, for the WHO, refers to the content, design and creative strategies used to target and persuade. In the case of packaged foods, appeals to fun, cartoon and licensed characters, and 'kid-sized' packaging (and so forth) all form part of the power of child-targeted foods. Such packaging is, indeed, powerful: packaging has been identified as the "predominant" source of children's exposure to food and beverage advertising [46] (pp. 137). Whether "predominant" or simply highly dominant, multiple studies have documented the impact of packaging on children's food preferences and choices [10]. Children have been shown to prefer the taste of foods that have branded or licensed characters [50–52] or that come in colorful packaging [53]; eye tracking studies reveal that children (ages 6–9) pay more attention to products with cartoon characters [8]; and survey research documents that children (ages 10–14) rank packages with cartoons as more "fun" [54].

In our study, the most prevalent techniques of power used on packaging in both 2009 and 2017 were cartoon characters and child-appealing fonts, and their use increased over time ($p < 0.001$). By 2017, 85.6% of the products contained a cartoon character, and 94.7% were coded as having a child-appealing font. Licensed characters (such as Dora the Explorer and Spiderman) also maintained a consistent presence in both years tracked, decorating 17% of products in 2009 and 16% in 2017. Examples (from 2017) include Star Wars movie character licensing found on products ranging from yogurt tubes, fruit snacks, granola bars, cookies and cereals, to chicken nuggets and chicken soup; Finding Dory movie characters on juices, drinkable yogurt, yogurt tubes and baked snack cookies; and Frozen movie characters on cereal, yogurt tubes, fruit snacks, canned soup and tuna fish "snack kits"(canned tuna with mayonnaise and packaged crackers). Combined, the prevalence of these cartoon and licensed characters speaks to the degree to which media culture saturates children's lives—a premise underscored by a new development observed in the 2017 dataset. Roughly one of every six products had prominent character licensing in 2017—yet in some cases, the product existed solely because of character licensing (such as Limited-Edition Stars Wars cereal, Special Edition Minions cereal, and Special Edition Paw Patrol cereal). Stated differently, instead of affixing Minions or Paw Patrol characters onto a previously existing cereal (such as Cheerios or Shreddies), an entirely new limited-edition foodstuff based on the media character was created. Such products reveal the extent to which children's popular culture is being infused into food. Paw Patrol cereal only exists because of Paw Patrol, and this has considerable implications. Character licensing (on products or as stand-alone products) can be understood as what media scholar Jonathan Gray identifies as paratexts [55]. Paratexts are the peripherals around media and television texts, such as licensed merchandise and movie trailers and posters, which must be recognized as important parts of popular culture [55], including children's food marketing [56]. Gray does not discuss food, but products like Paw Patrol cereal, Beauty and the Beast goldfish crackers, Frozen-themed tuna fish (and so forth) are without question paratexts that feed into children's popular culture and fuel demand for these products. The problem with such character licensing extends beyond the nutritional quality of what children eat to broader questions related to the commercialization of childhood. Does tuna fish or cereal really need to be the vehicle for a movie advertisement? Conversely, should children's movie characters be promotional vehicles for food products? Given the poor nutritional quality of the foods analyzed, there are both ethical and health-related implications of this move: it is certainly *not* the best strategy for creating, in the words of the WHO, an "enabling food environment" [49] (pp. 6).

Co-consumption and Declining Techniques of Fun, Games, and Unusual Product Names and/or Flavors

Cartoon characters and bubble/child-appealing fonts increased over the time period tracked, as did parent appeals on the package, signaled through the use of health or nutrition claims (as discussed above). Parent appeals jumped 20% between 2009 and 2017, from 65.3 to 85.3% of products ($p < 0.001$). At the same time, several marketing techniques declined, including verbal claims to "fun" on product packaging (from 22.0% in 2009 to 15.6% in 2017; $p < 0.031$), the presence of games or activities on the package (29.7 to 11.5%; $p < 0.001$) and the use of unusual product names and/or flavors (54.5 to 12.3%; $p < 0.001$). The explanation for some of these changes lies, we suggest, in the (previously discussed) rising parental awareness of and concerns over health and nutrition and the clean label trend—coupled with parents' desire to provide foods that they think their children will enjoy and will want to eat. Previous qualitative research has documented that many parents do not care whether packaged foods have child-oriented cartoons, shapes or fun appeals so long as the food is healthy [12,13]. Cartoons make packaged foods appealing to children, and the health and nutrition claims make parents feel reassured about buying those products for their children. Most striking in our study is the significant drop in the technique of using unusual products names and/or flavors. In the 2009 dataset there were "Funshines biscuits", "Fun Pix" waffles, "bubble gum"-flavored pudding and yogurts and fruit-flavored snacks in flavors like "Kaboom Fruit Punch", ""Cyber Strawberry", "Cosmic Crush" and "Jungle Rush". Such names and flavors do not communicate "health" to parents, nor are they transparent about what the food is, as is demanded by the clean label trend. There is an artificiality to "Fun Pix", bubblegum pudding, Kaboom Fruit Punch (etc.)—it does not sound like "real" food—and therefore it is unsurprising that these kinds of products largely disappeared by 2017. Moreover, research shows that older children reject packaging appeals that they believe may be too "kiddie" for them: these children do not wish to be associated with anything they feel is too childlike [50,57]. As such, the drop in the unusual product names and flavors might also reflect a marketing strategy to broaden the ages of the child audience that the product might appeal to. Also declining over the time tracked is the number of "kid-sized" products, which we speculate might reflect greater environmental awareness of consumers when it comes to excess packaging.

4.4. Strengths and Limitations

This is the first Canadian study to track transformations in child-targeted foods over time. Study strengths are the detailed examination and comparison of both nutrition and marketing appeals across 8 years, analyzing a comprehensive dataset of child-targeted products, using the same stores for data collection, visiting the data collection sites multiple times (to ensure all relevant products were captured), and data verification by multiple research assistants to ensure accuracy. Another strength is using two evaluative criteria to assess nutrition—one criteria that represents "best practices" at the time of the 2009 data collection, and one that represents "best practices" in 2017—because this approach reinforces that the poor nutritional quality of child-targeted foods is not simply a matter of "stricter" contemporary nutrition standards. Additionally, this study provides important, granular detail on the specific techniques used to capture children's attention when it comes to packaged foods, and the changing prevalence of those techniques. Such detail provides valuable—and much needed—insight into the power of child-targeted packaged foods. Finally, the findings provide further evidence of the need to regulate packaging as part of national and international efforts to mitigate the impact of unhealthy food and beverage marketing to children. Limitations are that, while large retailers carry the same national brands, not all stores have identical product offerings. Product variations exist between stores, which means that the reported findings may shift depending on the stores selected. Moreover, nutritional quality and marketing strategies are not necessarily generalizable to other countries, in which different products, product formulations and marketing strategies may be used. A final limitation is that the study provides insight into the products available for consumption but does not track actual sales or consumer intake of these products.

5. Conclusions

This study is the first to provide a detailed look into how child-targeted supermarket products in Canada have changed over time, both nutritionally and in terms of marketing appeals. It provides fascinating insight into the changing landscape of kids' supermarket foods, and evidence on the nutritional quality and prevalence of various marketing techniques. Our finding that 88% of child-targeted products (from both the 2009 and 2017 datasets) would not be permitted to be marketed to children reveals that the nutritional quality of these foods is not improving over time, despite the increasing number of (adult-directed) health and nutrition claims on packages—and despite the increasing research and policy focus on child nutrition. High sugar levels remain a persistent problem in child-targeted supermarket foods. Even though positive developments can be noted with respect to the declining use of more gamified elements of packaged foods (through unusual product flavors and names, or literal games on packages), the use of cartoon characters on packages increased over time. New developments in character licensing were also observed. The study findings are particularly timely from a policy perspective given that Canada, under its Healthy Eating Strategy, has committed to prohibit the marketing of foods high in sugar, sodium and saturated fat to children under age 13. The provisions for packaged foods have yet to be determined as part of this policy. This said, Health Canada's consultation with stakeholders on the proposed regulations on food marketing to children revealed that most health and academic stakeholders strongly supported the regulations including packaging and labelling, because of "its effectiveness in advertising to children" and because "it has been shown to be the top source of children's exposure to food and beverage advertising" [58] (pp. 2). Given the poor nutritional profile and compelling marketing appeals, this study reveals the critical need to consider the regulation of packaging—both in Canada and internationally—as part of the strategy for creating an "enabling food environment" for children [49].

Funding: This research was funded by the Canadian Institutes of Health Research Canada Research Chairs Program.

Acknowledgments: The author would like to acknowledge the Canada Research Chairs program for support of this research. She would also like to thank the superb doctoral candidate Natalie Scime for data analysis on suggestions for the manuscript, and to graduate students Madison Bischoff and Natasha Karim (for coding and data checking). Thank you to Elize Pauze for providing excellent statistical analysis.

Conflicts of Interest: The authors declare no conflict of interest.

References

1. Boyland, E.; Whalen, R.; Christiansen, P.; Mcgale, L.; Duckworth, J.; Halford, J.; Clark, M.; Rosenberg, G.; Vohra, J. *See It, Want It, Buy It, Eat It: How Food Advertising Is Associated with Unhealthy Eating Behaviours in 7–11 Year Old Children*; Cancer Research UK: London, UK, 2018.
2. Boyland, E.J.; Halford, J.C.G. Television advertising and branding. Effects on eating behaviour and food preferences in children. *Appetite* **2013**, *62*, 236–241. [CrossRef] [PubMed]
3. Sadeghirad, B.; Duhaney, T.; Motaghipisheh, S.; Campbell, N.R.C.; Johnston, B.C. Influence of unhealthy food and beverage marketing on children's dietary intake and preference: A systematic review and meta-analysis of randomized trials. *Obes. Rev.* **2016**, *17*, 945–959. [CrossRef] [PubMed]
4. Boyland, E.J.; Nolan, S.; Kelly, B.; Tudur-smith, C.; Jones, A.; Halford, J.C.G.; Robinson, E. Advertising as a cue to consume: A systematic review and meta-analysis of the effects of acute exposure to unhealthy food and nonalcoholic beverage advertising on intake in children. *Am. J. Clin. Nutr.* **2016**, *103*, 519–533. [CrossRef] [PubMed]
5. Cairns, G.; Angus, K.; Hastings, G.; Caraher, M. Systematic reviews of the evidence on the nature, extent and effects of food marketing to children. A retrospective summary. *Appetite* **2013**, *62*, 209–215. [CrossRef] [PubMed]
6. Hastings, G.; Stead, M.; McDermott, L.; Forsyth, A.; MacKintosh, A.M.; Godfrey, C.; Caraher, M.; Angus, K. *Review of Research on the Effects of Food Promotion to Children*; Centre for Social Marketing: Glasgow, UK, 2003.
7. Institute of Medicine *Food Marketing to Children and Youth*; The National Academies Press: Washington, DC, USA, 2006.

8. Osei-Assibey, G.; Dick, S.; MacDiarmid, J.; Semple, S.; Reilly, J.J.; Ellaway, A.; Cowie, H.; McNeill, G. The influence of the food environment on overweight and obesity in young children: A systematic review. *BMJ Open* **2012**, *2*, e001538. [CrossRef] [PubMed]
9. World Health Organization. Set of Recommendations on the Marketing of Foods and Non-Alcoholic Beverages to Children. Available online: http://apps.who.int/iris/bitstream/handle/10665/44416/9789241500210_eng.pdf;jsessionid=4DA284276CF8B522B7F886DBDF6776D8?sequence=1 (accessed on 10 January 2019).
10. Smith, R.; Kelly, B.; Yeatman, H.; Boyland, E. Food Marketing Influences Children's Attitudes, Preferences and Consumption: A Systematic Critical Review. *Nutrients* **2019**, *11*, 875. [CrossRef] [PubMed]
11. Federal Trade Commission. Marketing Food to Children and Adolescents: A Review of Industry Expenditures, Activities, and Self-Regulation. Available online: https://www.ftc.gov/sites/default/files/documents/reports/marketing-food-children-and-adolescents-review-industry-expenditures-activities-and-self-regulation/p064504foodmktingreport.pdf (accessed on 10 January 2019).
12. Den Hoed, R.C.; Elliott, C. Parents' views of supermarket fun foods and the question of responsible marketing. *Young Consum.* **2013**, *14*, 201–215. [CrossRef]
13. Elliott, C. Parents' Choice: Examining Parent Perspectives on Regulation and Child-Targeted Supermarket Foods. *Food Cult. Soc.* **2013**, *16*, 437–455. [CrossRef]
14. Elliott, C. Marketing Fun Foods: A Profile and Analysis of Supermarket Food Messages Targeted at Children. *Can. Public Policy* **2008**, *34*, 259–274. [CrossRef]
15. Elliott, C. 'Big Food' and 'gamified' products: Promotion, packaging, and the promise of fun. *Crit. Public Health* **2015**, *25*, 348–360. [CrossRef]
16. Hebden, L.; King, L.; Kelly, B.; Chapman, K.; Innes-Hughes, C. A Menagerie of Promotional Characters: Promoting Food to Children through Food Packaging. *J. Nutr. Educ. Behav.* **2011**, *43*, 349–355. [CrossRef] [PubMed]
17. Harris, J.L.; Schwartz, M.B.; Brownell, K.D. Marketing foods to children and adolescents: Licensed characters and other promotions on packaged foods in the supermarket. *Public Health Nutr.* **2010**, *13*, 409–417. [CrossRef] [PubMed]
18. Elliott, C. Assessing fun foods: Nutritional content and analysis of supermarket foods targeted at children. *Obes. Rev.* **2008**, *9*, 368–377. [CrossRef] [PubMed]
19. Schwartz, M.B.; Vartanian, L.R.; Wharton, C.M.; Brownell, K.D. Examining the Nutritional Quality of Breakfast Cereals Marketed to Children. *J. Am. Diet. Assoc.* **2008**, *108*, 702–705. [CrossRef] [PubMed]
20. Soo, J.; Letona, P.; Chacon, V.; Barnoya, J.; Roberto, C.A. Nutritional quality and child-oriented marketing of breakfast cereals in Guatemala. *Int. J. Obes.* **2016**, *40*, 39–44. [CrossRef] [PubMed]
21. Elliott, C. Packaging health: Examining "better-for-you" foods targeted at children. *Can. Public Policy* **2012**, *38*, 265–281. [CrossRef]
22. Chapman, K.; Nicholas, P.; Banovic, D.; Supramaniam, R. The extent and nature of food promotion directed to children in Australian supermarkets. *Health Promot. Int.* **2006**, *21*, 331–339. [CrossRef] [PubMed]
23. Elliott, C.; Scime, N.V. Nutrient profiling and child-targeted supermarket foods: Assessing a "made in Canada" policy approach. *Int. J. Environ. Res. Public Health* **2019**, *16*, E639. [CrossRef] [PubMed]
24. Elliott, C. Packaging Fun: Analyzing Supermarket Food Messages Targeted at Children. *Can. J. Commun.* **2012**, *37*, 303–318. [CrossRef]
25. Center for Science in the Public Interest. Guidelines for Responsible Food Marketing to Children. Available online: https://cspinet.org/sites/default/files/attachment/marketingguidelines.pdf (accessed on 1 January 2011).
26. World Health Organization. WHO Regional Office for Europe Nutrient Profile Model. Available online: http://www.euro.who.int/__data/assets/pdf_file/0005/270716/Nutrient-children_web-new.pdf?ua=1 (accessed on 12 October 2018).
27. Harrison, K.; Marske, A. Nutritional content of foods advertised during the television programs children watch most. *Am. J. Public Health* **2005**, *95*, 1568–1574. [CrossRef]
28. IBM Corp. *IBM SPSS Statistics for Windows, Version 25.0*; IBM Corp.: Armonk, NY, USA, 2017.
29. Statacorp. *Stata Statistical Software: Release 15*; StataCorp LLC: College Station, TX, USA, 2017.
30. BeverageDaily.com PepsiCo's Smart Spot spreads to Canada. Available online: https://www.beveragedaily.com/Article/2005/01/24/PepsiCo-s-Smart-Spot-spreads-to-Canada (accessed on 6 April 2019).
31. McNeal, J. *The Kids Market: Myths and Realities*; Paramount Market Publishing: Ithaca, NY, USA, 1999.

32. Calloway, E.E.; Ranjit, N.S.; Roberts-Gray, S.; Romo-Palafox, J.; McInnis, C.; Briley, M. Exploratory Cross-Sectional Study of Factors Associated with the Healthfulness of Parental Responses to Child Food Purchasing Requests. *Matern. Child Health J.* **2016**, *20*, 1569–1577. [CrossRef] [PubMed]
33. Papoutsi, G.S.; Nayga, R.M.; Lazaridis, P.; Drichoutis, A.C. Fat Tax, Subsidy or Both? The Role of Information and Children's Pester Power in Food Choice. *J. Econ. Behav. Organ.* **2015**, *117*, 196–208. [CrossRef]
34. Lapierre, M.A.; Brown, A.M.; Houtzer, H.V.; Thomas, T.J. Child-directed and nutrition-focused marketing cues on food packaging: Links to nutritional content. *Public Health Nutr.* **2017**, *20*, 765–773. [CrossRef] [PubMed]
35. Aerts, G.; Smits, T. Child-targeted on-pack communications in Belgian supermarkets: Associations with nutritional value and type of brand. *Health Promot. Int.* **2019**, *34*, 71–81. [CrossRef] [PubMed]
36. Giménez, A.; de Saldamando, L.; Curutchet, M.R.; Ares, G. Package design and nutritional profile of foods targeted at children in supermarkets in Montevideo, Uruguay. *Cad. Saude Publica* **2017**, *33*, 1–11. [CrossRef] [PubMed]
37. Maubach, N.; Hoek, J.; McCreanor, T. An exploration of parents' food purchasing behaviours. *Appetite* **2009**, *53*, 297–302. [CrossRef] [PubMed]
38. Cook, D.T. The missing child in consumption theory. *J. Consum. Cult.* **2008**, *8*, 219–243. [CrossRef]
39. Cook, D.T. Semantic provisioning of children's food: Commerce, care and maternal practice. *Childhood* **2009**, *16*, 317–334. [CrossRef]
40. Eyad, A.; King, K.S.; Bhavisha, P.; Chung, W.; Joseph, A.M.; Imad, A. Increasing incidence and altered presentation in a population-based study of pediatric celiac disease in North America. *J. Pediatr. Gastroenterol. Nutr.* **2017**, *65*, 432–437.
41. Gupta, R.S.; Springston, E.E.; Warrier, M.R.; Smith, B.; Kumar, R.; Pongracic, J.; Holl, J.L. The prevalence, severity, and distribution of childhood food allergy in the United States. *Pediatrics* **2011**, *128*, e9–e17. [CrossRef]
42. Sicherer, S.H.; Muñoz-Furlong, A.; Godbold, J.H.; Sampson, H.A. US prevalence of self-reported peanut, tree nut, and sesame allergy: 11-year follow-up. *J. Allergy Clin. Immunol.* **2010**, *125*, 1322–1326. [CrossRef] [PubMed]
43. GlobalData. Consumer Research Suggests that the Free-from Food Trend Is Here to Stay. Available online: https://www.foodprocessing-technology.com/comment/free-from-food-trend/ (accessed on 16 April 2019).
44. Shoup, M. How to Define Clean Label? 'There Isn't Any One Singular Definition,' Says Hartman Group. Available online: https://www.foodnavigator-usa.com/Article/2019/02/28/How-to-define-clean-label-There-isn-t-any-one-singular-definition (accessed on 28 February 2019).
45. Elliott, C. The Nutritional Quality of Gluten-Free Products for Children. *Pediatrics* **2018**, *142*, e20180525. [CrossRef] [PubMed]
46. Franco-Arellano, B.; Labonté, M.È.; Bernstein, J.T.; L'Abbé, M.R. Examining the nutritional quality of Canadian packaged foods and beverages with and without nutrition claims. *Nutrients* **2018**, *10*, 832. [CrossRef] [PubMed]
47. Kaur, A.; Scarborough, P.; Matthews, A.; Payne, S.; Mizdrak, A.; Rayner, M. How many foods in the UK carry health and nutrition claims, and are they healthier than those that do not? *Public Health Nutr.* **2016**, *19*, 988–997. [CrossRef]
48. Al-Ani, H.H.; Devi, A.; Eyles, H.; Swinburn, B.; Vandevijvere, S. Nutrition and health claims on healthy and less-healthy packaged food products in New Zealand. *Br. J. Nutr.* **2016**, *116*, 1087–1094. [CrossRef]
49. World Heath Organization. A Framework for Implementing the Set of Recommendations on the Marketing of Foods and Non-Alcoholic Beverages to Children. Available online: http://apps.who.int/iris/bitstream/handle/10665/80148/9789241503242_eng.pdf?sequence=1 (accessed on 10 January 2019).
50. Elliott, C.D. Healthy Food Looks Serious: How Children Interpret Packaged Food Products. *Can. J. Commun.* **2009**, *34*, 359–380. [CrossRef]
51. Letona, P.; Chacon, V.; Roberto, C.; Barnoya, J. Effects of licensed characters on children's taste and snack preferences in Guatemala, a low/middle income country. *Int. J. Obes.* **2014**, *38*, 1466–1469. [CrossRef]
52. McGale, L.S.; Halford, J.C.G.; Harrold, J.A.; Boyland, E.J. The Influence of Brand Equity Characters on Children's Food Preferences and Choices. *J. Pediatr.* **2016**, *177*, 33–38. [CrossRef]
53. Elliott, C.; Den Hoed, R.; Conlon, M. Food branding and young children's taste preferences: A reassessment. *Can. J. Public Heal.* **2013**, *104*, e364–e368. [CrossRef]

54. Pires, C.; Agante, L. Encouraging children to eat more healthily: The influence of packaging. *J. Consum. Behav.* **2011**, *10*, 161–168. [CrossRef]
55. Gray, J. *Show Sold Separately: Promos, Spoilers, and Other Media Paratexts*; New York University Press: New York, NY, USA, 2010.
56. Asquith, K. Join the Club: Food Advertising, 1930s Children's Popular Culture, and Brand Socialization. *Pop. Commun.* **2014**, *12*, 17–31. [CrossRef]
57. Ogle, A.D.; Graham, D.J.; Lucas-Thompson, R.G.; Roberto, C.A. Influence of Cartoon Media Characters on Children's Attention to and Preference for Food and Beverage Products. *J. Acad. Nutr. Diet.* **2017**, *117*, 265–270. [CrossRef] [PubMed]
58. Health Canada. Overview of Stakeholder Comments on Version 1.0 of Health Canada's Draft Guide to the Application of the Child Health Protection Act (Bill S-228). Available online: https://files.constantcontact.com/.../faf560b9-3f4c-48af-8212-0a2924eeaf37.pdf (accessed on 17 June 2019).

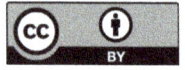 © 2019 by the author. Licensee MDPI, Basel, Switzerland. This article is an open access article distributed under the terms and conditions of the Creative Commons Attribution (CC BY) license (http://creativecommons.org/licenses/by/4.0/).

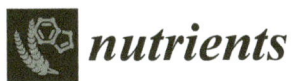

Article

Exposure to Food and Beverage Advertising on Television among Canadian Adolescents, 2011 to 2016

Christine D. Czoli [1,2], Elise Pauzé [1] and Monique Potvin Kent [1,*]

[1] School of Epidemiology and Public Health, University of Ottawa, Ottawa, ON K1G 5Z3, Canada; christine.czoli@gmail.com (C.D.C.); epauz022@uottawa.ca (E.P.)
[2] Heart and Stroke Foundation, Ottawa, ON K1Z 8R9, Canada
* Correspondence: mpotvink@uottawa.ca; Tel.: +1-(613)-562-5800 (ext. 7447)

Received: 20 January 2020; Accepted: 3 February 2020; Published: 7 February 2020

Abstract: Adolescents represent a key audience for food advertisers, however there is little evidence of adolescent exposure to food marketing in Canada. This study examined trends in Canadian adolescents' exposure to food advertising on television. To do so, data on 19 food categories were licensed from Nielsen Media Research for May 2011, 2013, and 2016 for the broadcasting market of Toronto, Canada. The average number of advertisements viewed by adolescents aged 12–17 years on 31 television stations during the month of May each year was estimated using television ratings data. Findings revealed that between May 2011 and May 2016, the total number of food advertisements aired on all television stations increased by 4%, while adolescents' average exposure to food advertising decreased by 31%, going from 221 ads in May 2011 to 154 in May 2016. In May 2016, the advertising of fast food and sugary drinks dominated, relative to other categories, accounting for 42% and 11% of all exposures, respectively. The findings demonstrate a declining trend in exposure to television food advertising among Canadian adolescents, which may be due to shifts in media consumption. These data may serve as a benchmark for monitoring and evaluating future food marketing policies in Canada.

Keywords: food advertising; adolescents; public health; sugary drinks; policy; obesity

1. Introduction

The advertising of unhealthy foods and beverages influences the dietary behavior of children and youth and is a likely contributor to obesity and diet related non-communicable diseases [1]. Several comprehensive reviews of the literature have concluded that commercial food advertising is associated with childhood obesity, influencing the food preferences of children, consumption patterns, and purchase requests [1–6]. While limited, there is some evidence linking adolescents' television advertising exposure to their food choices and consumption patterns [1,7], as well as adiposity [1]. Thus, public health experts and policymakers have expressed concerns about food marketing aimed at adolescents [8,9].

In Canada, the prevalence of obesity has increased dramatically since the late 1970s [10]. While this trend appears to have stabilized in the last decade [11], 34% of Canadian youth aged 12–17 years have excess weight or obesity and their diets remain poor [12]. For instance, research has shown that large proportions of Canadian youth do not meet national dietary guidelines [13–15]. Furthermore, Canadian adolescents (aged 14–18 years) obtain approximately 55% of their daily energy intake from ultra-processed foods (i.e., manufactured food products containing many ingredients extracted from foods or synthesized as well as additives and few whole foods or typical culinary ingredients) which usually contain excessive amounts of sugar, fat and sodium [16]. Of particular concern is youth consumption of beverages with free sugars ("sugary drinks"), which provide energy, but no nutritional value [17]. In 2004, 17% and 16% of daily calories among Canadian adolescent boys and girls, respectively, were derived from sweetened drinks (including regular soft drinks and fruit drinks), milk and fruit juice [18]. Taken together, these dietary patterns are problematic due to the high intake of energy-dense yet nutrient-poor foods, as well as the associated displacement of more nutritious foods, such as fruits, vegetables, and legumes [16].

Adolescents represent a key target audience for advertisers of foods and beverages [19]. Canadian youth are significant consumers of media, with adolescents aged 12–17 years watching an average of 16.4 h of television per week [20]. In addition, adolescence marks a transition in which children become direct consumers, acquiring the ability to purchase goods with their own money [8]. In the United States (US), marketing expenditures directed at adolescents exceed $1 billion annually [21]. Despite declines in food marketing expenditures for television over time, television remains the dominant medium for such expenditures [22]. Furthermore, as part of integrated marketing campaigns, television advertising is used concurrently with other forms of marketing to maximize the overall impact of ad campaigns on consumer behavior [23,24]. It is therefore important to monitor food advertising on television. This is also critical for informing policies aimed at protecting adolescents from unhealthy food advertising.

In the province of Quebec, commercial advertising is restricted to children under 13 years old, while in the rest of the country, unhealthy food advertising to children under 12 years old is self-regulated by the food and beverage industry [25,26]. Recently, the Government of Canada came close to adopting a law restricting unhealthy food marketing to children [27]. This law, however, like the existing law in Quebec, would not have protected adolescents aged 13 and over [28]. To our knowledge, there is little research examining food and beverage marketing exposure among Canadian adolescents [29]. This represents a critical evidence gap, given that such data are needed to consider marketing restrictions to adolescents, which are increasingly acknowledged as uniquely vulnerable to marketing [30,31]. To fill this gap, the current study sought to examine Canadian adolescents' exposure to food and beverage advertising on television over time. Given the significant contribution of sugary drinks to the caloric intake of Canadian adolescents, and its documented contribution to weight gain [32,33], an in-depth examination of sugary drink advertising was also conducted.

2. Materials and Methods

Data for food and beverage television advertisements that aired in May 2011, 2013, and 2016 on 34 television stations were licensed from Nielsen Media Research (a marketing research company). As national advertising ratings data are not available in Canada, data were licensed for the Toronto Extended Market (i.e., the city of Toronto and adjacent urban areas all located in the province of Ontario), as it constitutes the largest broadcast market in the country. The month of May was chosen to avoid major holidays that could influence advertising budgets and usual exposure. For each month, data for four weeks of 24 h television programming were analyzed (1 May to 28 May in 2011, 29 April to 26 May in 2013, and 1 May to 28 May in 2016), and included advertising data for 19 food/beverage categories defined by Nielsen, which are known to be frequently advertised to young people [21,34] (Table 1). The three years examined were selected as this study constitutes a secondary analysis of data used for previously funded research [35,36].

Table 1. Definitions of Nielsen food/beverage categories included in the study.

Food/Beverage Category	Definition
Cakes	All cakes and puddings, including items that are ready to eat or require additional preparation (excludes frozen pastry and pie shells)
Candy	Confectionary made from sugar, water, flavoring and food coloring (excludes candy with chocolate)
Cereal	Ready-to-eat products marketed as breakfast food (excludes infant cereals and oatmeal)
Cheese	Cheese products in various formats, e.g., brick, string or slice (excludes cottage cheese)
Chocolate	Individually wrapped chocolate and candy bars (excludes boxed chocolate and candy with chocolate)
Compartment snacks	Pre-packaged products comprise of two or more ingredients in separate compartments sold as portable snacks or meals
Cookies	Small baked sweet biscuits
Ice cream	Includes ice cream, frozen yogurt, sherbet, sorbet and frozen treats made from these foods
Pizza	Pizza not sold in restaurants
Portable snacks	Cereal, protein or fruit bars and squares, and fruit snacks
Snack foods	Savory snacks such as chips, pretzels, cheese puffs, and meat-based snacks like jerky (excludes crackers)
Fast food restaurants	Foods sold at restaurants where ordering is conducted at a counter or drive-through, where menu boards are placed above the counter, and the table is cleaned up by the customer
Restaurants	Restaurants that serve prepared food and beverages that are ordered from a menu once seated and are consumed on the premises
Yogurt	Yogurt in tub, tube, and drink form (excludes frozen yogurt)
Juices, drinks and nectars	Sweetened and unsweetened juices and beverages that come in liquid, frozen, concentrated, and powdered forms (excludes water, milk and alternatives, tea and coffee drinks, cocktail mixers, and alcoholic beverages)
Energy drinks	Drink products that are primarily consumed for the purpose of boosting one's mental and physical stimulation
Soft drinks (regular)	Any non-alcoholic carbonated drink
Soft drinks (diet)	Diet versions of soft drinks
Sports drinks	Drink products that are primarily consumed to rehydrate the body and replace electrolytes lost during physical activity

2.1. Analysis

Nielsen data includes information for all advertisements aired and viewed by an audience for a specified time period. Television viewership data are collected among a stratified probability sample of households that is proportional to the population in which each member, whose demographic characteristics are known, wears a portable device that records when and what they are watching on television [37]. Data are weighted based on age, sex, household size, geography and other characteristics, and estimates of audience viewership at the television extended market level are calculated by Nielsen, and can be examined by specific demographic groups, such as adolescents aged 12 to 17 years. Nielsen data expresses advertising exposure in terms of a "rating", representing the estimated percentage of the population (or specific demographic group) that viewed a specific advertisement. As has been done previously [38,39], ratings for all advertisements viewed by adolescents were summed for each food/beverage category. Rating sums were then divided by 100 to determine the average number of advertisements seen by individual adolescents. An in-depth analysis was conducted to examine adolescents' exposure to advertising for beverages with free sugars, given its contribution to the caloric intake of Canadian youth and associated public health concern [18]. While "sugary drinks" contain a broad range of beverage categories [40], the current analysis was limited to the following beverage categories defined by Nielsen: juices, regular soft drinks, sports drinks, and energy drinks.

Of the 34 stations available in 2011, 3 were excluded from the study because Nielsen ceased to record these stations during the examined period. Adolescents' exposure to food and beverage advertising on the remaining 31 television stations was assessed for each time point (May 2011, 2013, and 2016), overall and by food category. Television stations included in the analysis are listed in Supplementary Table S1. Food/beverage advertising exposure was also examined by television station type, including children specialty stations (Teletoon and YTV), adolescent specialty stations (Much Music and MTV), and generalist stations (all others). Teletoon and YTV were considered child specialty stations as their programming is predominantly intended for children under 13 years. Adolescent specialty stations were classified as such because a large share of their programming focused on either popular music and comedy shows that appeal to youth (i.e., Much; e.g., Playlist, Simpsons, Everybody Hates Chris, Tosh.0) or adolescent-targeted sitcoms and reality TV shows (i.e., MTV; e.g., Degrassi, Student Bodies, 16 and Pregnant, Teen Mom). The number of food advertisements that aired on all stations and adolescents' exposure were described using frequencies and the percent changes between May 2011 and May 2016 were calculated. Nielsen Spotwatch software was used to extract television advertising exposure data among adolescents and analyses were conducted using IBM SPSS v.25.

2.2. Ethical Approval

As this study used licensed media data, ethical approval was not required.

3. Results

3.1. Food and Beverage Advertisements Aired on Television

A total of 84,700, 82,432, and 87,825 advertisements for foods and beverages aired on all television stations in May 2011, 2013, and 2016, respectively. Between May 2011 and 2016, the total number of food and beverage advertisements aired increased by 4% (see Table 2). With respect to frequency of advertising, an average of 97.6 and 101.2 advertisements aired per station per day in 2011 and 2016, respectively. The largest increases in the number of food and beverage advertisements aired were for cakes (+713%), candy (+345%), regular soft drinks (+254%), snack foods (+160%), and sports drinks (+179%). The five food/beverage categories that were most heavily advertised in May 2011 included fast food (34% of total ads), chocolate (12%), yogurt (9%), cereal (9%), and cheese (7%). In May 2016, these were fast food (41% of total ads), chocolate (8%), restaurants (7%), snack foods (6%), and cheese (6%) (May 2016).

Table 2. Number of television food and beverage advertisements aired, in May 2011, 2013 and 2016.

Food/Beverage Category	Total Advertisements Aired			% Change in Ad Frequency May 2011 to 2016
	May 2011 n (%)	May 2013 n (%)	May 2016 n (%)	
Cakes	52 (0.1)	3 (<0.1)	423 (0.5)	+713%
Candy	814 (1.0)	4893 (5.9)	3623 (4.1)	+345%
Cereal	7349 (8.7)	3044 (3.7)	2992 (3.4)	−59%
Cheese	5931 (7.0)	3731 (4.5)	4924 (5.6)	−17%
Chocolate	10,001 (11.8)	12,165 (14.8)	7140 (8.1)	−29%
Compartment snacks	-	352 (0.4)	1 (<0.1)	-
Cookies	3875 (4.6)	2333 (2.8)	1597 (1.8)	−59%
Ice cream	1318 (1.6)	2387 (2.9)	2626 (3.0)	+99%
Pizza	2332 (2.8)	1258 (1.5)	1498 (1.7)	−36%
Portable snacks	2397 (2.8)	1892 (2.3)	1739 (2.0)	−27%
Snack foods	2158 (2.5)	4850 (5.9)	5609 (6.4)	+160%
Fast food	28,508 (33.7)	26,861 (32.6)	35,652 (40.6)	+25%
Restaurants	5686 (6.7)	4506 (5.5)	5918 (6.7)	+4%
Yogurt	7660 (9.0)	4777 (5.8)	2810 (3.2)	−63%
Juices	3491 (4.1)	4615 (5.6)	4845 (5.5)	+39%
Energy drinks	765 (0.9)	804 (1.0)	857 (1.0)	+12%
Soft drinks (regular)	1199 (1.4)	3878 (4.7)	4247 (4.8)	+254%
Soft drinks (diet)	804 (0.9)	-	318 (0.4)	−60%
Sports drinks	360 (0.4)	83 (0.1)	1006 (1.1)	+179%
TOTAL	84,700 (100)	82,432 (100)	87,825 (100)	+4%

Source: Nielsen Media Research, May 2011, 2013, 2016.

3.2. Adolescents' Exposure to Food and Beverage Advertising on Television

On average, adolescents were exposed to 221, 180 and 154 food and beverage advertisements in May 2011, 2013 and 2016, respectively. Between May 2011 and 2016, adolescents' exposure to food and beverage advertising decreased by 31%. As shown in Table 3, this trend differed by food/beverage category: despite decreases in exposure for several categories, large increases were observed for cakes (+340%), candy (+193%), sports drinks (+155%), and regular soft drinks (+111%). The five food/beverage categories to which adolescents were most exposed in May 2011 included fast food (34% of total exposure), cereal (10%), chocolate (10%), yogurt (9%), and cheese (8%). In May 2016, these categories were fast food (42% of total exposure), cheese (7%), cereal (7%), candy (6%), and juices (5%).

Table 3. Adolescent exposure to food and beverage television advertisements in May 2011, 2013 and 2016.

Food/Beverage Category	Average Number of Advertisements Viewed by Adolescents (Aged 12–17 Years)			% Change in Ad Exposure (n) May 2011 to 2016
	May 2011 n (%)	May 2013 n (%)	May 2016 n (%)	
Cakes	0.15 (<0.1)	-	0.66 (0.4)	+340%
Candy	3.40 (1.5)	9.62 (5.3)	9.96 (6.5)	+193%
Cereal	22.70 (10.3)	8.24 (4.6)	10.21 (6.6)	−55%
Cheese	17.18 (7.8)	10.24 (5.7)	10.58 (6.9)	−38%
Chocolate	22.55 (10.2)	21.54 (11.9)	7.62 (5.0)	−66%
Compartment snacks	-	0.67 (0.4)	-	-
Cookies	10.09 (4.6)	5.19 (2.9)	2.60 (1.7)	−74%
Ice cream	2.88 (1.3)	3.93 (2.2)	3.94 (2.6)	+37%
Pizza	6.24 (2.8)	2.76 (1.5)	1.31 (0.9)	−79%
Portable snacks	9.35 (4.2)	4.11 (2.3)	5.14 (3.3)	−45%
Snack foods	3.40 (1.5)	7.53 (4.2)	6.67 (4.3)	+96%
Fast food	74.76 (33.8)	68.00 (37.7)	64.05 (41.7)	−14%
Restaurants	12.50 (5.7)	10.83 (6.0)	8.14 (5.3)	−35%
Yogurt	19.19 (8.7)	10.31 (5.7)	5.06 (3.3)	−74%
Juices	10.10 (4.6)	10.20 (5.7)	8.36 (5.4)	−17%
Energy drinks	1.65 (0.8)	1.71 (0.9)	0.91 (0.6)	−45%
Soft drinks (regular)	2.69 (1.2)	5.36 (3.0)	5.67 (3.7)	+111%
Soft drinks (diet)	1.68 (0.8)	-	0.83 (0.5)	−51%
Sports drinks	0.75 (0.3)	0.25 (0.1)	1.91 (1.2)	+155%
TOTAL	221.26 (100)	180.49 (100)	153.62 (100)	−31%

Source: Nielsen Media Research, May 2011, 2013, 2016.

Changes in adolescents' exposure to food and beverage advertising also differed by television station type. For instance, in May 2016, 75% of adolescents' total exposure was derived from generalist stations (i.e., stations not specifically targeted at children or adolescents), while 24% and 1% were derived from children's specialty and teen specialty stations, respectively. While adolescents' exposure to food advertising showed little change between May 2011 and May 2016 on children's specialty stations (−7%), the magnitude of change in exposure on teen specialty stations (−76%) and generalist stations (−34%) was considerably greater (Table 4).

Table 4. Adolescent exposure to food and beverage television advertisements, in May 2011, 2013 and 2016, by food category and television station type.

Food/Beverage Category	Average Number of Advertisements Viewed by Adolescents (Aged 12–17 Years)											
	Children's Specialty Stations (n = 2)				Teen Specialty Stations (n = 2)				Generalist Stations (n = 27)			
	May 2011	May 2013	May 2016	% Change May 2011 to 2016	May 2011	May 2013	May 2016	% Change May 2011 to 2016	May 2011	May 2013	May 2016	% Change May 2011 to 2016
Cakes	-	-	-	-	-	-	-	-	0.15	-	0.66	340%
Candy	2.04	4.35	7.89	+287%	0.29	0.45	1.67	476%	1.08	4.82	2.07	92%
Cereal	7.32	2.81	7.23	−1%	-	-	-	-	15.38	5.43	2.99	−81%
Cheese	4.74	2.76	4.06	−14%	0.36	-	-	-	12.08	7.47	6.52	−46%
Chocolate	0.87	1.72	1.60	+84%	1.01	0.33	0.14	−86%	20.66	19.49	5.87	−72%
Compartment snacks	-	-	-	-	-	-	-	-	-	0.67	-	-
Cookies	1.71	0.55	0.17	−90%	0.82	0.25	-	-	7.56	4.39	2.43	−68%
Ice cream	0.43	1.56	0.63	+47%	-	-	-	-	2.45	2.36	3.31	35%
Pizza	0.23	-	0.39	+70%	-	-	-	-	6.01	2.76	0.92	−85%
Portable snacks	4.01	1.19	2.83	−29%	-	-	-	-	5.35	2.92	2.31	−57%
Snack foods	0.12	-	0.48	+300%	0.27	0.35	0.16	−41%	3.01	7.18	6.03	100%
Fast food	11.64	8.51	8.36	−28%	2.23	0.83	0.91	−59%	60.88	58.67	54.77	−10%
Restaurants	0.91	1.15	0.11	−88%	0.13	0.26	0.08	−38%	11.47	9.43	7.95	−31%
Yogurt	4.39	1.56	1.94	−56%	0.44	0.78	0.03	−93%	14.36	7.97	3.10	−78%
Juices	1.29	0.55	1.15	−11%	0.29	0.57	-	-	8.52	9.09	7.21	−15%
Energy drinks	-	0.18	0.06	∞	0.25	0.31	0.07	−72%	1.40	1.22	0.79	−44%
Soft drinks (regular)	0.39	0.70	0.51	+31%	0.60	1.24	0.26	−57%	1.71	3.41	4.89	186%
Soft drinks (diet)	-	-	-	-	-	-	-	-	1.68	-	0.83	−51%
Sports drinks	-	-	-	-	0.26	-	0.01	−96%	0.49	0.25	1.89	286%
TOTAL	40.09	27.58	37.41	−7%	6.94	5.36	1.67	−76%	174.24	147.54	114.54	−34%

Notes: Children's specialty stations included Teletoon and YTV. Teen specialty stations included Much Music and MTV. All other stations were classified as generalist stations; Source: Nielsen Media Research, May 2011, 2013, 2016.

3.3. Beverages with Free Sugars

When juices, regular soft drinks, sports drinks and energy drinks were considered together, the total number of television advertisements for beverages with free sugars increased by 88% between May 2011 (n = 5815) and May 2016 (n =10,955). In addition, adolescents' exposure to advertisements for beverages with free sugars increased by 11% between May 2011 (n = 15.19) and May 2016 (n = 16.85). However, exposure in May 2016 (n = 16.85) was lower than in May 2013 (n = 17.52). As shown in Figure 1, decreases in exposure were observed for juices (−17%) and energy drinks (−45%), while increases were observed for regular soft drinks (+111%) and sports drinks (+155%). In 2016, beverages with free sugars represented the second-most heavily advertised food/beverage category among those examined in May 2016, increasing in relative importance from May 2011 (seventh-most heavily advertised category), and May 2013 (third-most heavily advertised category). Correspondingly, beverages with free sugars represented the second-highest levels of exposure among adolescents in May 2016 (11% of total exposure), following that for fast food, increasing in relative importance from 2011 (ranked sixth with respect to exposure) and 2013 (ranked third with respect to exposure).

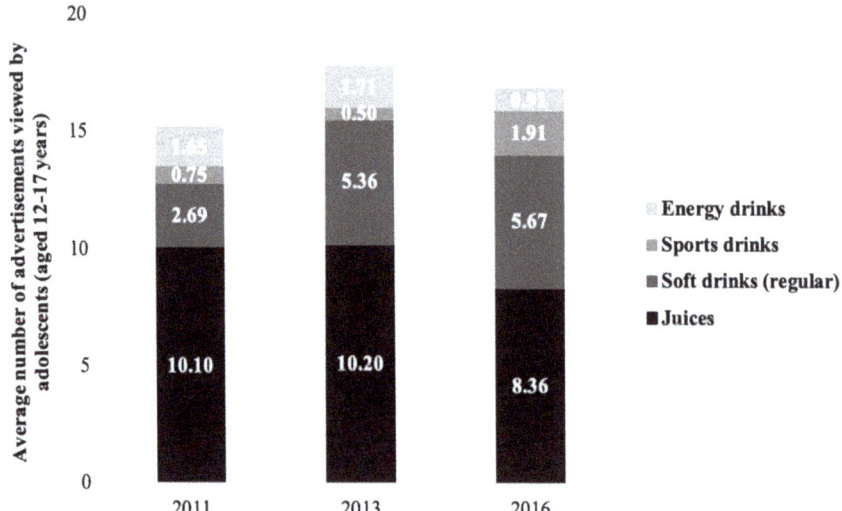

Figure 1. Adolescent exposure to television advertisements for beverages with free sugars, May 2011, 2013 and 2016. Source: Nielsen Media Research, May 2011, 2013, 2016.

4. Discussion

The study findings indicate a decline in exposure to food/beverage advertising on television between May 2011 and May 2016 among Canadian youth. This decline was observed despite relatively little change in the total number of food/beverage advertisements aired over the study period. Given that exposure to television advertising is a function of time spent watching television and the frequency of aired advertising, the findings suggest that the observed change may be due to changes in media preferences and consumption among adolescents. Indeed, according to the Canadian Radio-television and Telecommunications Commission (CRTC), Canadians' weekly viewing of television has decreased from 2011/12 to 2015/16, with the largest decrease among teens aged 12–17 years [20]. Trends in food-related advertising expenditures, given recent shifts in expenditures that favor digital marketing via websites, social media, and mobile applications, also appear to support this interpretation [22]. Despite the observed decline, our findings show that Canadian adolescents are still exposed to more than 150 food and beverage television advertisements per four-week period, which may result in annual exposures of 1800 on television alone. As such, broadcast television remains an important source of food advertising exposure among Canadian adolescents. Its continued monitoring is therefore warranted.

Trends over time in commercial food advertising exposure among adolescents differed by specific food/beverage categories. While some foods and beverages, such as cakes and sports drinks, showed considerable growth over time (+340% and +155%, respectively), they contributed little to adolescents' total exposure to food/beverage advertising (<1 advertisement exposure in May 2016, respectively). In contrast, categories such as regular soft drinks showed growth over time (+111%), while also contributing more to exposure among youth (6 advertisement exposures in May 2016, up from 3 in May 2011). Finally, while advertising exposure to cereal and cheese decreased over the time period examined (−55% and −38%, respectively), they remained within the five food/beverage categories to which adolescents were most exposed. These findings highlight the importance of regular monitoring of trends in commercial food advertising with respect to both changes within food/beverage categories over time as well as their relative contribution to total exposure. Continued monitoring may also yield greater insights into the variation of commercial food advertising on television and inform the interpretation of observed trends in exposure over time.

Advertising for fast food dominated relative to other categories, remaining by far the top category with respect to the quantity of television advertising as well as exposure among adolescents over the examined period. Specifically, in May 2016, advertisements for fast food accounted for almost half (42%) of all commercial food advertising exposure among adolescents, as examined in this study. These findings are consistent with analyses examining television advertising exposure among adolescents in the US [8,38]. Findings from the current study also show an increase over time in youth advertising exposure to beverages containing free sugars. When considered together, these sugary drinks represented a significant food/beverage category, with marked increases over time in the quantity of television advertising, as well as in levels of exposure among adolescents, second only to fast food. These findings contrast with declining trends in children's advertising exposure on television to sugary drinks in both Canada and the US in recent years [41–43] and may mark a shift in targeted advertising of older demographic groups. Increased advertising exposure to sugary drinks is concerning, given that consumption of these beverages has been associated with weight gain [32,33] and is a risk factor for various chronic diseases [40]. The dominance of adolescents' advertising exposure to both fast food and sugary drinks is consistent with elements of the current marketplace. First, it reflects commercial food and beverage marketing expenditures: of the more than $1 billion spent annually on marketing directed at adolescents in the US [21], approximately two-thirds of this is for fast food and sugary drinks [22]. Second, the findings are consistent with this subpopulation's consumer profile: in addition to influencing family purchases [1], adolescents are direct consumers with access to their own money, and items like fast food and beverages are within their purchasing power [8].

Findings from the current study have several policy implications. First, our study revealed that Canadian adolescents are exposed to a considerable volume of food and beverage advertisements, including sugary drinks, on broadcast television. As such, policymakers should consider protecting adolescents when crafting laws restricting unhealthy food marketing directed to children. Given that most (75%) of adolescents' exposure occurred on generalist stations, statutory restrictions should also apply to programs watched by large numbers of children and adolescents, regardless of the intended audience of a given station or program [24]. As it has been done for children under 13 years of age [9], additional research is needed to understand how various food advertising restrictions on broadcast television may impact adolescents' exposure. In the United Kingdom, for instance, the restriction of unhealthy food and beverage advertising before 9 pm has been proposed as an alternative to current restrictions based on television audience measurements [44]. However, research on time-based restrictions of alcohol advertising suggests that this may in fact lead to higher advertising exposure among youth [45]. As such, more research is needed to inform policy in this area.

Second, concerns have been raised that restrictions on unhealthy food and beverage marketing to children may result in unintended consequences in the form of increased marketing targeting adolescents. While such changes have been observed in the US [38], it is not clear whether they may follow in the Canadian context if statutory restrictions exclusively targeting children under 13 years were to be adopted. Continued monitoring of food and beverage marketing to both children and adolescents is warranted. Finally, given that adolescents consumption of broadcast television is declining [20], future research or monitoring should also examine youth's exposure to food advertising during television or video content viewed on YouTube, online streaming platforms and on smart televisions whose connection to the internet allow advertisers to use meta-data and advanced analytics to target specific demographic groups [46]. While no such study has yet to be conducted, food and beverage advertising during television content viewed online is likely to mirror the predominantly unhealthy nature of food advertising on broadcast television and other media [29,38,39]. Given the increased viewing of television content online, statutory restrictions of unhealthy food and beverage advertising to children and youth should apply to these digital platforms.

To our knowledge, the current study is the first to examine trends over time in food and beverage advertising and exposure among Canadian adolescents. A significant strength of the study is its use of objective exposure data, rather than data based on potential exposure or self-reported measures. The study findings likely underestimate adolescents' exposure to food and beverage advertising on television, given that not all food and beverage categories were included in the study and exposure to food marketing embedded within television programs (e.g., product placements and sponsorship of broadcasted sporting events) are not captured in the analyzed data [47,48]. Adolescents' exposure to sugary drink advertising, particularly soft drinks, may also be underestimated as these products are often featured within restaurant advertising because of exclusive marketing agreements that exist between restaurant chains and large beverage manufacturers [49]. Furthermore, some television stations were excluded from the analysis to ensure comparability for data collected across different time periods. For example, TSN, a popular sports station, was excluded because data was not collected by Nielsen for May 2016. However, data collected for TSN in May 2011 suggests that adolescents were exposed to considerable advertising for various food and beverages, and in particular, for sports drinks. Since television ratings data are only available in aggregate, statistical testing could not be conducted to determine whether differences in exposure between May 2011 and May 2016 were statistically significant. The study is also limited by its lack of nutritional analysis of advertised foods and beverages, which would have objectively determined their nutritional quality. However, nearly all the examined food and beverage categories represented largely "unhealthy" foods. Indeed, this bias in food marketing is reflected in youth-targeted marketing expenditures, which are dominated by fast food restaurants, beverages, breakfast cereals, and snack foods, with fruits and vegetables accounting for less than 1% of expenditures [22]. Finally, data were analyzed for the broadcast market of Toronto for the month of May in each examined year; thus, the extent to which the findings represent trends over the entire calendar year and markets across Canada is unclear. Given seasonal variations in advertising, with some products being advertised for only parts of the year, recorded changes in advertising by food category may not be representative of annual trends.

5. Conclusions

The current study demonstrates a declining trend over time in exposure to food and beverage television advertising among Canadian adolescents. This decline was observed despite no considerable changes in the quantity of commercial food advertisements on television, suggesting that this trend may be due to shifts in adolescents' media preferences and consumption. Adolescents' commercial food advertising on television is dominated by advertisements for fast food and increasingly, for beverages with free sugars. These data highlight the need to include adolescents in statutory food marketing restrictions in Canada. They may serve as a benchmark for monitoring and evaluating future food and beverage marketing policies in the country.

Supplementary Materials: The following are available online at http://www.mdpi.com/2072-6643/12/2/428/s1, Table S1: List of television stations included in the study.

Author Contributions: Conceptualization C.D.C., E.P. and M.P.K. Methodology C.D.C., E.P. and M.P.K. Formal Analysis C.D.C. Writing—Original Draft Preparation, C.D.C. Writing—Review & Edition, C.D.C., E.P. and M.P.K. All authors have read and agreed to the published version of the manuscript.

Funding: This research received no external funding.

Acknowledgments: Financial support for researchers/authors was provided by Canadian Institutes of Health Research (CIHR)—Heart and Stroke Foundation (HSF) Health System Impact Fellowship (CDC).

Conflicts of Interest: In 2018, E.P. received a small honorarium from the Stop Marketing to Kids Coalition for providing expert advice.

References

1. McGinnis, J.M.; Gootman, J.; Kraak, V.I. *Food Marketing to Children and Youth: Threat or Opportunity?* The National Academies Press: Washington, DC, USA, 2006.
2. Hastings, G.; McDermott, L.; Angus, K.; Stead, M.; Thomson, S. *The Extent, Nature and Effects of Food Promotion to Children: A Review of the Evidence*; World Health Organization: Geneva, Switzerland, 2006.
3. Cairns, G.; Angus, K.; Hastings, G.; Caraher, M. Systematic reviews of the evidence on the nature, extent and effects of food marketing to children. A retrospective summary. *Appetite* **2013**, *62*, 209–215. [CrossRef] [PubMed]
4. Sadeghirad, B.; Duhaney, T.; Motaghipisheh, S.; Campbell, N.R.C.; Johnston, B.C. Influence of unhealthy food and beverage marketing on children's dietary intake and preference: A systematic review and meta-analysis of randomized trials. *Obes. Rev.* **2016**, *17*, 945–959. [CrossRef] [PubMed]
5. Norman, J.; Kelly, B.; Boyland, E.; McMahon, A.T. The impact of marketing and advertising on food behaviours: Evaluating the evidence for a causal relationship. *Curr. Nutr. Rep.* **2016**, *5*, 139–149. [CrossRef]
6. Smith, R.; Kelly, H.; Yeatman, H.; Boyland, E. Food marketing influences children's attitudes, preferences and consumption: A systematic critical review. *Nutrients* **2019**, *11*, 875. [CrossRef]
7. Scully, M.; Wakefield, M.; Niven, P.; Chapman, K.; Crawford, D.; Pratt, I.S.; Baur, L.A.; Flood, V.; Morley, B. Association between food marketing exposure and adolescents' food choices and eating behaviors. *Appetite* **2012**, *58*, 1–5. [CrossRef]
8. Powell, L.M.; Szczypka, G.; Chaloupka, F.J. Adolescent exposure to food advertising on television. *Am. J. Prev. Med.* **2007**, *33*, S251–S256. [CrossRef]
9. Harris, J.L.; Sarda, V.; Schwartz, M.B.; Brownell, K.D. Redefining "child-directed advertising" to reduce unhealthy television food advertising. *Am. J. Prev. Med.* **2013**, *44*, 358–364. [CrossRef]
10. Public Health Agency of Canada; The Canadian Institute for Health Information. Obesity in Canada. 2011. Available online: https://secure.cihi.ca/free_products/Obesity_in_canada_2011_en.pdf. (accessed on 9 November 2018).
11. Rodd, C.; Sharma, A.K. Recent trends in the prevalence of overweight and obesity among Canadian children. *CMAJ* **2016**, *188*, E313–E320. [CrossRef]
12. Statistics Canada. Table 13-10-0795-01 Measured Children and Youth Body Mass Index (BMI) (World Health Organization Classification), by Age Group and Sex, Canada and Provinces, Canadian Community Health Survey-Nutrition. 2019. Available online: https://www150.statcan.gc.ca/t1/tbl1/en/tv.action?pid=1310079501&pickMembers%5B0%5D=1.1&pickMembers%5B1%5D=2.3&pickMembers%5B2%5D=3.1&pickMembers%5B3%5D=5.5 (accessed on 9 November 2018).
13. Garriguet, D. Canadians' eating habits. *Health Rep.* **2007**, *18*, 17–32.
14. Garriguet, D. Sodium consumption at all ages. *Health Rep.* **2007**, *18*, 47–52.
15. Langlois, K.; Garriguet, D. Sugar consumption among Canadians of all ages. *Health Rep.* **2011**, *22*, 23–27. [PubMed]
16. Moubarac, J.C. *Ultra-Processed Foods in Canada: Consumption, Impact on Diet Quality and Policy Implications*; University of Montreal: Montreal, QC, Canada, 2017; Available online: https://www.heartandstroke.ca/-/media/pdf-files/canada/media-centre/hs-report-upp-moubarac-dec-5-2017.ashx (accessed on 6 November 2018).

17. World Health Organization. *Guideline: Sugars Intake for Adults and Children*; World Health Organization: Geneva, Switzerland, 2015; Available online: http://apps.who.int/iris/bitstream/handle/10665/149782/9789241549028_eng.pdf;jsessionid=DB27D7FF33CEE9A8E0A544505A81CC41?sequence=1 (accessed on 2 November 2018).
18. Garriguet, D. Beverage consumption of children and teens. *Health Rep.* **2008**, *19*, 17–22. [PubMed]
19. Story, M.; French, S. Food advertising and marketing directed at children and adolescents in the US. *Int. J. Behav. Nutr. Phys. Act.* **2004**, *1*, 3. [CrossRef]
20. The Canadian Radio-television and Telecommunications Commission (CRTC). *Communications Monitoring Report*; CRTC: Ottawa, ON, Canada, 2017. Available online: https://crtc.gc.ca/eng/publications/reports/policymonitoring/2017/index.htm (accessed on 2 November 2018).
21. Federal Trade Commission. A Review of Food Marketing to Children and Adolescents: Follow-Up Report. 2012. Available online: https://www.ftc.gov/sites/default/files/documents/reports/review-food-marketing-children-and-adolescents-follow-report/121221foodmarketingreport.pdf (accessed on 2 November 2018).
22. Powell, L.M.; Harris, J.L.; Fox, T. Food marketing expenditures aimed at youth: Putting the numbers in context. *Am. J. Prev. Med.* **2013**, *45*, 453–461. [CrossRef] [PubMed]
23. Luxton, S.; Reid, M.; Mavondo, F. Integrated marketing communication capability and brand performance. *J. Advert.* **2015**, *44*, 37–46. [CrossRef]
24. World Health Organization Regional Office for Europe. *Evaluating Implementation of the WHO Set of Recommendations on the Marketing of Foods and Non-Alcoholic Beverages to Children. Progress, Challenges and Guidance for Next Steps in WHO European Region*; WHO Regional Office for Europe: Copenhagen, Denmark, 2018; Available online: http://www.euro.who.int/__data/assets/pdf_file/0003/384015/food-marketing-kids-eng.pdf?ua=1 (accessed on 14 October 2019).
25. Office de la Protection du Consommateur. *Advertising Directed at Children under 13 Years of Age. Guide to Application of Sections 248 and 249 Consumer Protection Act*; Office de la Protection du Consommateur: Québec, QC, Canada, 2012. Available online: https://www.opc.gouv.qc.ca/fileadmin/media/documents/consommateur/sujet/publicite-pratique-illegale/EN_Guide_publicite_moins_de_13_ans_vf.pdf (accessed on 29 January 2019).
26. Ad Standards. *The Canadian Children's Food and Beverage Advertising Initiative: 2018 Compliance Report*; Ad Standards: Toronto, ON, Canada, 2019; Available online: https://adstandards.ca/wp-content/uploads/2020/01/AdStandards-CAI-Compliance-Report-18-EN.pdf (accessed on 29 January 2019).
27. Parliament of Canada. Bill S-228—An Act to Amend the Food and Drugs Act (Prohibiting Food and Beverage Marketing Directed at Children). 2017. Available online: https://www.parl.ca/DocumentViewer/en/42-1/bill/S-228/third-reading (accessed on 25 September 2018).
28. Duggan, K. Liberals Plan to Amend Junk Food Ad Bill: Petitpas Taylor. *iPolitics*, 12 December 2017. Available online: https://ipolitics.ca/2017/12/12/liberals-plan-amend-junk-food-ad-bill-petitpas-taylor/ (accessed on 16 October 2019).
29. Potvin Kent, M.; Pauzé, E.; Roy, E.-A.; De Billy, N.; Czoli, C. Children and adolescents' exposure to food and beverage marketing in social media apps. *Pediatr. Obes.* **2019**, *14*, e12508. [CrossRef] [PubMed]
30. Penchmann, C.; Levine, L.; Loughlin, S.; Leslie, F.M. Impulsive and self-conscious: Adolescents' vulnerability to advertising and promotion. *J. Public Policy Mark.* **2005**, *24*, 202–221. [CrossRef]
31. Leslie, F.M.; Levine, L.J.; Loughlin, S.E.; Penchmann, C. *Adolescents Psychological & Neurobiological Development: Implications for Digital Marketing*; Centre for Digital Democracy and Berkeley Media Studies Group: Berkeley, CA, USA, 2009; Available online: http://digitalads.org/sites/default/files/publications/digitalads_leslie_et_al_nplan_bmsg_memo.pdf (accessed on 6 February 2020).
32. Luger, M.; Lafontan, M.; Bes-Rastrollo, M.; Winzer, E.; Yumuk, V.; Farpour-Lambert, N. Sugar-sweetened beverages and weight gain in children and adults: A systematic review from 2013 to 2015 and a comparison with previous studies. *Obes. Facts.* **2017**, *10*, 674–693. [CrossRef]
33. Malik, V.S.; Pan, A.; Willett, W.C.; Hu, F.B. Sugar-sweetened beverages and weight gain in children and adults: A systematic review and meta-analysis. *Am. J. Clin. Nutr.* **2013**, *98*, 1084–1102. [CrossRef]
34. Kelly, B.; Vandevijvere, S.; SeeHoe, N.; Adams, J.; Allemandi, L.; Bahena-Espina, L.; Barquera, A. Global benchmarking of children's exposure to television advertising of unhealthy food and beverages across 22 countries. *Obes. Rev.* **2019**, *20*, 116–128. [CrossRef]

35. Potvin Kent, M.; Smith, J.R.; Pauzé, E.; L'Abbé, M. The effectiveness of the food and beverage industry's self-established Uniform Nutrition Criteria at improving the healthfulness of food advertising viewed by Canadian children on television. *Int. J. Behav. Nutr. Phys. Act.* **2018**, *15*, 57. [CrossRef] [PubMed]
36. Potvin Kent, M.; Martin, C.; Kent, E.A. Changes in the volume, power and nutritional quality of foods marketed to children on television in Canada 2006-2011. *Obesity* **2014**, *22*, 2053–2060. [CrossRef] [PubMed]
37. Numeris. A Guide to Numeris' Meter Panel. 2018. Available online: http://en.numeris.ca/participants/meter-panel (accessed on 15 November 2018).
38. Powell, L.M.; Szczypka, G.; Chaloupka, F.J. Trends in exposure to television food advertisements among children and adolescents in the United States. *Arch. Pediatr. Adolesc. Med.* **2010**, *164*, 794–802. [CrossRef] [PubMed]
39. Fleming-Milici, F.; Harris, J.L. Television food advertising viewed by preschoolers, children and adolescents: Contributors to differences in exposure for black and white youth in the United States. *Pediatr. Obes.* **2018**, *13*, 103–110. [CrossRef] [PubMed]
40. Jones, A.C.; Veerman, J.L.; Hammond, D. The Health and Economic Impact of a Tax on Sugary Drinks in Canada (Summary). 2017. Available online: https://www.heartandstroke.ca/-/media/pdf-files/canada/media-centre/the-health-and-economic-impact-of-a-sugary-drink-tax-in-canada-summary.ashx?la=en&hash=69765598FF624EE7D8586EBAD7BCF96835F3FA10 (accessed on 14 October 2019).
41. Potvin Kent, M.; Wanless, A. The influence of the Children's Food and Beverage Advertising Initiative: Change in children's exposure to food advertising on television in Canada between 2006–2009. *Int. J. Obes.* **2014**, *38*, 558–562. [CrossRef]
42. Frazier, W.C.; Harris, J.L. *Trends in Television Food Advertising to Young People: 2017 Update*; Rudd Centre for Food Policy and Obesity: University of Connecticut, Hartford, USA, 2018; Available online: http://www.uconnruddcenter.org/files/Pdfs/RuddReport_TVFoodAdvertising_6_14.pdf (accessed on 8 November 2018).
43. King, L.; Hebden, L.; Grunseit, A.; Kelly, B.; Chapman, K.; Venugopal, K. Industry self-regulation of television food advertising: Responsible or responsive? *Int. J. Pediatr. Obes.* **2011**, *6*, e390–e398. [CrossRef]
44. Department of Health and Social Care: Global Public Health Directorate: Obesity, Food and Nutrition. *Childhood Obesity: A Plan for Action (Chapter 2)*; Department of Health and Social Care: London, UK, 2018. Available online: https://assets.publishing.service.gov.uk/government/uploads/system/uploads/attachment_data/file/718903/childhood-obesity-a-plan-for-action-chapter-2.pdf (accessed on 1 January 2020).
45. Ross, C.S.; De Bruijn, A.; Jernigan, D. Do time restrictions on alcohol advertising reduce youth exposure? *J. Public Aff.* **2013**, *13*, 123–129. [CrossRef]
46. World Health Organization's Regional Office for Europe. *Tackling Food Marketing to Children in a Digital World: Trans-Disciplinary Perspectives*; WHO Europe: Copenhagen, Denmark, 2016; Available online: http://www.euro.who.int/__data/assets/pdf_file/0017/322226/Tackling-food-marketing-children-digital-world-trans-disciplinary-perspectives-en.pdf?ua=1 (accessed on 1 January 2020).
47. Elsey, J.W.B.; Harris, J.L. Trends in food and beverage television brand appearances viewed by children and adolescents from 2009 to 2014 in the USA. *Public Health Nutr.* **2016**, *19*, 1928–1933. [CrossRef]
48. Sherriff, J.; Griffiths, D.; Daube, M. Cricket: Notching up runs for food and alcohol companies? *Aust. N. Z. J. Public Health* **2010**, *34*, 19–23. [CrossRef]
49. Coalition Poids. *Sugar-Sweetened Beverage Marketing Unveiled*; Coalition Poids: Montreal, QC, Canada, 2012; Available online: http://cqpp.qc.ca/app/uploads/2018/08/Report_Marketing-Sugar-Sweetened-Beverage_Volume2-Price_2012-03_petit.pdf (accessed on 15 November 2018).

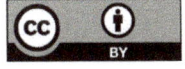 © 2020 by the authors. Licensee MDPI, Basel, Switzerland. This article is an open access article distributed under the terms and conditions of the Creative Commons Attribution (CC BY) license (http://creativecommons.org/licenses/by/4.0/).